Manual of Diagnostic Radiology

Manual of Diagnostic Radiology

Joseph A. Pierro, M.D.

Department of Radiology
Saint Elizabeth's Hospital Medical Center
Western Reserve Care System
Youngstown, Ohio

Bruce M. Berens, M.D.

Department of Radiology
Saint Elizabeth's Hospital Medical Center
Western Reserve Care System
Youngstown, Ohio

William L. Crawford, M.D.

Department of Radiology
Saint Elizabeth's Hospital Medical Center
Youngstown, Ohio

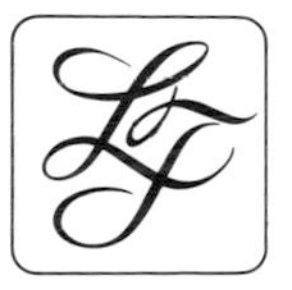

Lea & Febiger Philadelphia • London 1989

Lea & Febiger
600 Washington Square
Philadelphia, PA 19106-4198
U.S.A.
(215) 922-1330

Lea & Febiger (UK) Ltd.
145a Croydon Road
Beckenham, Kent BR3 3RB
U.K.

Library of Congress Cataloging-in-Publication Data

Pierro, Joseph A.
Manual of diagnostic radiology.

Includes index.
1. Diagnosis, Radioscopic—Handbooks, manuals, etc.
I. Berens, Bruce M. II. Crawford, William L.
(William Lawrence), 1944- . III. Title.
[DNLM: 1. Radiography—handbooks. WN 39 P623m]
RC78.P49 1989 616.07′57 88-32598
ISBN 0-8121-1219-9

PRINTED IN THE UNITED STATES OF AMERICA

Print number: 5 4 3 2 1

To our wives,
Joanne and Teresa

To our children,
Nicole and Eric

To our parents and families

PREFACE

The educational process has one fundamental premise: an individual must grasp simple basic concepts before complex issues can be appreciated or understood. In medical education, for information to be useful in the clinical setting it must be concise and easily accessible.

Radiology is a field of medicine that is integrated with every discipline; however, it is a field of study that does not receive the necessary attention in the curriculum of most medical schools. Thus, a need for a manual of clinical radiology is very real. Medical students and residents need access to basic radiologic information quickly and do not have the time, energy, or enthusiasm to wade through cumbersome radiology textbooks.

This resource presents normal basic radiographic anatomy and provides a reference of common radiographic pathology and applicable differential diagnoses.

This text is not intended to be an all-inclusive reference; the ultimate goal is to provide distilled information in an easy portable source. To understand radiology, one must see radiographs. It is not our aim to show every feasible presentation regarding a certain pathologic entity, but to give the individual a workable base of knowledge.

Youngstown, Ohio

Joseph A. Pierro
Bruce M. Berens
William L. Crawford

ACKNOWLEDGMENTS

We wish to thank the Radiology departments of Saint Elizabeth's Hospital Medical Center and Western Reserve Care System; LouAnn Davis; Kathleen Dlabick, photography; and Sharon Sharo, cover design.

J.A.P.
B.M.B.
W.L.C.

CONTENTS

Chapter 3. CHEST

Chapter 4. ABDOMEN AND GASTROINTESTINAL TRACT

1

Head

1.01 INTERPRETATION OF THE NORMAL SKULL

A. The routine examination of the skull consists of four standard views.
   1. An inclined PA view known as the Caldwell projection
   2. An occipital view known as the Towne view
   3. Right lateral view
   4. Left lateral view
B. An additional view of the base of the skull may be obtained if necessary and is known as the submentovertex.
   1. Evaluation of the skull requires an understanding of normal anatomy. See normal skull series provided.
C. Approach to skull evaluation
   1. Establish a routine method that is most comfortable for you.
   2. Always examine the soft tissues (utilizing a "hot" light) to identify soft tissue swelling or other soft tissue disease.
   3. Always look for the presence of symmetry.
   4. Examine the configuration of the skull.
   5. Look for the presence of normal physiologic calcifications and possible displacement of these structures.
      a. Pineal gland
      b. Choroid plexus
      c. Falx cerebri and tentorium cerebelli
      d. Habenular commissure
      e. Posterior commissure
   6. Differentiation between normal vascular grooves and skull fractures
   7. Evaluation of the sella turcica
      a. AP measurement is approximately 10 mm +/− 4 mm
      b. Depth measurement is approximately 8 mm +/− 4 mm
      c. Width measurement is approximately 14 mm +/− 4 mm
D. Normal anatomic structures
   1. Sutures
      a. Normal sutures include coronal, sagittal, lambdoidal, sphenoparietal, squamosal, and sphenofrontal.
      b. They have a serrated, irregular appearance and follow a predictable course.
   2. Arterial and venous vascular markings
      a. Markings follow a smooth, undulating, branching course with a somewhat predictable pattern.
   3. Dural venous sinus
      a. May produce smooth radiolucent pathways on the inner table of the skull
   4. Venous lakes
      a. Irregular round areas of radiolucency located within the diploë
   5. Gyral markings
      a. Prior to age 16, the convolutions of the brain may produce irregular elliptical areas of increased and decreased density. These markings are diffusely located throughout the skull. If these markings are present in an adult, they are suggestive of elevated intracranial pressure.
   6. Major foramina of the skull and their contents
      a. Superior orbital fissure

(1) Cranial nerve III (oculomotor)
(2) Cranial nerve IV (trochlear)
(3) Cranial nerve V (ophthalmic branch of trigeminal)
(4) Cranial nerve VI (abducens)
(5) Orbital branch of middle meningeal artery
(6) Ophthalmic veins

b. Foramen rotundum
  (1) Cranial nerve V2 (maxillary branch of trigeminal)
c. Foramen ovale
  (1) Cranial nerve V3 (mandibular branch of trigeminal)
  (2) Accessory meningeal artery
d. Foramen spinosum
  (1) Middle meningeal artery
e. Foramen lacerum
  (1) Vidian nerve
  (2) Meningeal branch of ascending pharyngeal artery
  (3) Carotid artery overlying the foramen
f. Carotid canal
  (1) Internal carotid artery
g. Jugular foramen
  (1) Cranial nerve IX (glossopharyngeal)
  (2) Cranial nerve X (vagus)
  (3) Cranial nerve XI (accessory)
  (4) Meningeal branches of occipital and pharyngeal arteries
  (5) Inferior petrosal sinus
h. Hypoglossal canal
  (1) Cranial nerve XII (hypoglossal)
  (2) Meningeal branch of ascending pharyngeal artery
i. Stylomastoid foramen
  (1) Cranial nerve VII (facial)
j. Foramen magnum
  (1) Medulla oblongata
  (2) Spinal roots of cranial nerve XI (accessory)
  (3) Vertebral arteries
  (4) Anterior and posterior spinal arteries

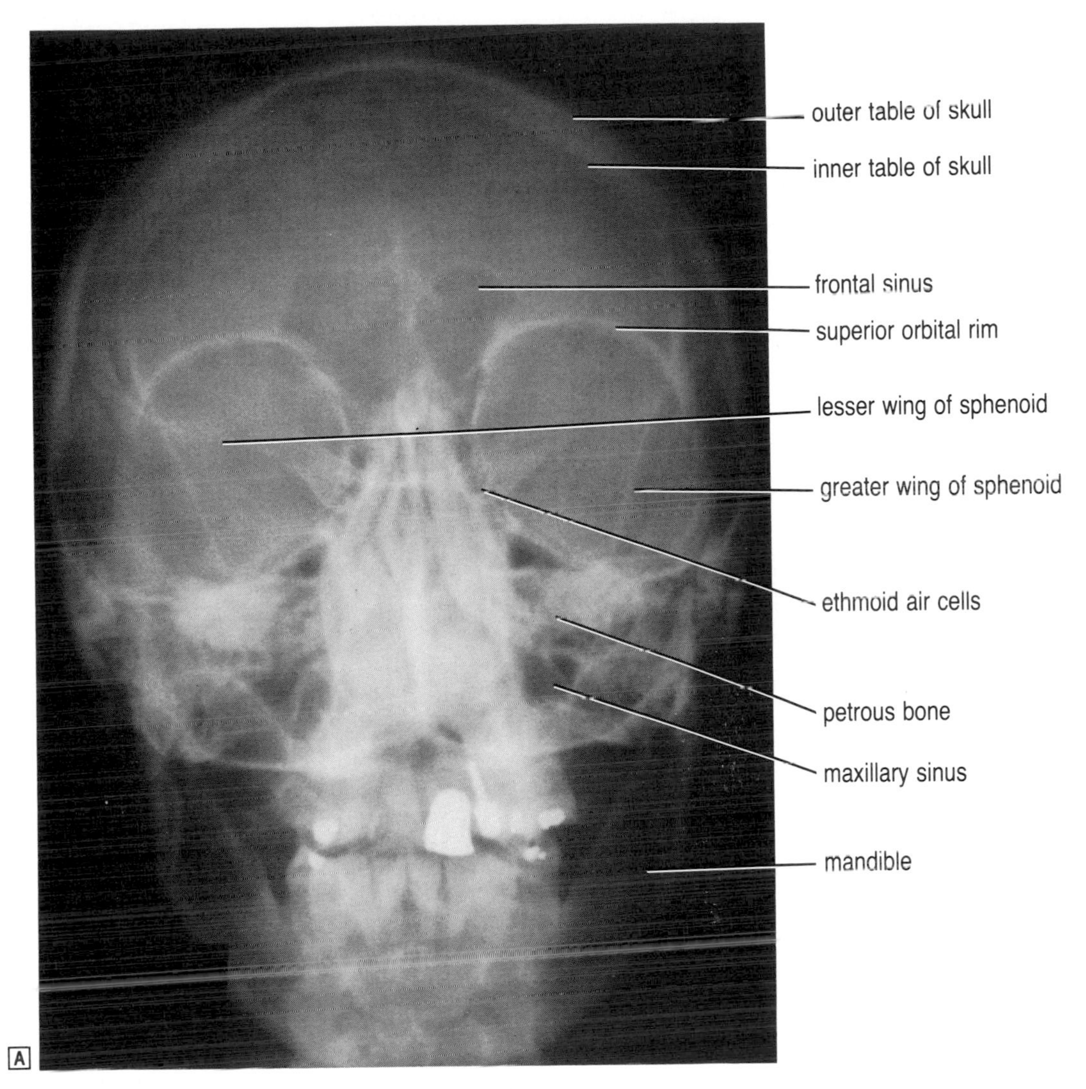

Figure 1.01. *A,* Interpretation of the normal skull.

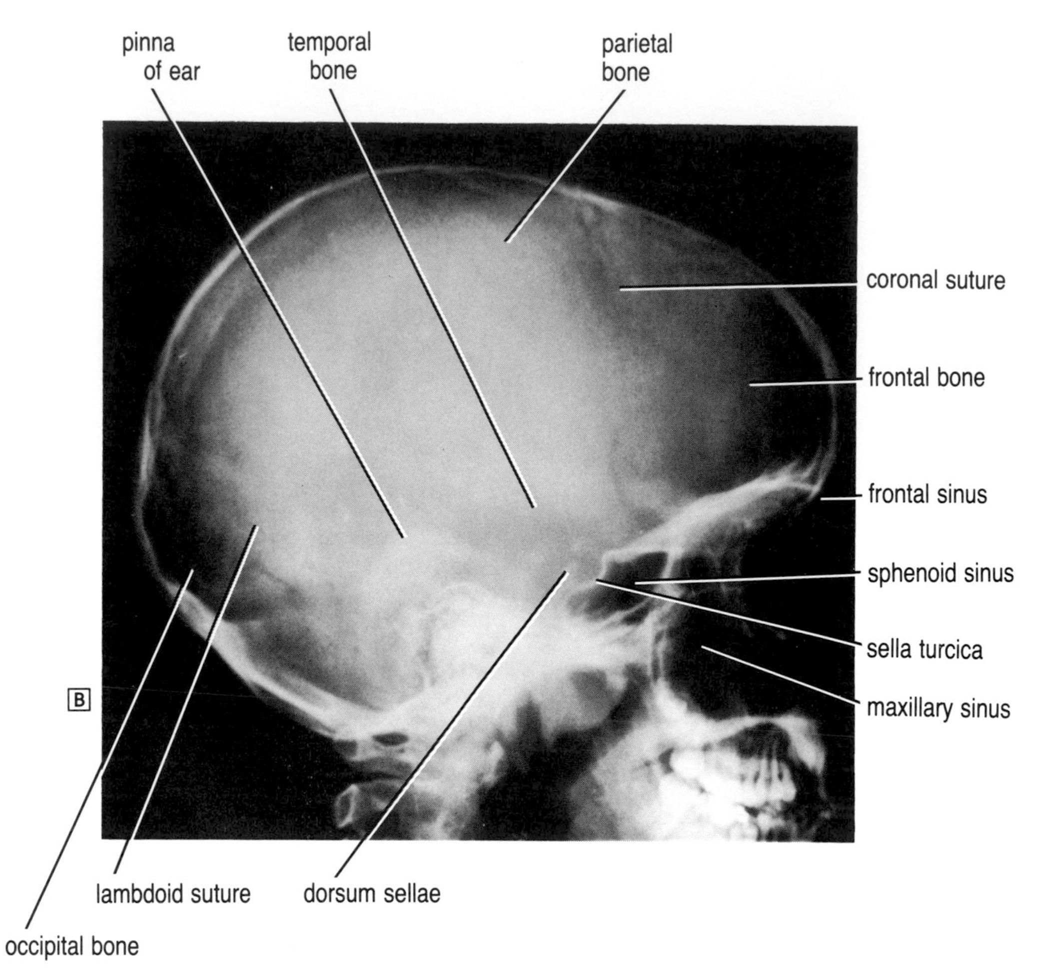

Figure 1.01. *B,* Interpretation of the normal skull.

1.02 SKULL FRACTURE

A. Differentiation between vascular grooves and fractures
   1. Vascular grooves are smooth, undulating radiolucent channels that demonstrate gradual branching and follow predictable patterns.
   2. Skull fractures appear as sharp, straight radiolucent lines that often demonstrate sharp angles. There is a lack of symmetry with the other side of the skull.
   3. Linear skull fracture is the most common type of skull fracture.
   4. Depressed fractures are more clinically significant, and the area involved is more radiodense due to superimposition of bone fragments.
   5. The presence of soft tissue swelling may allow you to localize the site of trauma.
   6. Linear skull fractures of the parietal region indicate the possibility of an epidural hemorrhage due to laceration of the middle meningeal artery.
   7. The presence of underlying brain injury does not correlate with the presence or absence of a skull fracture. If significant head injury has occurred, CT examination of the head without contrast is the best imaging modality to utilize (see Secs. 1.09 to 1.15, Trauma).
   8. Plain films of the skull may not demonstrate basilar skull fractures. They should be suspected if blood is visualized behind the tympanic membrane or is leaking from the external ear canal. CT evaluation is helpful.

B. Complications of skull fracture
   1. Acute hemorrhage (see Sec. 1.10 to 1.15)
      a. Epidural hematoma
      b. Subdural hematoma
      c. Brain contusion
      d. Subarachnoid hemorrhage
   2. Pneumocephalus
   3. Infection
      a. Brain abscess
      b. Meningitis
      c. Osteomyelitis of skull
   4. Cerebrospinal fluid leak
      a. Rhinorrhea
   5. Leptomeningeal cyst
      a. Trauma may result in a tear of the dura resulting in protrusion of arachnoid and cerebrospinal fluid with resultant cyst formation.

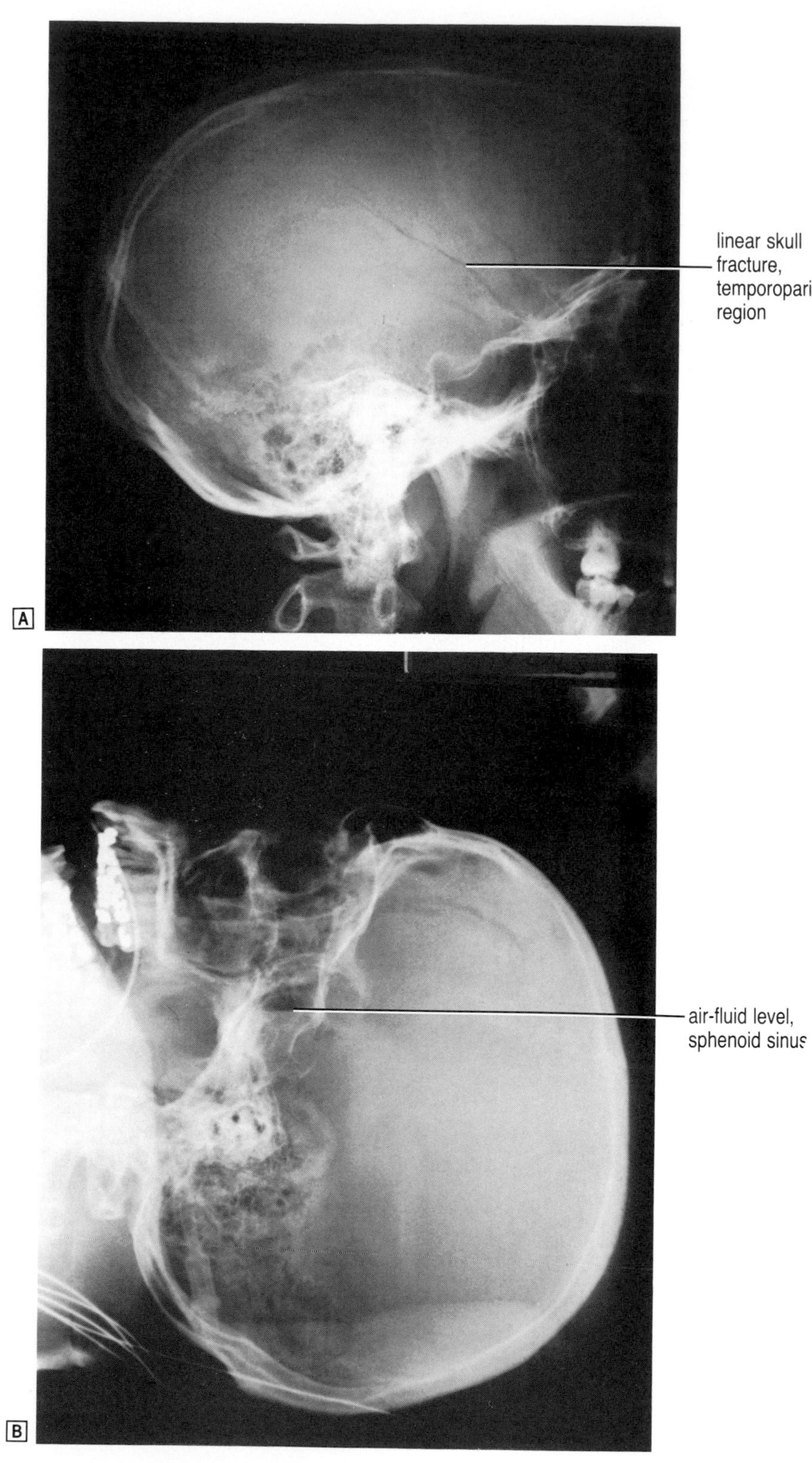

Figure 1.02. *A,* Skull fracture. *B,* Skull fracture.

1.03 MULTIPLE LUCENT LESIONS OF THE SKULL

A. Differential diagnosis
   1. Metastatic disease
      a. Hematogenous spread to the skull
      b. Usually osteolytic lesions, less likely osteoblastic
      c. Neoplasms that metastasize to the skull
         (1) Breast
         (2) Prostate
         (3) Lung
         (4) Renal
         (5) Thyroid
   2. Multiple myeloma
      a. Visualized as multiple well-defined "punched out" lytic areas (see Sec. 6.24)
   3. Hyperparathyroidism (see Sec. 6.27)
   4. Histiocytosis X
   5. Osteomyelitis

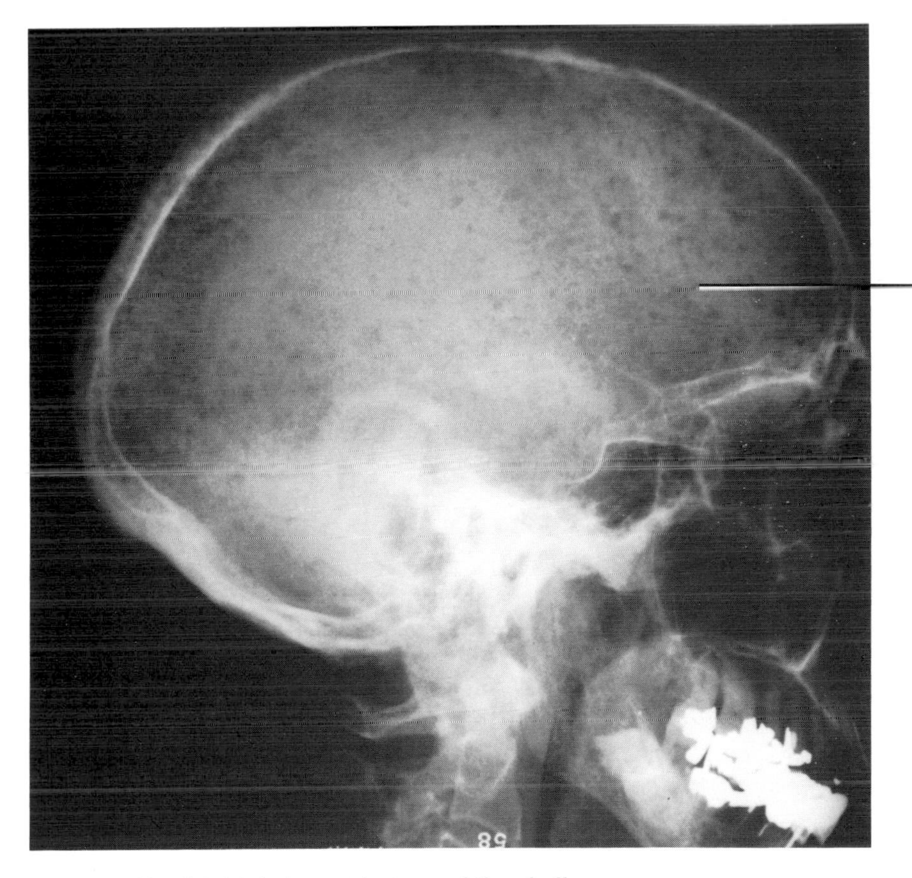

Figure 1.03. Multiple lucent lesions of the skull.

1.04 NASAL BONE FRACTURE

A. Two nasal bones join in the midline to form the nasal bridge. In adults the nasal bones are fused together.
   1. Detection of nasal fractures requires an understanding of normal anatomy.
   2. Certain structures may mimic fractures.
      a. Nasofrontal suture is visualized as a transverse lucency located at the junction of the nasal bones and frontal bone.
      b. Nasomaxillary suture and nasociliary nerve are visualized as a lucency that parallels the long axis of the nasal bones.
   3. Always examine the soft tissues for the presence of soft tissue swelling.
   4. Fracture of the anterior nasal spine may occur along with nasal bone fractures or by itself.
   5. Nasal bone fractures may be associated with additional facial trauma.

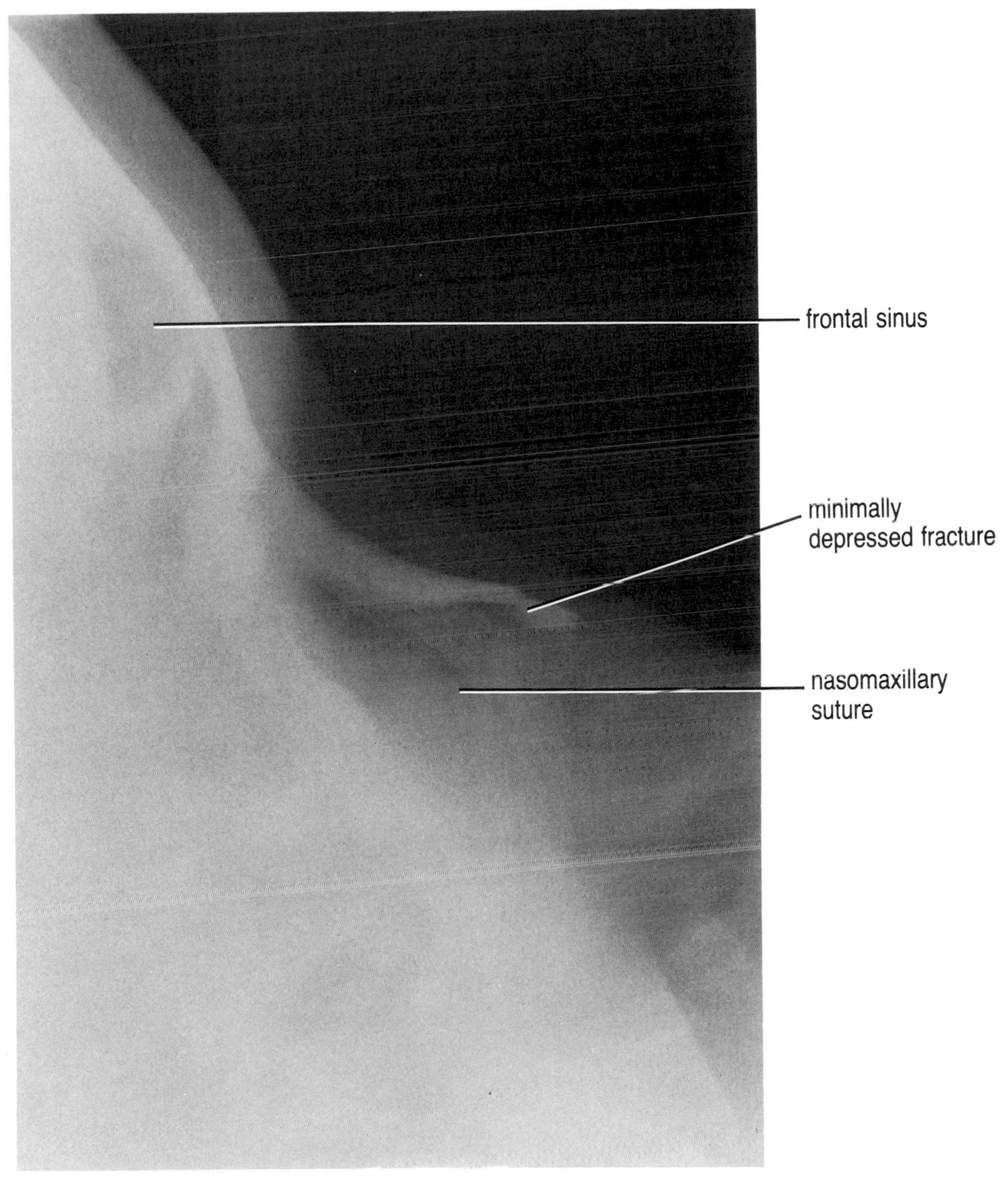

Figure 1.04. Nasal bone fracture.

1.05 OPACIFICATION OF MAXILLARY SINUS

Paranasal sinuses consist of the frontal, maxillary, ethmoid, and sphenoid. Routine examination includes a posteroanterior view, Water's view, Caldwell view, and a lateral view. A submentovertex view may also be obtained if necessary.

A. Differential diagnosis of an opacified maxillary sinus
   1. Trauma—acute hemorrhage within the sinus; look for associated fracture and fluid level.
   2. Sinusitis—a fluid level may also be present
   3. Artifactual opacification—overlying soft tissue swelling secondary to trauma
   4. Retention cyst
   5. Polyp
   6. Epistaxis
   7. Neoplasm
   8. Wegener's granulomatosis

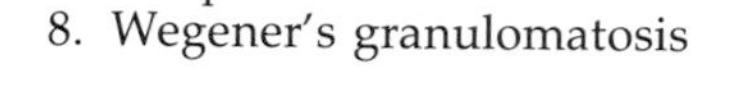

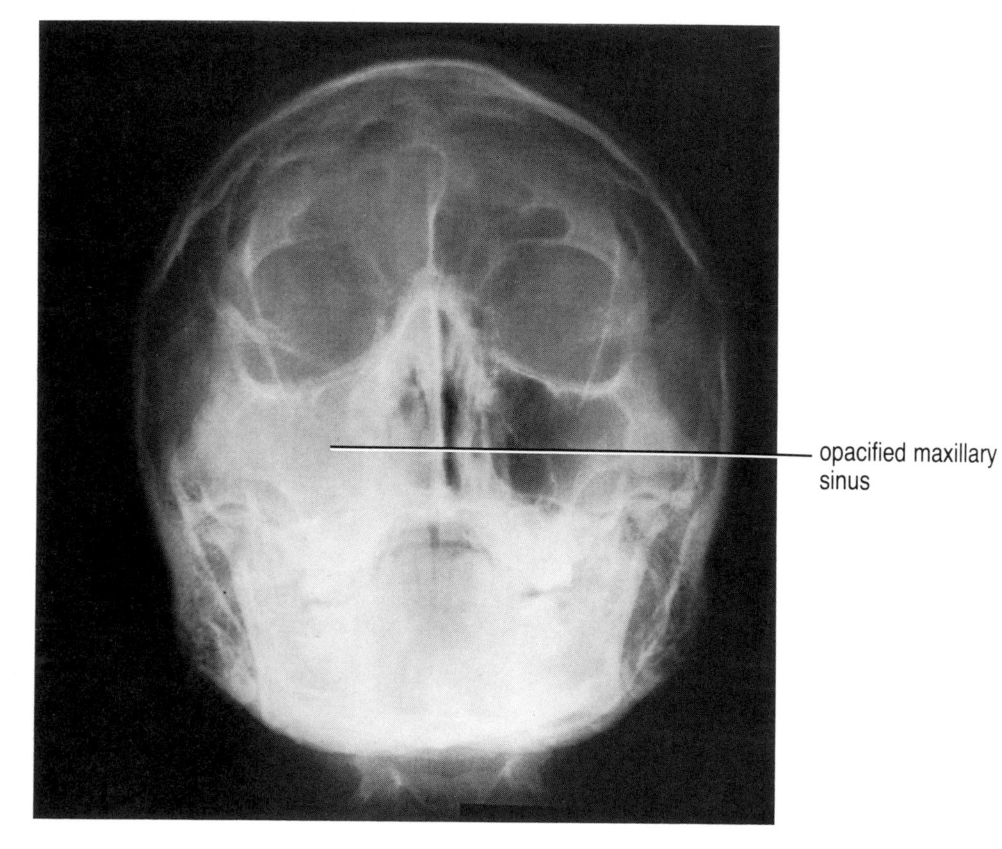

Figure 1.05. Opacification of maxillary sinus.

1.06 MANDIBULAR FRACTURE

A. Mandibular fracture is one of the most common fractures of the face.
B. Application of a force to cause fracture at one site often results in additional fracture sites.
C. Dislocation of the temporomandibular joint may occur with mandibular trauma. Condyles are usually dislocated anteriorly and superiorly.

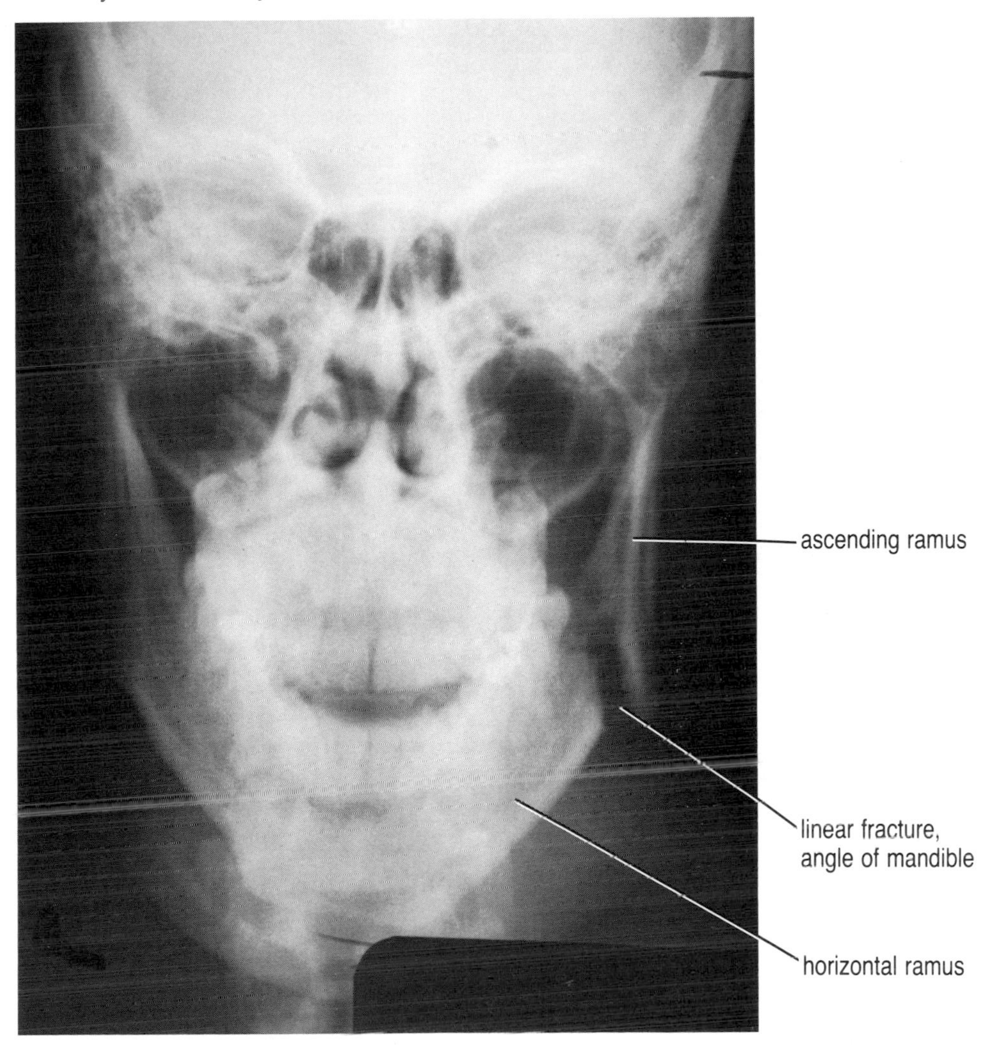

Figure 1.06. Mandibular fracture.

1.07 BLOW-OUT FRACTURE OF THE ORBIT

A. Results from a direct force applied to the orbit
B. Routine orbital views include a Water's view, Caldwell view, and lateral view.
   1. There is a fracture of the orbital floor while the inferior orbital rim remains intact.
   2. Fracture may also involve the medial orbital wall. Extension into the ethmoid air cells may result in orbital emphysema.
   3. Entrapment of orbital contents may result in sensory deficit involving the infra-orbital nerve distribution, enophthalmos, diplopia, and limitation of extraocular eye movements.
   4. Fracture is visualized radiographically as a soft tissue mass extending below the orbit into the superior aspect of the maxillary antrum.
C. Plain film tomography and CT evaluation provide additional information in the presence of facial trauma.

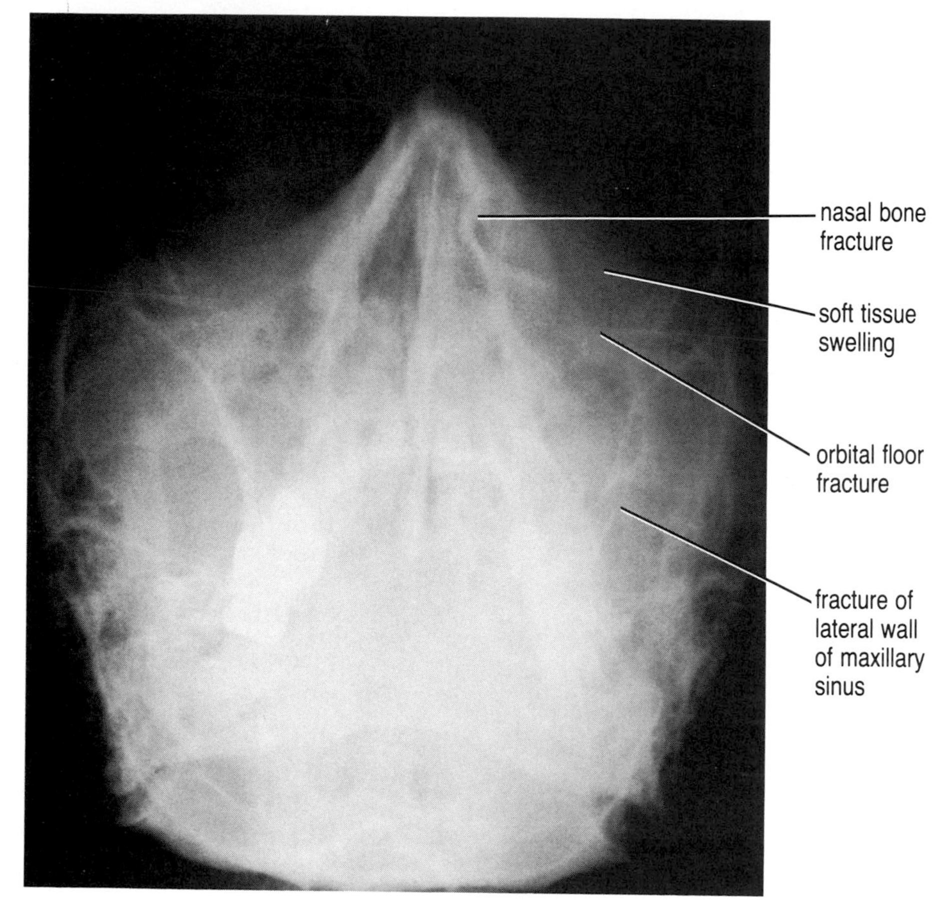

Figure 1.07. Blow-out fracture of the orbit.

1.08 FACIAL FRACTURES: LE FORT CLASSIFICATION

A. Le Fort fractures are complex facial fractures due to direct trauma along planes of weakness in the facial bones.
B. The fractures are symmetrical across the face.
C. Routine views of the face include a Water's view, Caldwell view, and lateral view.
D. CT evaluation provides additional detailed information.
   1. Le Fort I fracture
      a. This is a complete transverse fracture that extends through the maxilla and the inferior portion of the nasal cavity. This fracture line occurs superior to the hard palate and results in a freely movable palate.
      b. There is usually opacification of the maxillary sinuses.
   2. Le Fort II fracture
      a. This is also known as the pyramidal fracture.
      b. This fracture appears as an inverted "V." The fracture line extends above the bridge of the nose in the region of the nasofrontal suture. The fracture line then extends obliquely through the inferior aspect of the orbit and continues through the maxillary antrum and terminates within the zygoma. This fracture also has a symmetrical appearance bilaterally.
      c. The cribriform plate may also be fractured with this injury resulting in cerebrospinal fluid rhinorrhea.
      d. Opacification of the maxillary sinuses occurs.
   3. Le Fort III fracture
      a. This is a severe injury that results in craniofacial dysjunction.
      b. The fracture line extends across the nasal bridge in the region of the nasofrontal suture. The fracture line extends laterally through the orbit and the zygomatic arches.
      c. Because of the severe force necessary to create this injury, it is usually associated with a Le Fort II fracture.
      d. The midportion of the face becomes completely separated from the skull.
      e. It is a symmetrical fracture bilaterally with opacification of the maxillary sinuses.
      f. This is also associated with fracture of the cribriform plate.

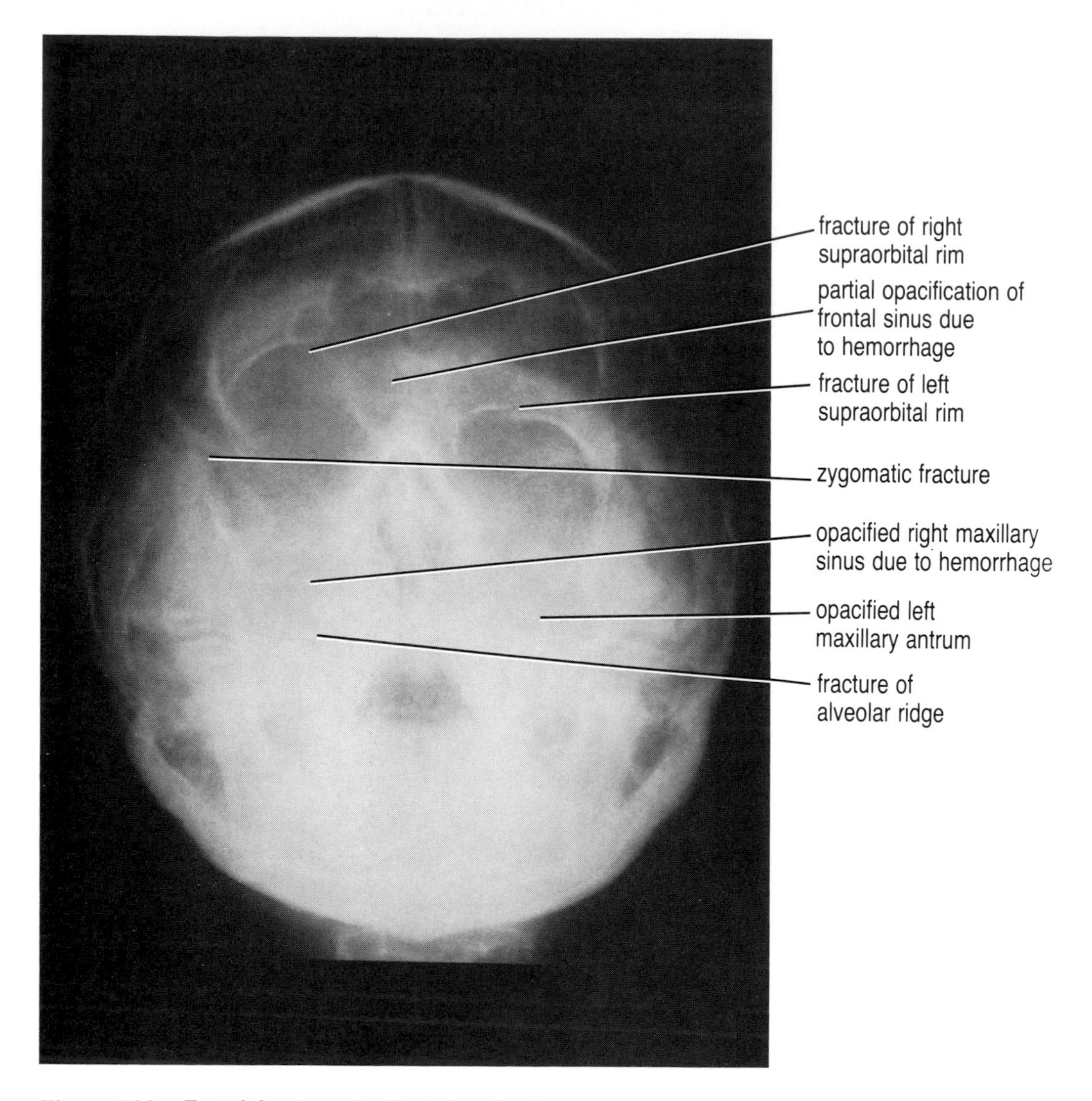

Figure 1.08. Facial fracture: Le Fort classification.

1.09 CT OF THE HEAD: NORMAL ANATOMY AND EVALUATION

A. CT of the head
  1. Computed tomography without infusion of contrast is an excellent method of evaluation of the brain in the event of trauma, cerebral vascular accident (CVA), emergence of neurologic impairment, or altered mental status.
  2. Infusion of contrast provides additional information and is indicated if brain metastases, primary brain tumor, abscess, vascular lesions such as arteriovenous malformation, or aneurysm are suspected.
  3. The administration of contrast is not without risk. An "allergic reaction" may result in complete respiratory or cardiovascular collapse.
  4. The routine examination consists of approximately 12 axial scans from the level of the foramen magnum to the top of the cerebral convexities.
  5. Newer-generation CT scanners allow evaluation of the brain in sagittal and coronal views.
  6. The ability to identify different structures is based on the relative attenuation of the x-ray beam. For example, calcification appears "white" (high attenuation) because it attenuates the x-ray beam. On the other hand, cerebrospinal fluid or fat appears "black" (low attenuation) because the x-ray beam is not attenuated to the same degree.

B. CT evaluation
  1. An individual must understand axial anatomy. See normal scans provided.
  2. Look for the presence of symmetry. Compare one side of the brain with the other.
  3. High-attenuation areas (white) include calcification and acute hemorrhage.
  4. Low-attentuation areas (black) include cerebrospinal fluid, fat, and areas of encephalomalacia.
  5. An individual must understand the difference between an acute process and an old, remote process.
     a. Acute process: Cerebral edema may often cause effacement (nonvisualization of the sulci on one side), or may appear as an area of low density (low attenuation). Cerebral edema may produce a mass effect on normal structures, i.e., ventricular system, or may produce a midline shift.
     b. Old process: An area of low attenuation (black) often may represent an area of encephalomalacia from previous infarction or trauma. No edema, mass effect, or midline shift is seen. Compensatory hypertrophy of an ipsilateral ventricle may occur.

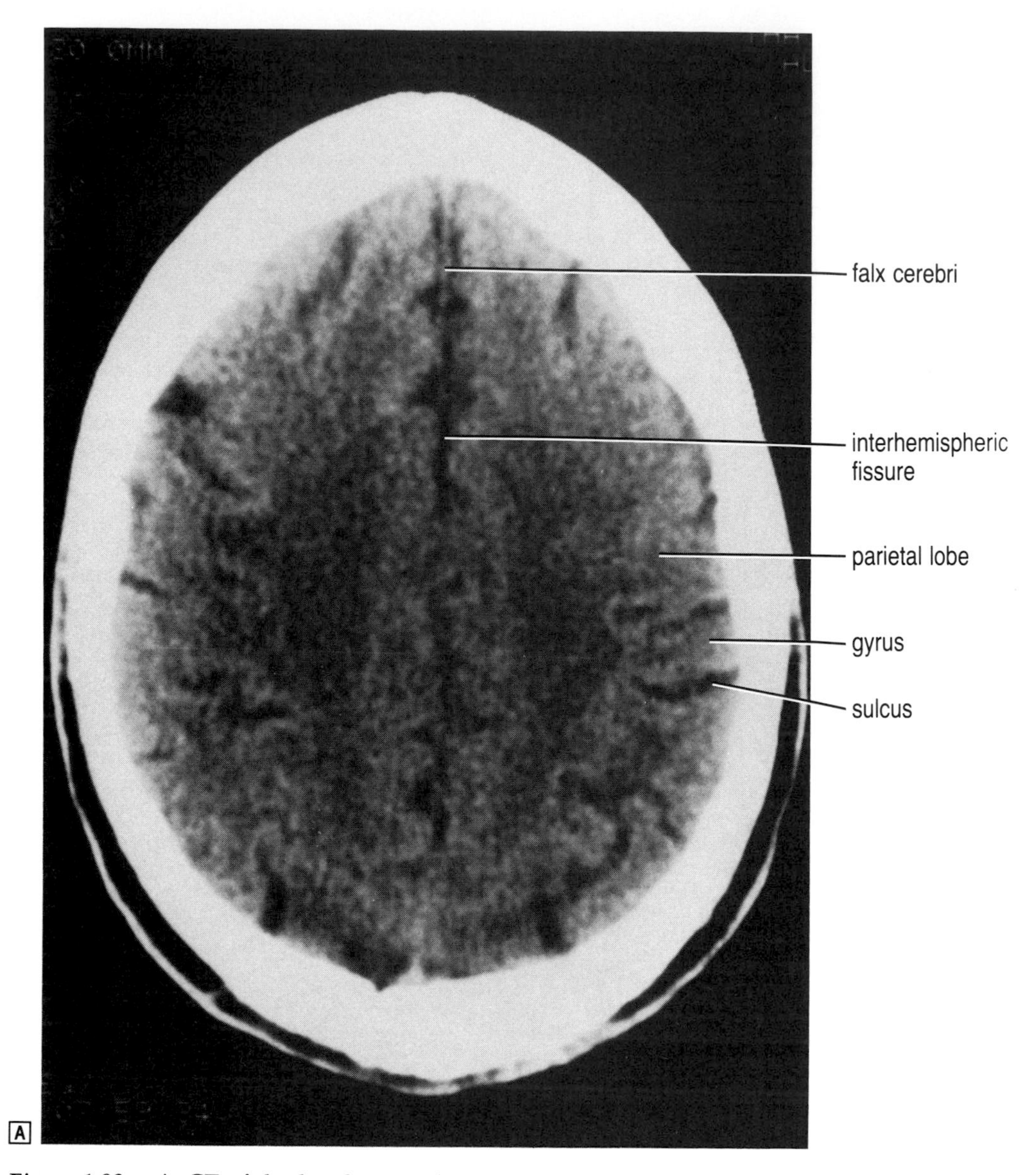

Figure 1.09. *A,* CT of the head: normal anatomy and evaluation.

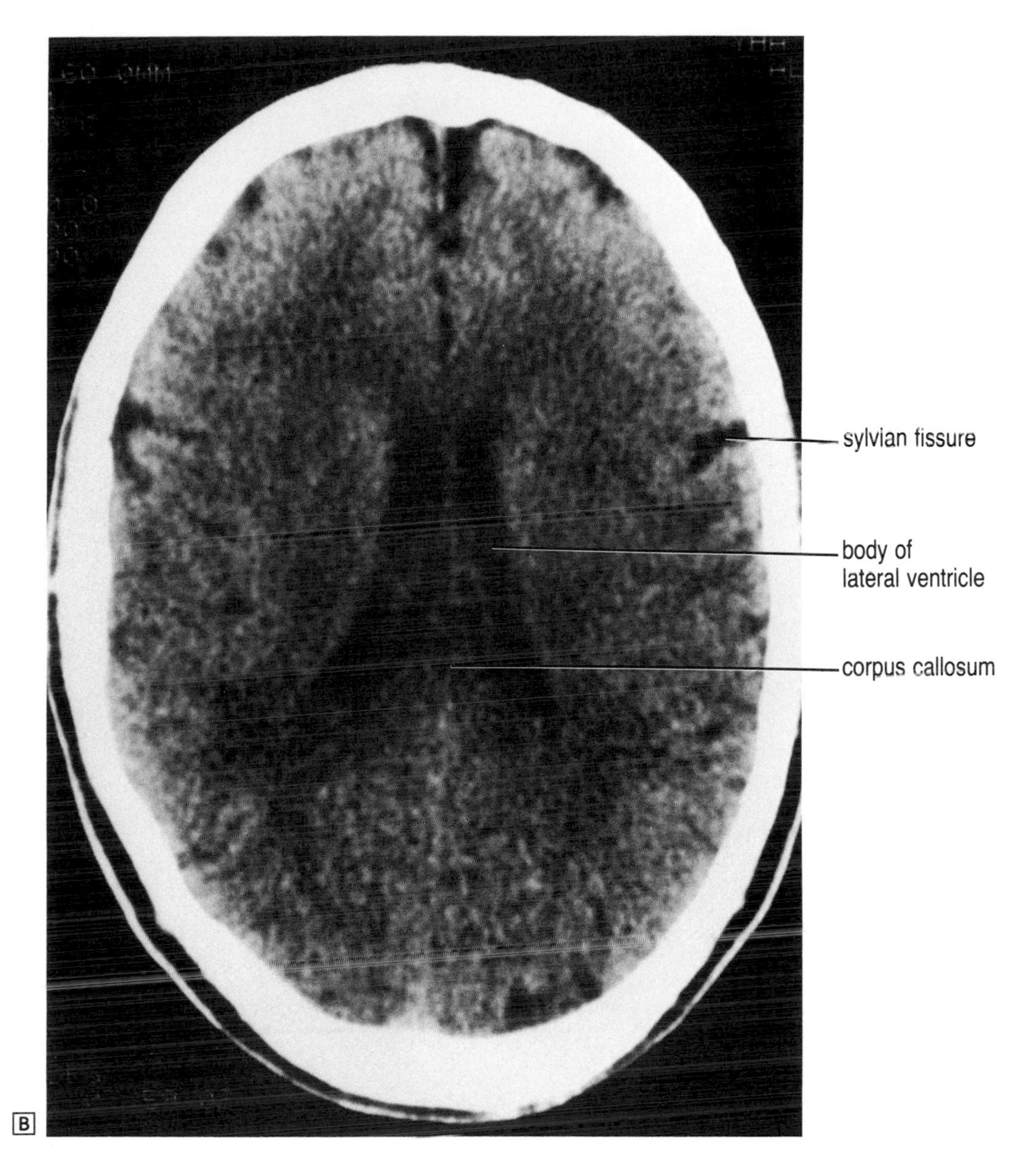

Figure 1.09. *B*, CT of the head: normal anatomy and evaluation.

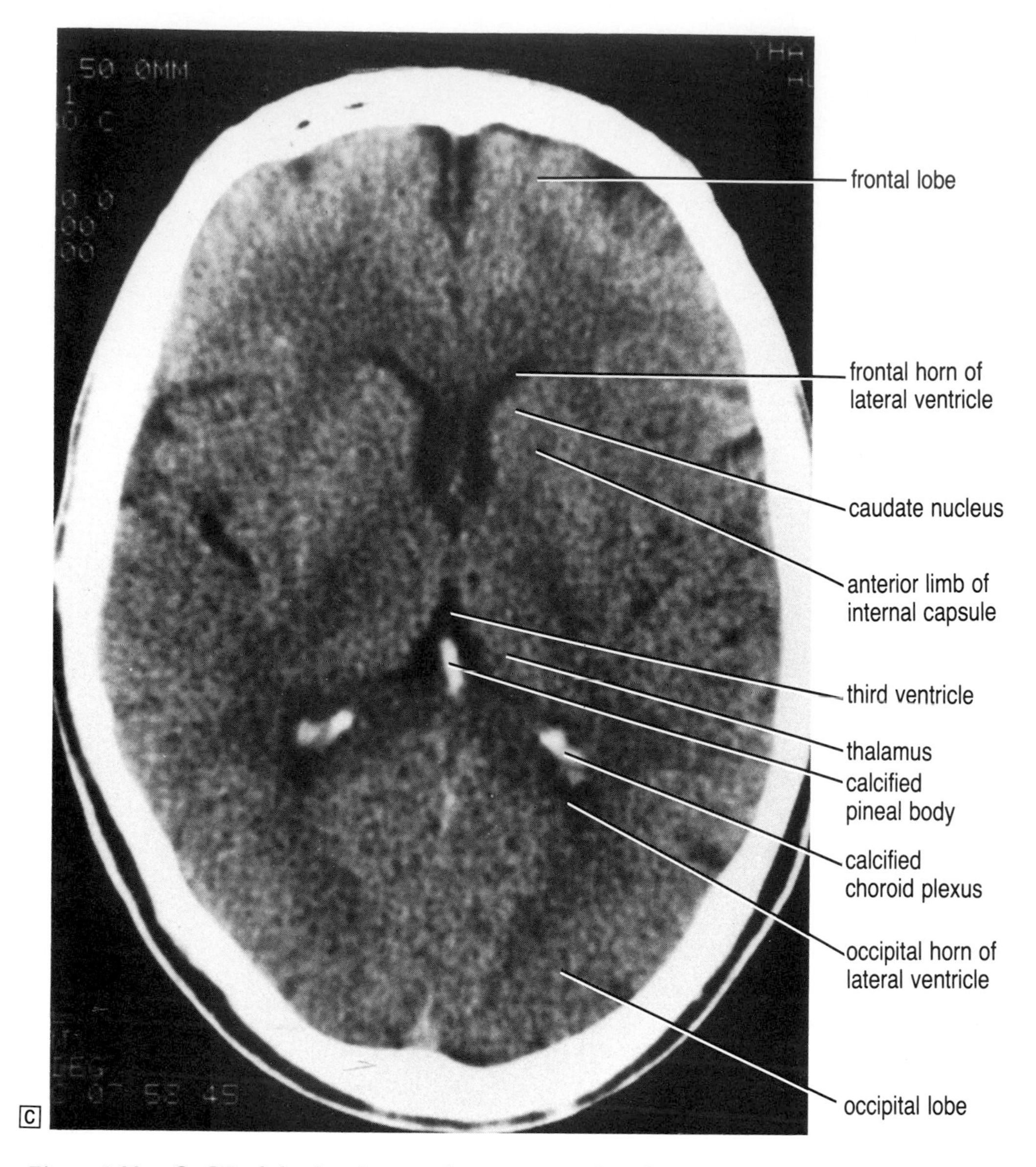

Figure 1.09. C, CT of the head: normal anatomy and evaluation.

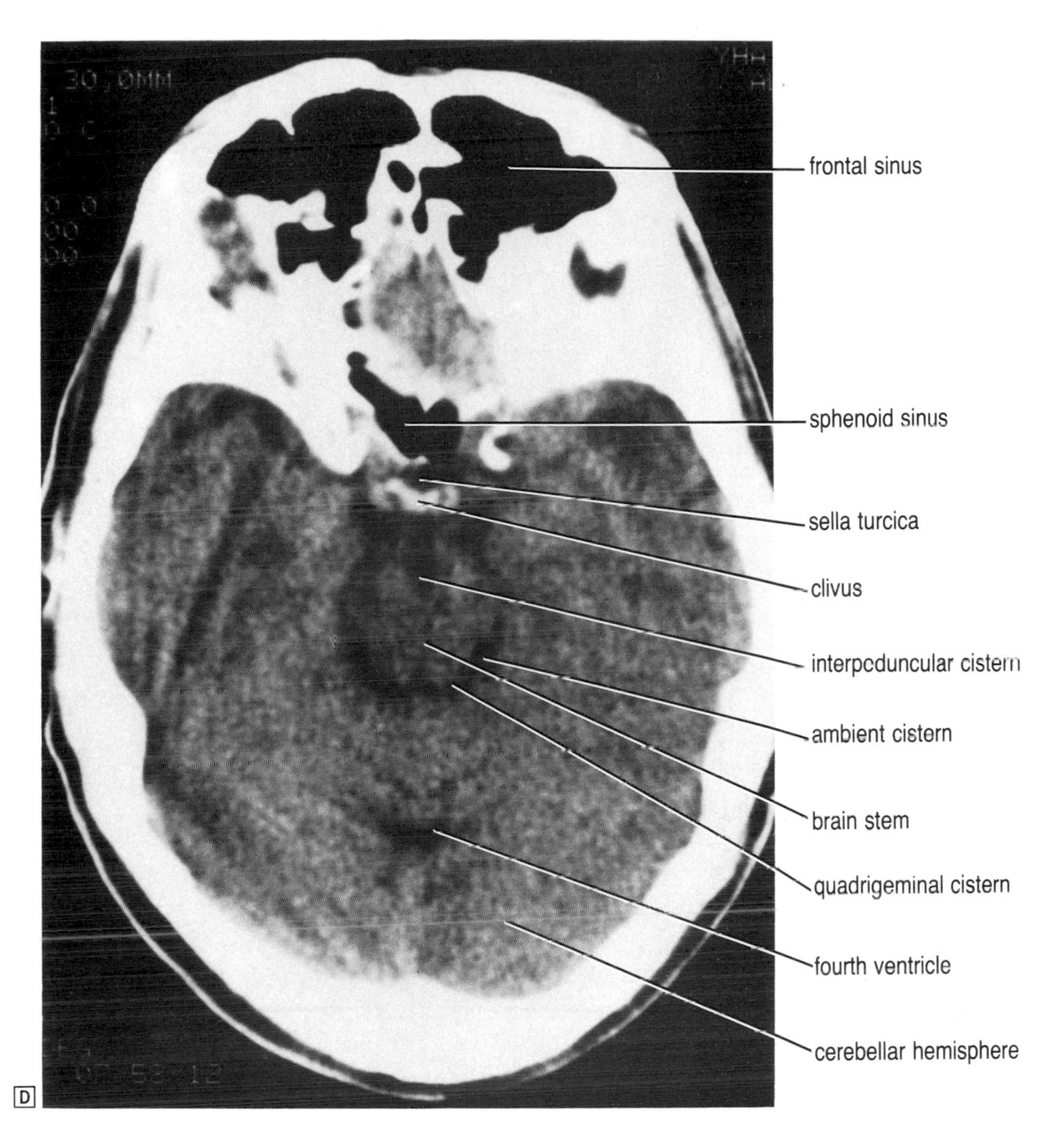

Figure 1.09. *D,* CT of the head: normal anatomy and evaluation.

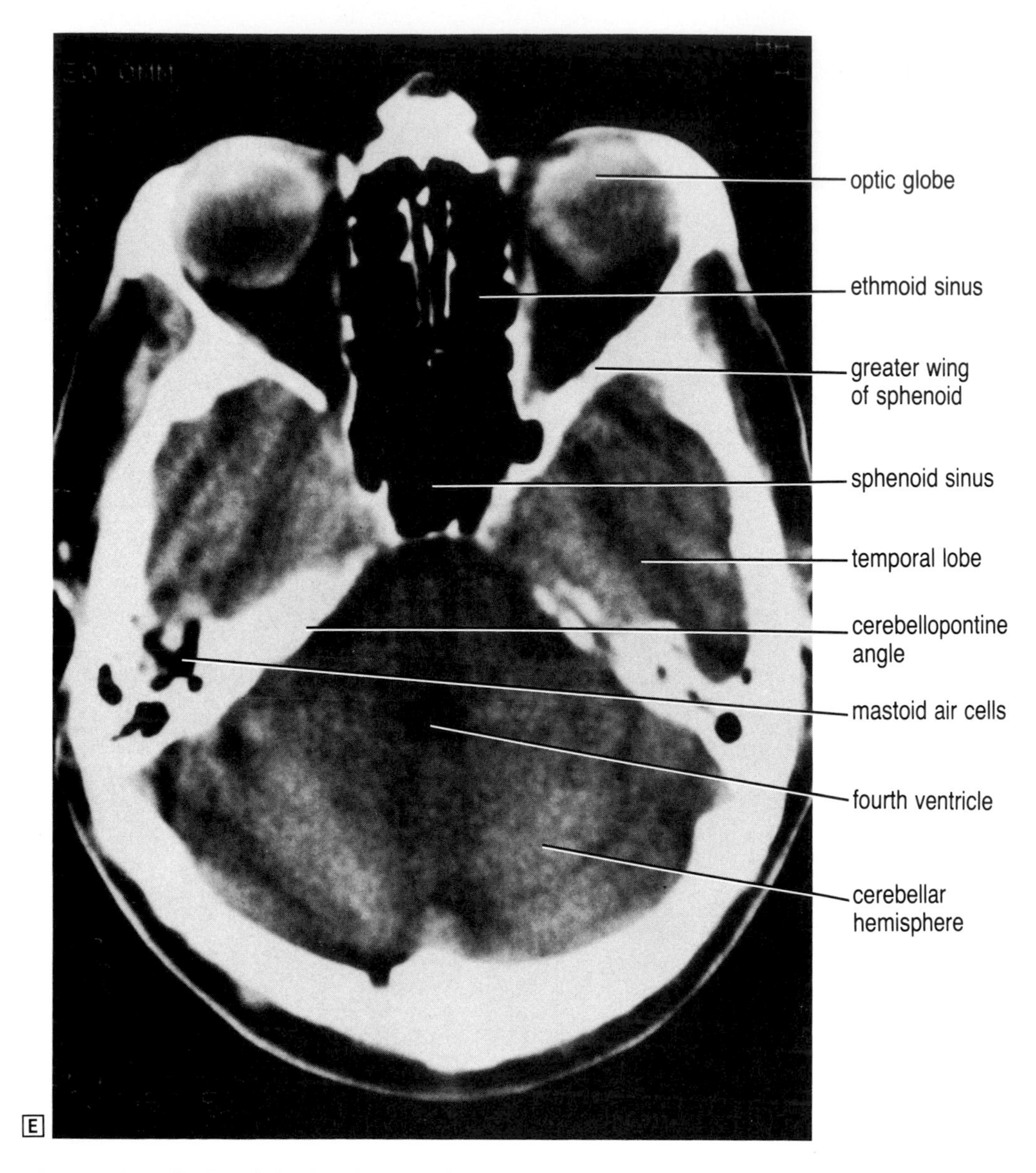

Figure 1.09. *E,* CT of the head: normal anatomy and evaluation.

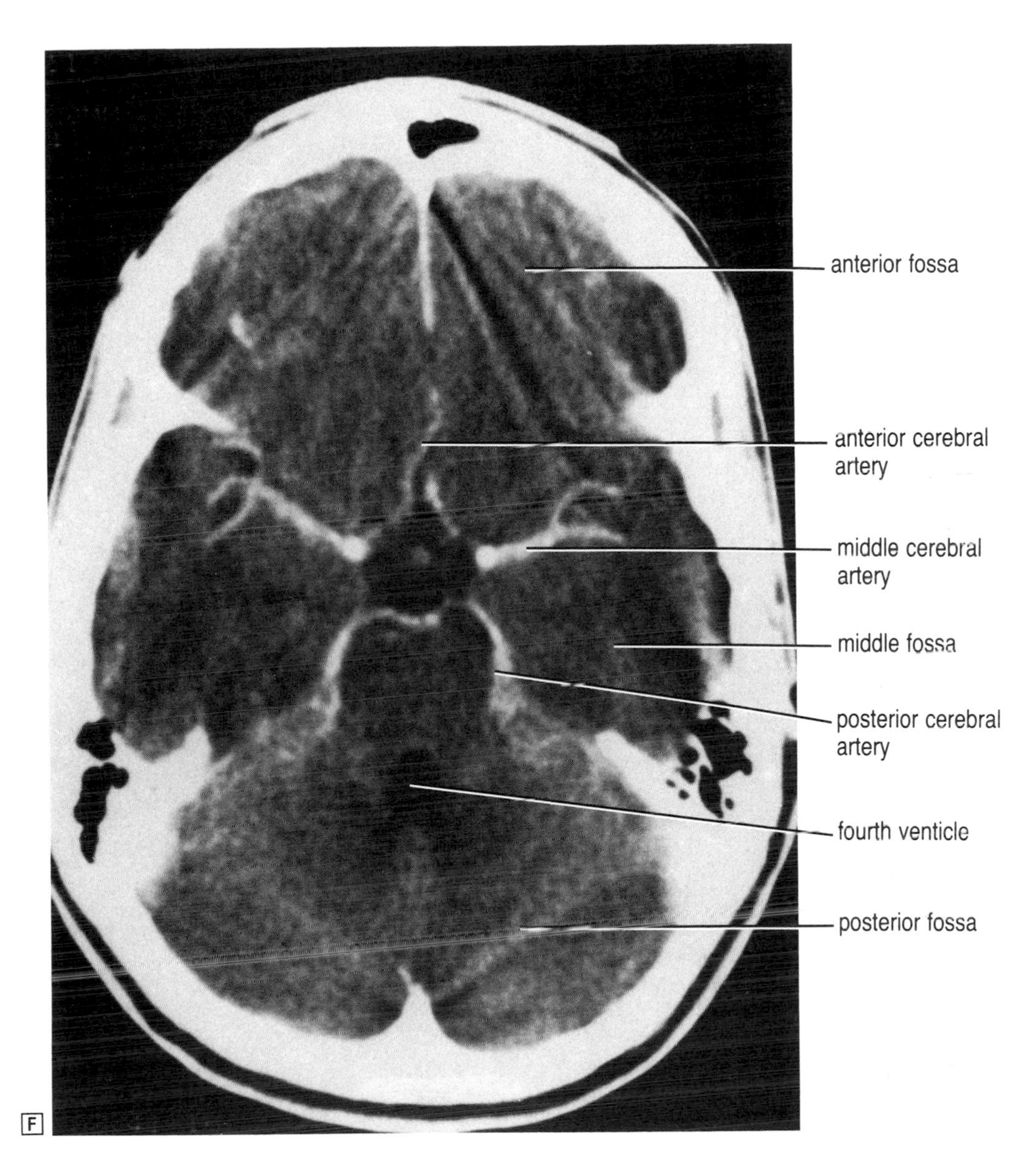

Figure 1.09. *F*, CT of the head: normal anatomy and evaluation.

1.10 CT OF HEAD TRAUMA: BRAIN CONTUSION

A. Brain contusion
  1. Results from impact of brain parenchyma against the skull. Capillary damage results in small parenchymal hemorrhage. The periphery of the convexities is more susceptible to contusion.
  2. A coup injury is the result of direct impact of the brain parenchyma against the skull. This injury is most often seen in the frontal and temporal regions.
  3. With a contracoup injury, the contusion occurs on the opposite side of the impact.
  4. Brain contusion is the most frequent parenchymal bleed, and about one third of these contusions are multiple.

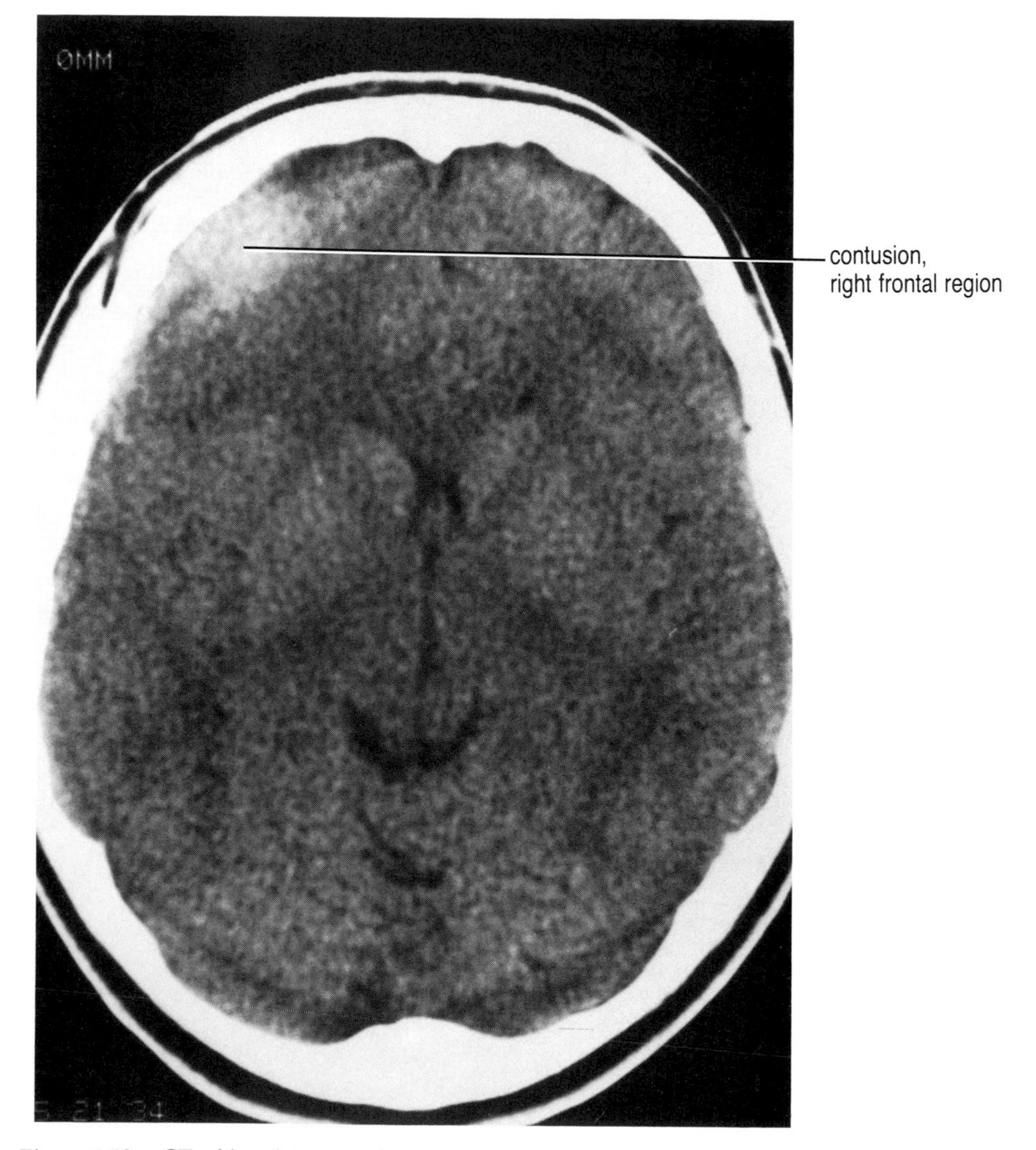

Figure 1.10. CT of head trauma: brain contusion.

1.11 CT OF HEAD TRAUMA: EPIDURAL HEMATOMA

A. Area of high attenuation (white), which has a biconvex appearance.
B. The epidural space is a potential space between the dura and cranium. The dura is attached at the suture margins; therefore, an epidural hematoma is limited in its distribution, unlike a subdural hematoma.
C. The temporoparietal region is the most common location due to laceration of the middle meningeal artery or vein.
D. Is often associated with a skull fracture in the area of the middle meningeal artery.
E. Following trauma there may or may not be loss of consciousness. Following a lucid interval there may be development of headache, emesis, confusion, or seizures.
F. Cerebral herniation and death may result if there is no intervention.

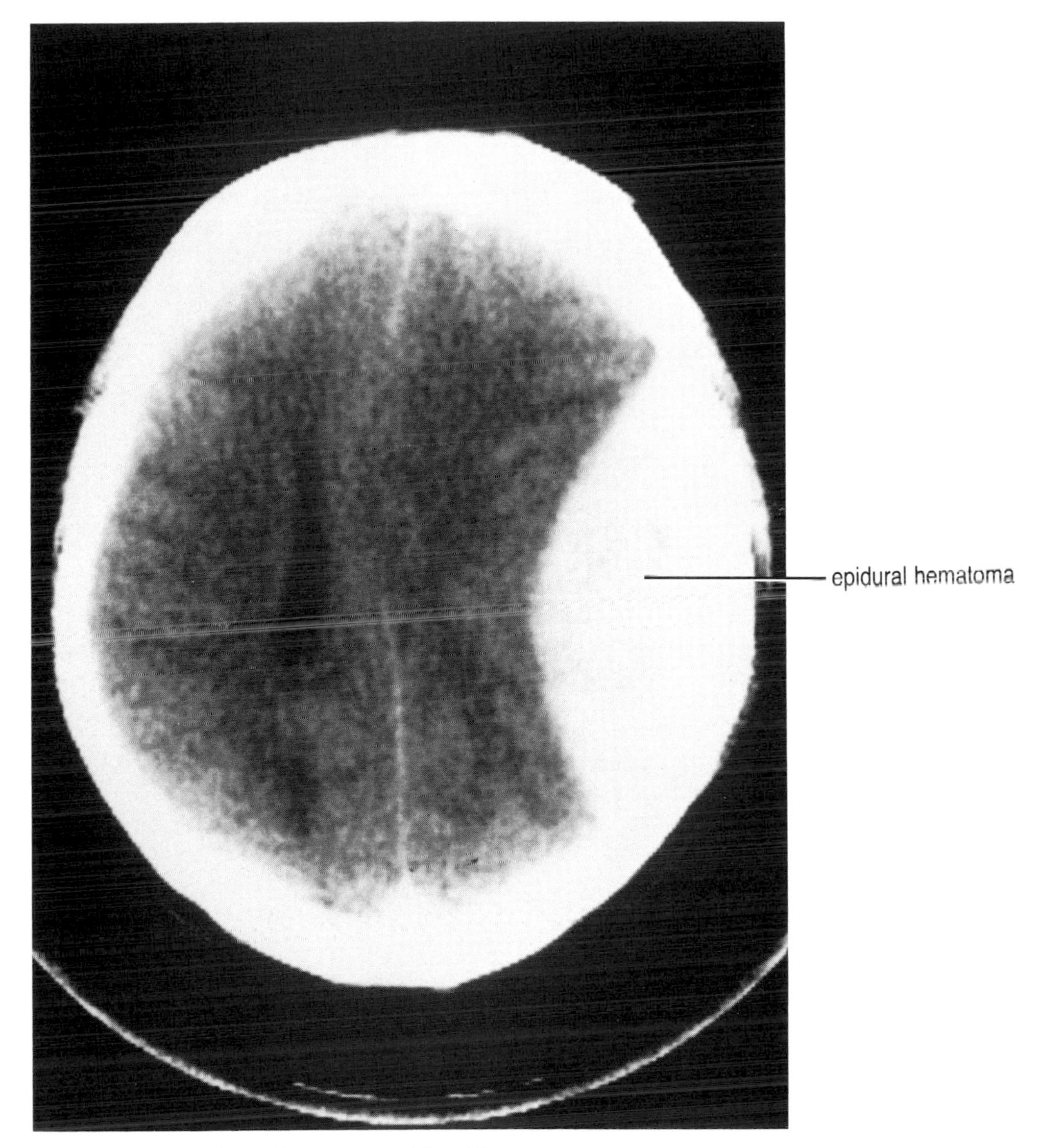

Figure 1.11. CT of head trauma: epidural hematoma.

1.12 CT OF HEAD TRAUMA: ACUTE SUBDURAL HEMATOMA

A. Area of high attenuation (white) that is crescent-shaped between the periphery of the brain and the inner table of the skull. Blood may extend along the entire length of the hemisphere, which is unlike an epidural hematoma. The blood follows the contour of the convexity.
B. The acute hemorrhage is venous blood.
C. Subdural space is located between the dura and the leptomeninges.
D. There is often associated mass effect with ventricular effacement or midline shift.
E. Symptoms develop at a variable interval following trauma. There may be headache, confusion, drowsiness, or impaired mentation.

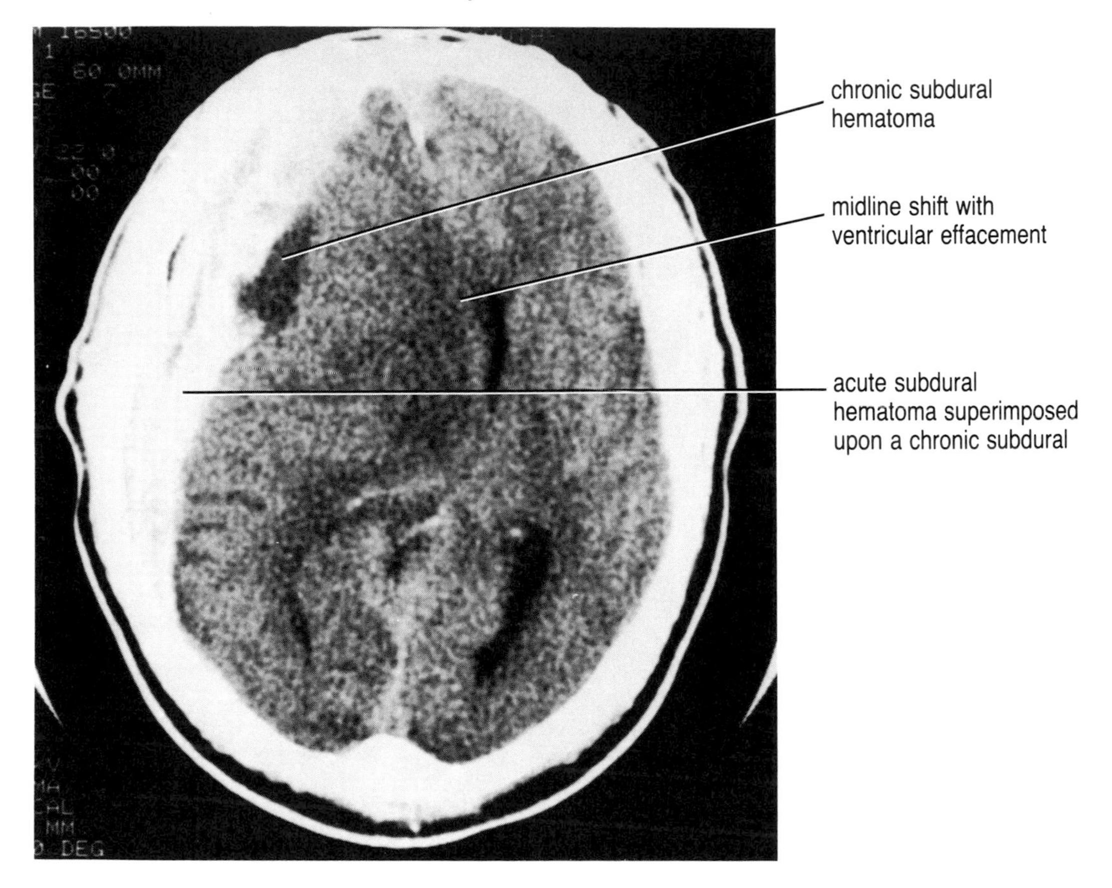

Figure 1.12. CT of head trauma: acute subdural hematoma.

1.13 CT OF HEAD TRAUMA; CHRONIC SUBDURAL HEMATOMA

A. Is the result of chronic accumulation of blood within the subdural space.
B. Is usually visualized as an area of decreased attenuation because the hemoglobin has been broken down over time.
C. The low-attenuation area follows the contour of the convexities the same as an acute subdural hematoma.
D. If new bleeding has occurred, there may be a fluid-fluid level with the acute blood layering in a dependent position because it is more dense.
E. There may or may not be a definite history of trauma. There is progressive development of headaches, confusion, and decreased mentation.

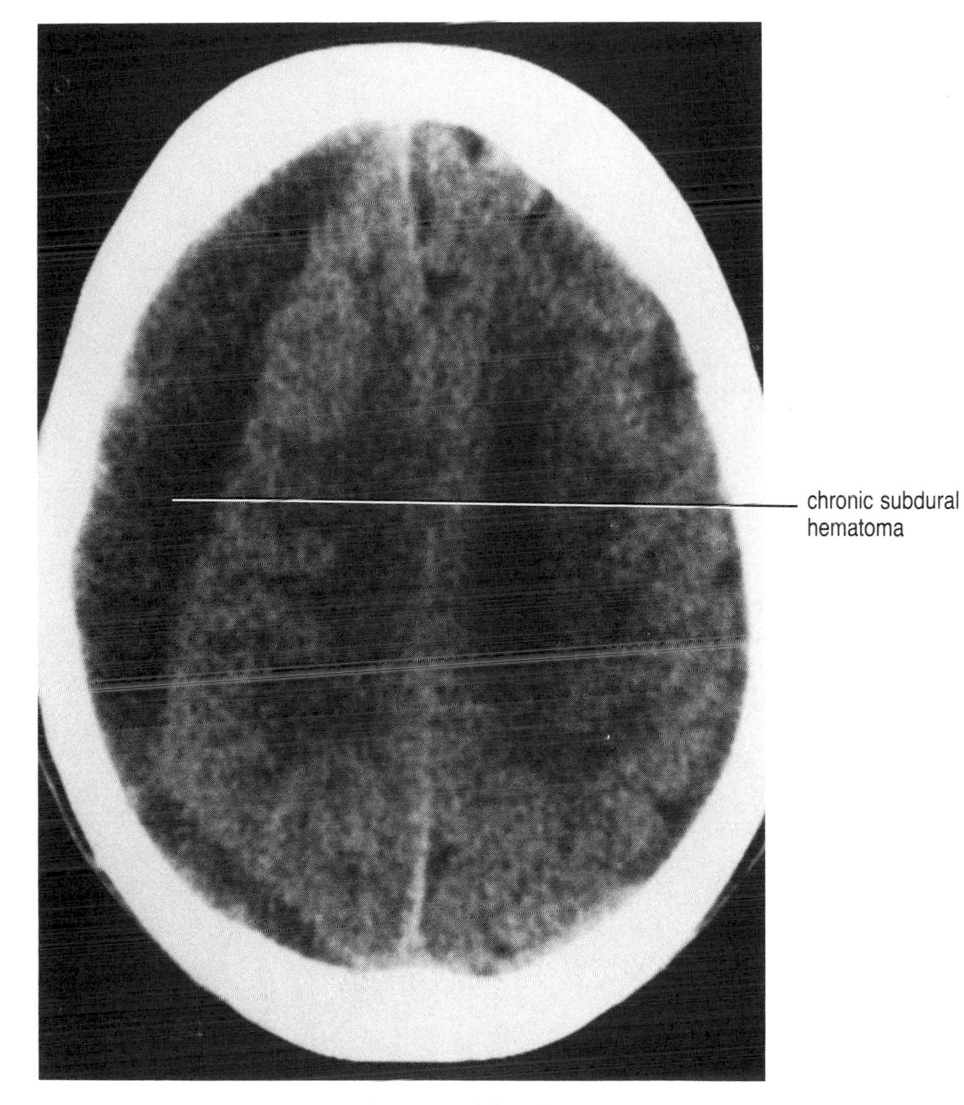

Figure 1.13. CT of head trauma: chronic subdural hematoma.

1.14 CT OF HEAD TRAUMA: SUBARACHNOID HEMORRHAGE

A. An acute subarachnoid hemorrhage is identified as an area of increased attenuation located within the subarachnoid space. The acute hemorrhage is often seen within the interhemispheric fissure, between sulci, within the sylvian fissure and cisterns.

B. After approximately seven days, the blood becomes isodense and is not visualized on CT.

C. A lumbar puncture may be diagnostic, demonstrating red blood cells.

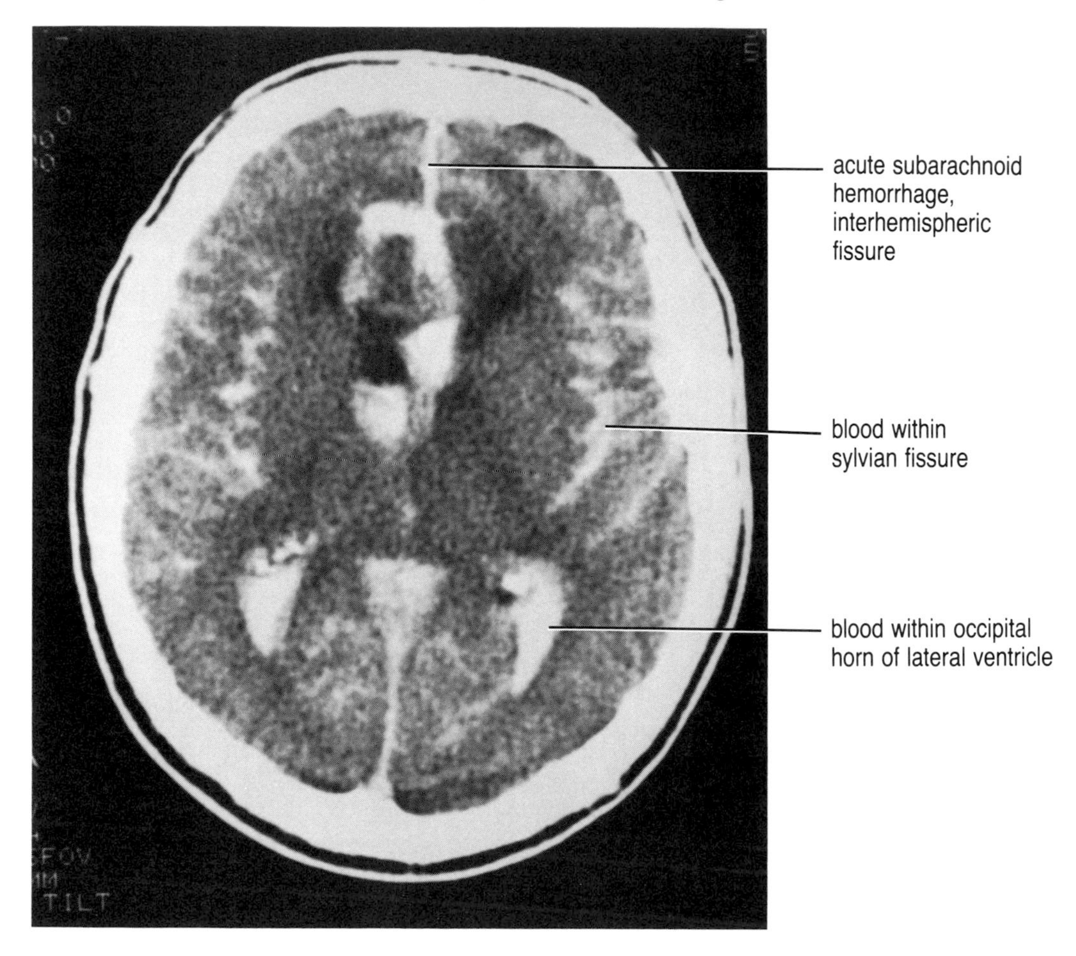

Figure 1.14. CT of head trauma: subarachnoid hemorrhage.

1.15 CT OF HEAD TRAUMA: INTRACEREBRAL HEMORRHAGE

A. Visualized on a noncontrast CT as an area of increased attenuation (white), located within the brain parenchyma, which is usually round or oval. The acute hemorrhage may decompress into the ventricular system.

B. Differential diagnosis of intracerebral hemorrhage
   1. Trauma (see Secs. 1.10 to 1.14)
   2. Hypertensive hemorrhage
   3. Anticoagulant therapy
   4. Aneurysm (see Sec. 1.18)
   5. Arteriovenous malformation
   6. Neoplasm (see Sec. 1.17)
   7. Hemorrhagic infarction
   8. Blood disorders (i.e., leukemia, thrombocytopenia purpura, aplastic anemia)

C. Hypertensive intracerebral hemorrhage
   1. Most common sites
      a. Basal ganglia
         (1) Basal ganglia consists of the caudate nucleus, putamen, globus pallidus, substantia nigra, and subthalamic nuclei.
         (2) Approximately 50% of all hypertensive hemorrhages involve the putamen.
      b. Thalamus
         (1) Next most common location
      c. Cerebellum
      d. Pons
   2. Symptoms
      a. No sex or age predilection
      b. Blacks affected more often than whites
      c. Bleed occurs while the individual is awake and active with symptoms gradually developing.
      d. Hemorrhage within the putamen may result in hemiplegia due to the proximity of the internal capsule.
      e. Hemorrhage within the thalamus may also lead to hemiplegia.
      f. Cerebellar involvement results in emesis, vertigo, and ataxia.
      g. The individual may complain of headache.

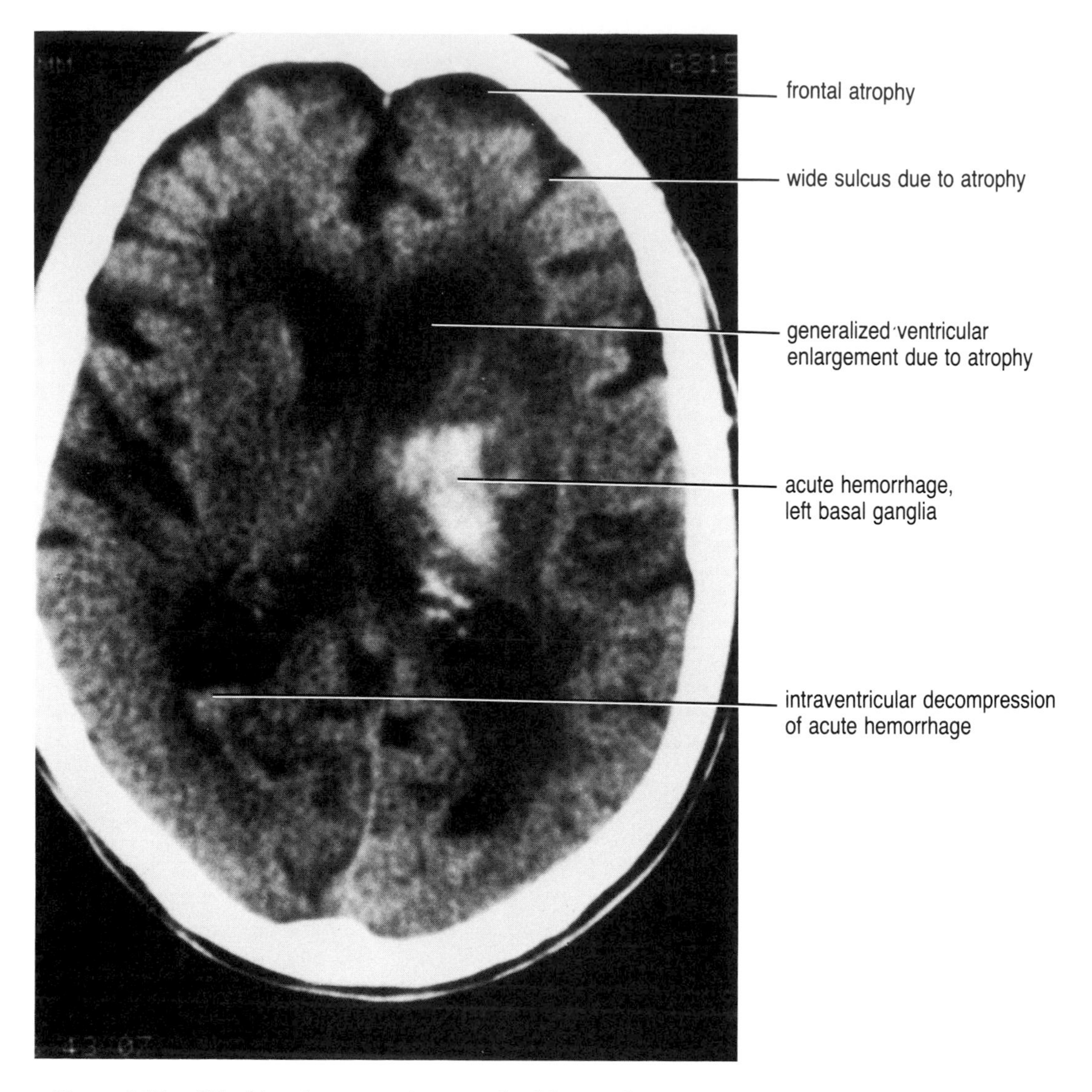

Figure 1.15. CT of head trauma: intracerebral hemorrhage.

1.16 INTRACRANIAL INFARCTION

A. Transient ischemic attack (TIA) is a reversible neurologic event that usually lasts from a few seconds to several minutes.
B. Reversible ischemic neurologic deficit (RIND) is a neurologic event that totally resolves after 24 hours.
C. Cerebral vascular accident (CVA) or stroke represents a nonreversible neurologic event.
D. Cerebral infarction may or may not be visualized during the first 24 to 48 hours on CT examination.
E. The importance of a noncontrast CT examination early in the acute phase allows differentiation between cerebral infarction and intracerebral hemorrhage. This allows the clinician to begin anticoagulation and antiplatelet therapy if indicated.
F. As the signs of infarction appear, they are generally located within the vascular supply of the middle cerebral artery (MCA), anterior cerebral artery (ACA), or posterior cerebral artery (PCA).
G. Signs of acute cerebral infarction on a noncontrast CT of the brain
   1. Area of decreased attenuation (darker than the remainder of the brain parenchyma) due to the presence of cerebral edema, localized to an area of vascular supply
   2. Asymmetry of the brain with effacement of sulci, possible mass effect upon the ventricular system, or midline shift.
   3. A hemorrhagic component may be visualized as an area of increased attenuation within the area of involvement. Approximately 25% of cerebral infarctions are hemorrhagic.
H. Symptoms have a variable expression based on the degree of involvement and the amount of collateral circulation.
I. Symptoms of internal carotid artery occlusion or middle cerebral artery occlusion
   1. Aphasia
   2. Contralateral hemiplegia
   3. Sensory deficits
   4. Homonymous hemianopia
J. Symptoms of anterior cerebral artery occlusion are more variable.
   1. Motor and sensory deficits involving the contralateral leg
   2. Contralateral upper extremity may be involved.
   3. Behavior may also be altered.
K. Symptoms of the vertebral-basilar system including the posterior cerebral artery. Some examples included depend on the area of supply compromised.
   1. Ataxia
   2. Nausea or vomiting
   3. Memory deficit
   4. Cortical blindness or visual field defects
   5. Numerous sensorimotor and cranial nerve disturbances
   6. Deafness
   7. Hemiplegia
L. From 10 to 14 days after the onset of symptoms a contrast-enhanced CT may demonstrate areas of enhancement that follow the contour of the gyri in the affected area. This is known as luxury perfusion and occurs because of the breakdown of the blood-brain barrier as a result of the injury.
M. Signs of remote cerebral infarction on a noncontrast CT of the brain
   1. An area of encephalomalacia (low attenuation) forms in the area of previous insult.
   2. There is no evidence of mass effect.
   3. Volume loss is present manifested by compensatory dilatation of the ipsilateral ventricle and prominence of sulci in the affected area.
N. Types of strokes
   1. Embolic stroke
      a. Rapid onset of symptoms
      b. Source of embolism most often cardiac in origin due to atrial fibrillation, subacute bacterial endocarditis, or mural thrombus

c. Also embolism from plaque formation in the internal carotid artery near the carotid bifurcation
d. Most often affects the middle cerebral vascular supply

2. Arteriosclerotic stroke
   a. Result of gradual thrombosis
   b. Demonstrates a more gradual progression of symptoms
   c. Occurs because of gradual luminal narrowing of a vessel that may ulcerate and undergo hemorrhage into the plaque resulting in occlusion
   d. Most common site of narrowing occurs in the proximal portion of the internal carotid artery near the carotid bifurcation
3. Hypertensive stroke (see Sec. 1.15)
4. Stroke secondary to ruptured aneurysm (see Sec 1.18)
5. Lacunar infarcts
   a. These are small focal areas of decreased attenuation representing infarcts of small end-arteries of the lenticulostriates, thalamostriates, and thalamoperforating and pontine perforating arteries.

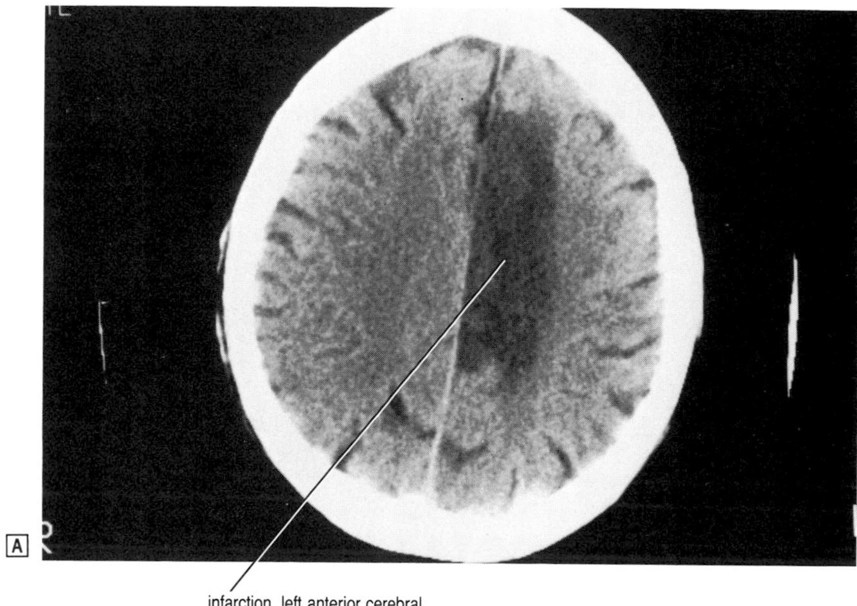

Figure 1.16. *A,* Intracranial infarction.

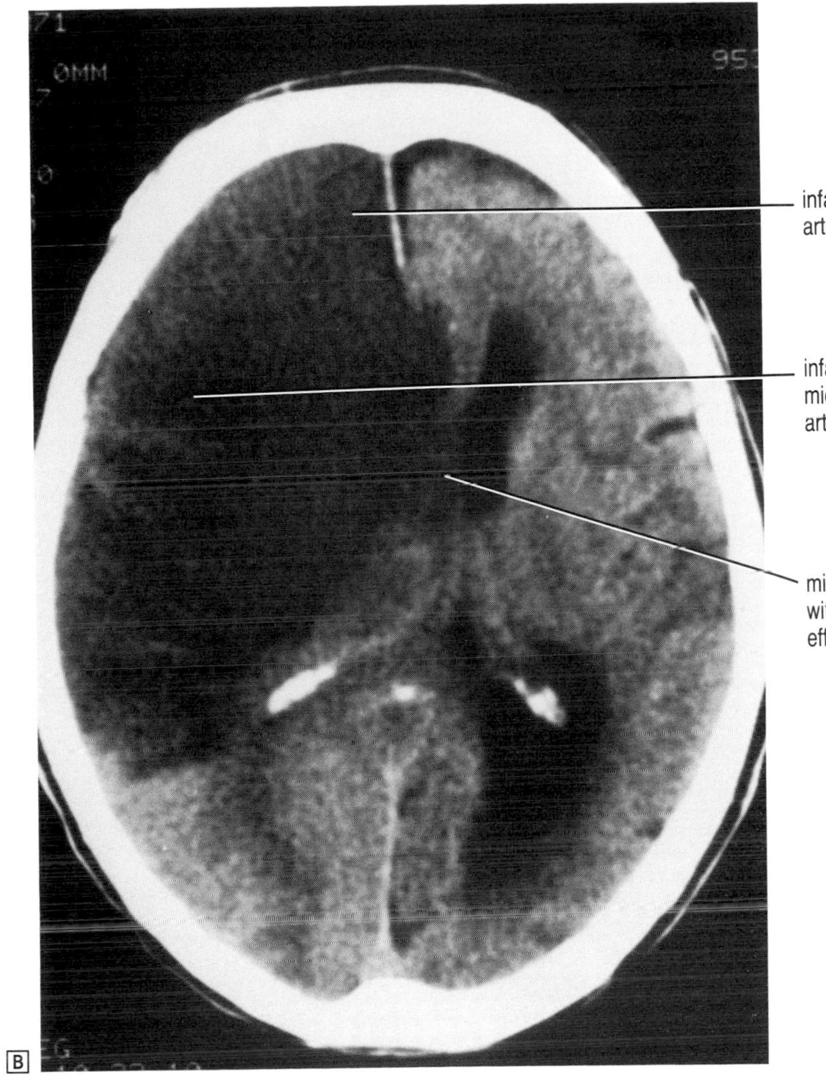

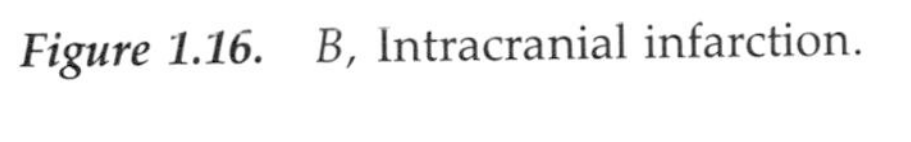
Figure 1.16. *B,* Intracranial infarction.

1.17 INTRACRANIAL NEOPLASMS

A. Intracranial neoplasms have a variable presentation with symptoms related to the area of the brain involved. Patients may suffer from headache, nausea, vomiting, gait disturbance, motor deficit, and personality changes.
B. A noncontrast study may demonstrate cerebral edema or the presence of mass effect.
C. Infusion of contrast is extremely important when intracranial neoplasms are suspected. Most tumors demonstrate enhancement following infusion of contrast.
D. Majority of brain tumors in adults are supratentorial
E. Majority of brain tumors in children are infratentorial
F. Brain metastases
   1. Account for approximately one third of intracranial neoplasms
   2. Primary neoplasm undergoes hematogenous spread to the brain.
   3. Most common primary site of involvement
      a. Lung
      b. Breast
      c. GI tract (colon)
      d. GU tract (kidney)
      e. Melanoma
   4. Noncontrast scans may demonstrate areas of low density representing edema involving white matter near the gray-white matter junction.
   5. May be solitary or multiple round lesions that demonstrate enhancement with contrast
G. Supratentorial neoplasms
   1. Gliomas
      a. Astrocytoma
         (1) Accounts for nearly 50% of intracranial neoplasms
         (2) Most often affects individuals in their 30s and 40s
         (3) Variable appearance based on whether it is low-grade or high-grade tumor
         (4) Most often involves the frontal and temporoparietal lobes
         (5) Usually a low dense lesion that demonstrates irregular contrast enhancement
      b. Glioblastoma multiforme
         (1) Accounts for approximately 25% of gliomas
         (2) Very high-grade tumor of astrocytic origin
         (3) Most often affects individuals in middle age
      c. Oligodendroglioma
         (1) Accounts for approximately 10% of gliomas
         (2) Most often seen in individuals in their 20s and 30s
         (3) Most often involves the frontal lobes
         (4) Majority of these neoplasms contain calcification
      d. Ependymoma
         (1) Most often located within the fourth ventricle, less likely present within the lateral ventricle. Neoplasm may project into the frontal and parietal lobes.
         (2) May be visualized as a well-defined, cystic mass with low attenuation
         (3) Approximately 50% demonstrate calcification.
      e. Choroid plexus papilloma
         (1) Is derived from the choroid plexus, which is located within the ventricular system
         (2) Neoplastic growth occurs within the ventricular system and may produce hydrocephalus, by means of excess CSF production.
         (3) May be seen in young children and adults
         (4) Lesion usually demonstrates enhancement with infusion of contrast.
   2. Meningioma
      a. Accounts for approximately 15% of intracranial neoplasms
      b. Usually visualized as a well-defined, round area of calcification (high attenuation) on noncontrast CT

c. May have surrounding rim of decreased attenuation representing cerebral edema
d. It is located adjacent to bone. Most common sites include parasagittal area of the frontal and parietal regions, sphenoid ridge, orbital roof, cerebellopontine angle, and tentorium cerebelli.

3. Ganglioglioma and ganglioneuroma
   a. These are rare neoplasms that most often affect individuals in their second and third decades of life.
   b. Most often located within the third ventricle and temporal lobes
   c. May contain calcification
   d. Usually enhance following infusion of contrast
4. Pinealoblastoma
   a. This is a rare and aggressive neoplasm that affects children and young adults.
   b. May also contain calcification and usually enhances following infusion of contrast

H. Infratentorial neoplasms
1. Medulloblastoma
   a. Is the second most common brain neoplasm in children
   b. Accounts for approximately 25% of brain neoplasms in children
   c. Lesion is found within the vermis of the cerebellum and fourth ventricle.
   d. Usually visualized as a well-defined round area of increased attenuation with a surrounding rim of cerebral edema (low attenuation)
   e. Owing to the location of the tumor, obstructive hydrocephalus may result producing nausea, vomiting, and headache.
   f. Presentation includes headache, vomiting, progressive gait disturbance, and papilledema.
2. Cerebellar astrocytoma
   a. The most common brain neoplasm in children
   b. Tumor found within the cerebellum
   c. Usually visualized as a cystic mass (low attenuation) that enhances with infusion of contrast
   d. Approximately 25% demonstrate calcification
   e. This lesion may also produce obstructive hydrocephalus
3. Hemangioblastoma
   a. Tumor occurs within the cerebellum and medulla oblongata
   b. Usually a cystic mass (low attenuation) that demonstrates ring-like enhancement with contrast
4. Ependymoma (see Supratentorial neoplasms)
5. Brain stem astrocytoma
6. Choroid plexus papilloma (see Supratentorial neoplasms)

I. Endocrine brain neoplasms
1. Craniopharyngioma
   a. The most common suprasellar neoplasm in children
   b. May also occur in adults
   c. CT demonstrates a suprasellar mass that may contain calcification and cystic components and that enhances with contrast.
   d. Children may present with hydrocephalus, obesity, and growth retardation.
   e. Adult manifestations include diminished gonadal function, diabetes insipidus, or panhypopituitarism.
   f. Tumor mass effect may produce visual field disturbances (i.e., bitemporal hemianopia).
2. Pituitary adenomas
   a. Account for approximately 10% of intracranial tumors
   b. Most adenomas involve the adenohypophysis (anterior lobe).
   c. CT evaluation reveals a suprasellar lesion.
   d. Enlargement of the tumor may compress the optic chiasm resulting in a visual field disturbance (i.e., bitemporal hemianopia).
3. Types of adenomas

a. Chromophobe adenoma
  (1) May be a nonfunctioning or hormone-secreting tumor
b. Eosinophilic adenoma
  (1) Produces an excess of growth hormone that results in giantism prior to puberty or acromegaly following puberty
  (2) Signs of acromegaly
    (a) Enlargement of hands, feet, mandible, and nose
    (b) Increased heel pad thickness (>22 mm).
    (c) Coarsening of facial features
    (d) Enlargement of frontal sinuses
    (e) Deepening of voice
    (f) Arthralgias
    (g) Hypertension
    (h) Diabetes
(c) Basophilic adenoma
  (1) Produces an excess of ACTH that results in Cushing's syndrome
  (2) Signs of Cushing's syndrome
    (a) Truncal obesity
    (b) Abdominal striae
    (c) Moon facies
    (d) Hypertension
    (e) Buffalo hump
    (f) Weakness
    (g) Amenorrhea
    (h) Ecchymoses
    (i) Osteoporosis
    (j) Hirsutism
d. Prolactin-secreting adenoma
  (1) Amenorrhea
  (2) Galactorrhea
  (3) Males demonstrate hypogonadism.

J. Tumors of the cerebellopontine angle
  1. Include meningioma, glioma, acoustic neuroma, and cholesteatoma
  2. These neoplasms involve the fifth, sixth, seventh, and eighth cranial nerves.
    a. Acoustic neuroma
      (1) Accounts for approximately 10% of all intracranial neoplasms and up to 80% of those tumors arising along the cerebellopontine angle
      (2) Occurs within the internal auditory canal and involves the eighth cranial nerve
      (3) Symptoms include dizziness, diminished hearing, and tinnitus.
    b. Neurofibromatosis (von Recklinghausen's disease)
      (1) May have bilateral acoustic neuromas
      (2) Is considered one of the phakomatoses
      (3) Autosomal dominant
      (4) Cutaneous manifestations consist of "café-au-lait" spots.
      (5) Neurofibromas (nerve sheath tumors) involve the dorsal nerve roots of the spinal cord.
      (6) Scoliosis and osteoporosis

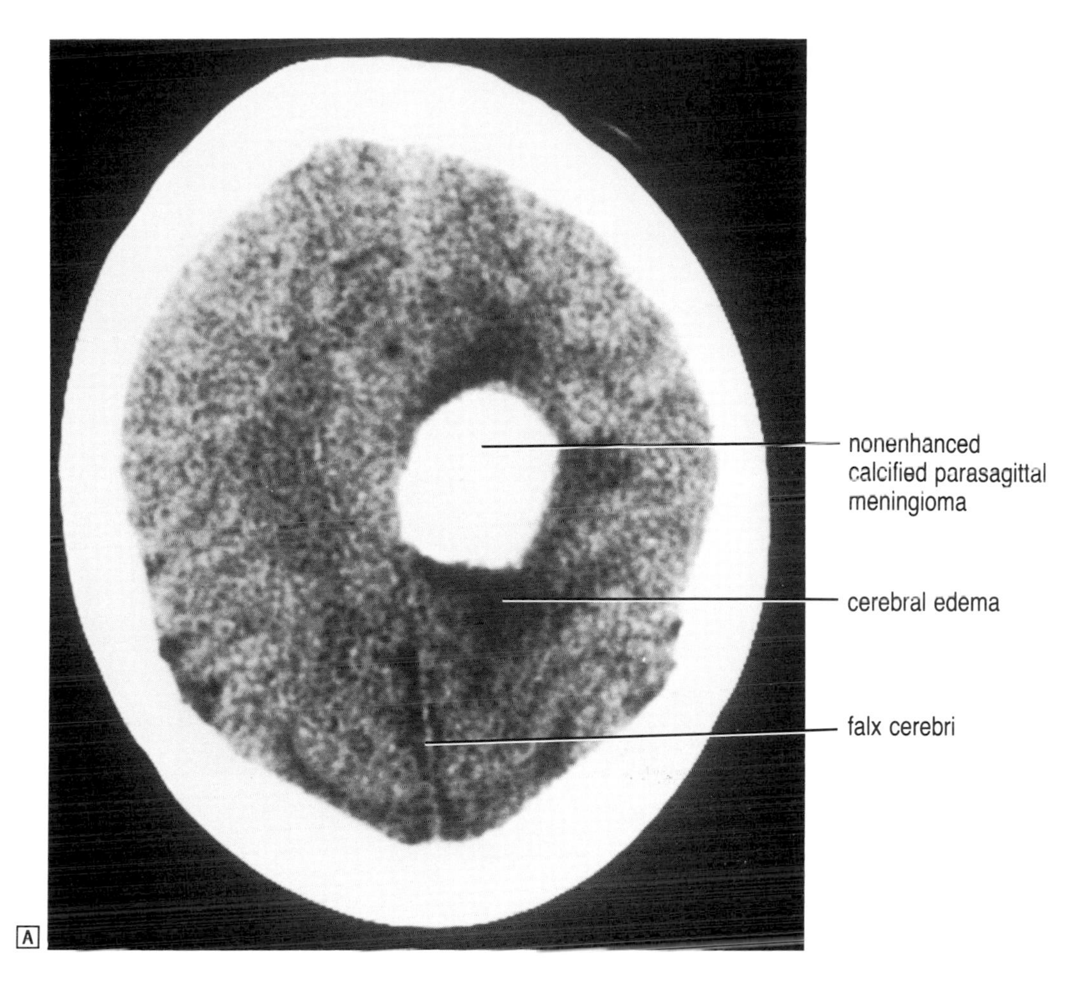

Figure 1.17. *A*, Intracranial neoplasms.

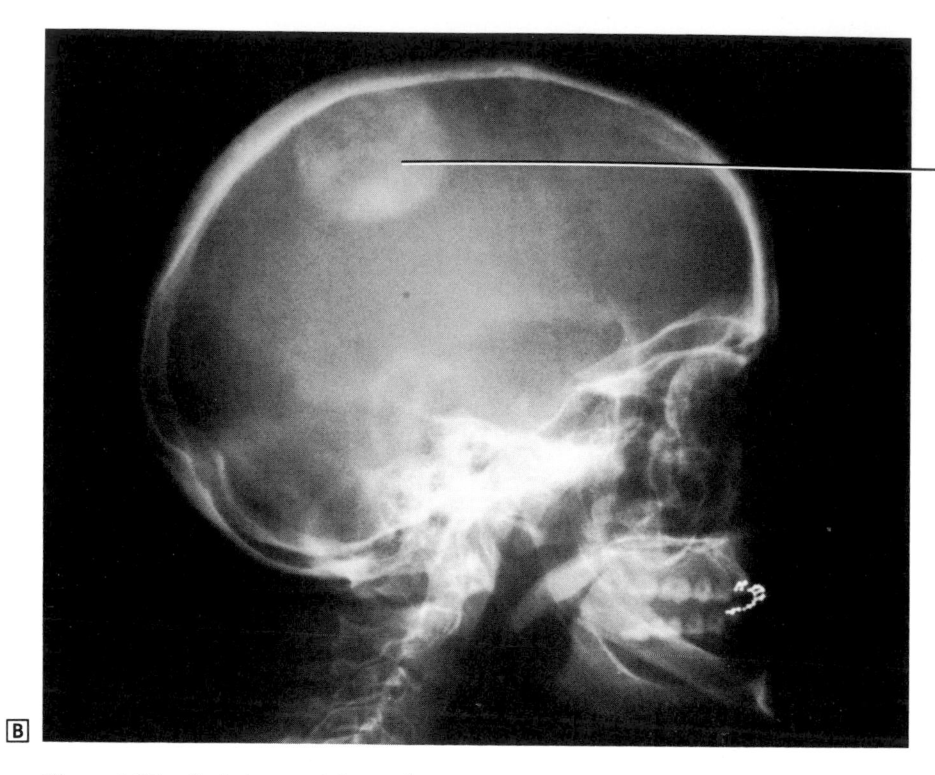

Figure 1.17. *B,* Intracranial neoplasms.

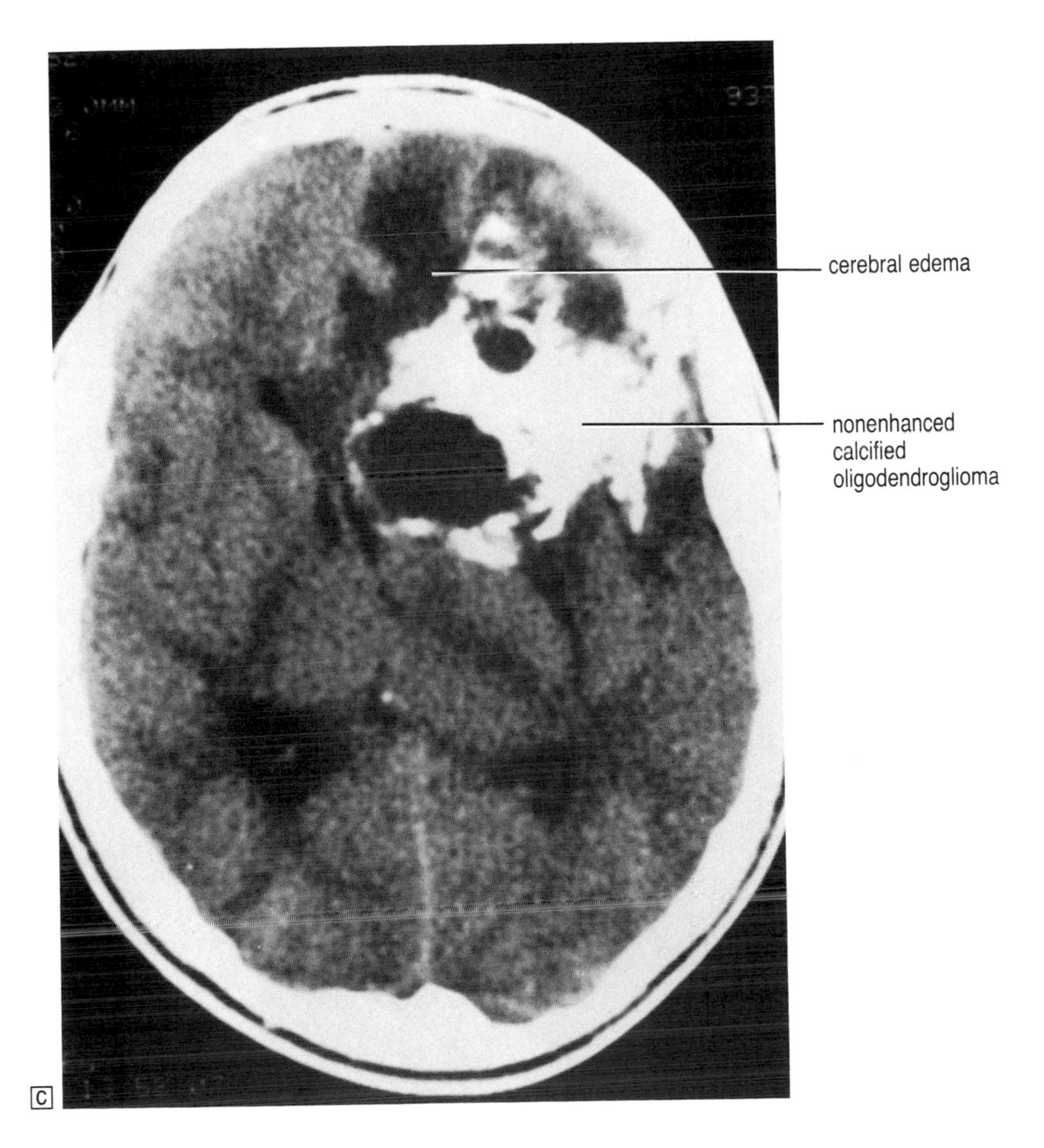

Figure 1.17. C, Intracranial neoplasms.

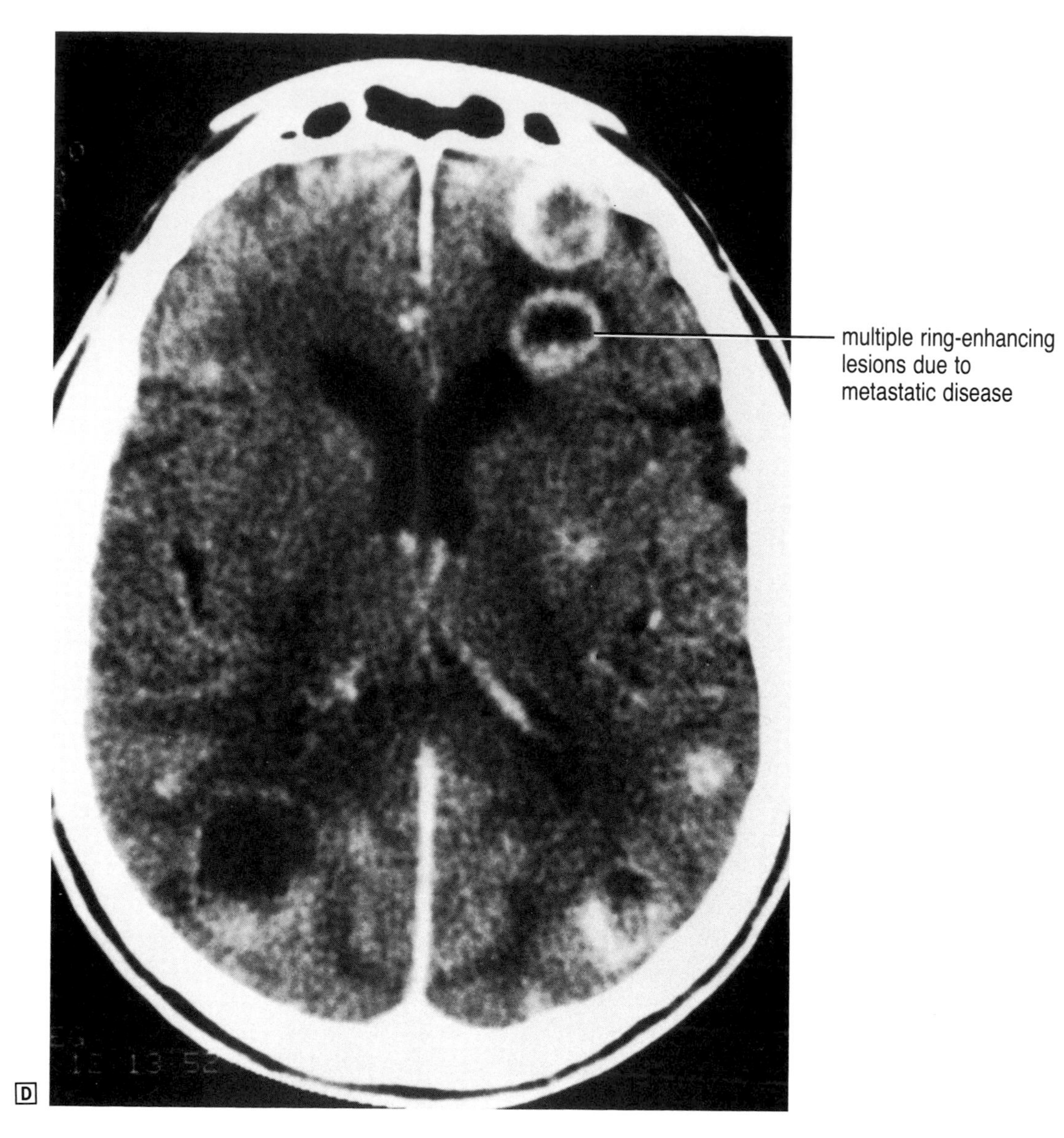

Figure 1.17. *D,* Intracranial neoplasms.

1.18 INTRACRANIAL ANEURYSMS

A. Types of aneurysms
   1. Congenital berry aneurysm
      a. Accounts for approximately 80% of all intracranial aneurysms
      b. A congenital, saccular aneurysm that forms as a result of a weakness in the arterial wall at bifurcation points around the circle of Willis
      c. Most common sites include the anterior communicating artery, posterior communicating artery, and middle cerebral artery
   2. Arteriosclerotic aneurysms
      a. Account for about 10% of intracranial aneurysms
   3. Inflammatory aneurysms
      a. Bacterial and mycotic
      b. Involve peripheral branching vessels of middle cerebral artery
   4. Traumatic aneurysms
      a. Also tend to be located peripherally

B. Conditions associated with aneurysms
   1. Polycystic kidney disease
   2. Coarctation of aorta
   3. Ehlers-Danlos syndrome
   4. Fibromuscular hyperplasia
   5. Systemic lupus erythematosus
   6. Moyamoya

C. Rupture of intracranial aneurysm
   1. Most often results in subarachnoid hemorrhage. Visualized as an area of increased attenuation (white) located within the interhemispheric fissure, between sulci and within the sylvian fissure and cisterns.
   2. May also result in parenchymal hemorrhage or interventricular hemorrhage
   3. Complications of a ruptured aneurysm include increased intracranial pressure, arterial spasm, cerebral infarction, and herniation of the brain.
   4. Symptoms include severe headache and onset of meningeal irritation.
   5. Most aneurysms rupture between the fifth and sixth decades of life.

D. Cerebral angiography should be used to confirm the diagnosis and localize the aneurysm. Most aneurysms fill via the carotid circulation. All the cerebral circulation should be visualized because 20% have additional aneurysms.

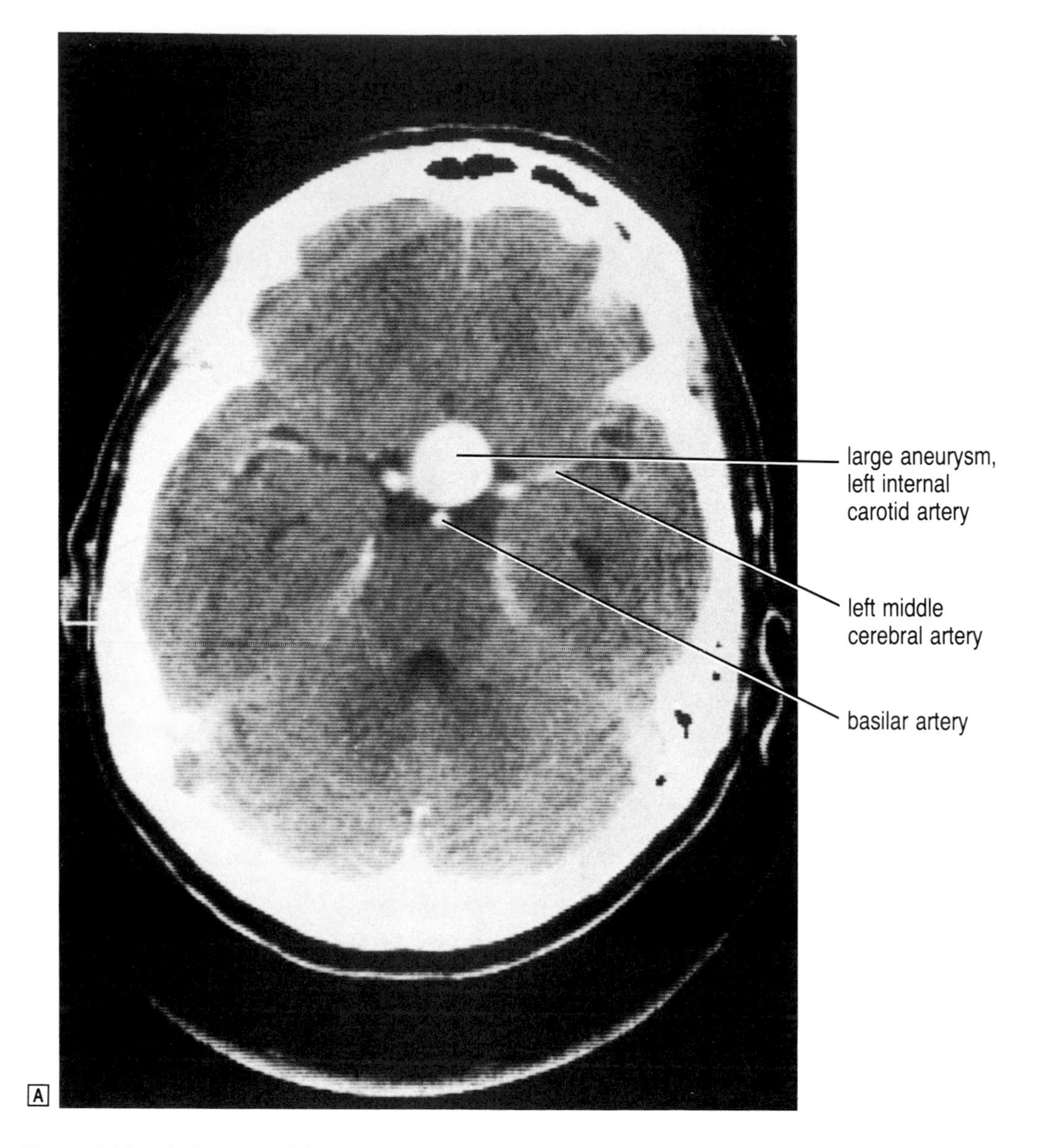

Figure 1.18. *A,* Intracranial aneurysms.

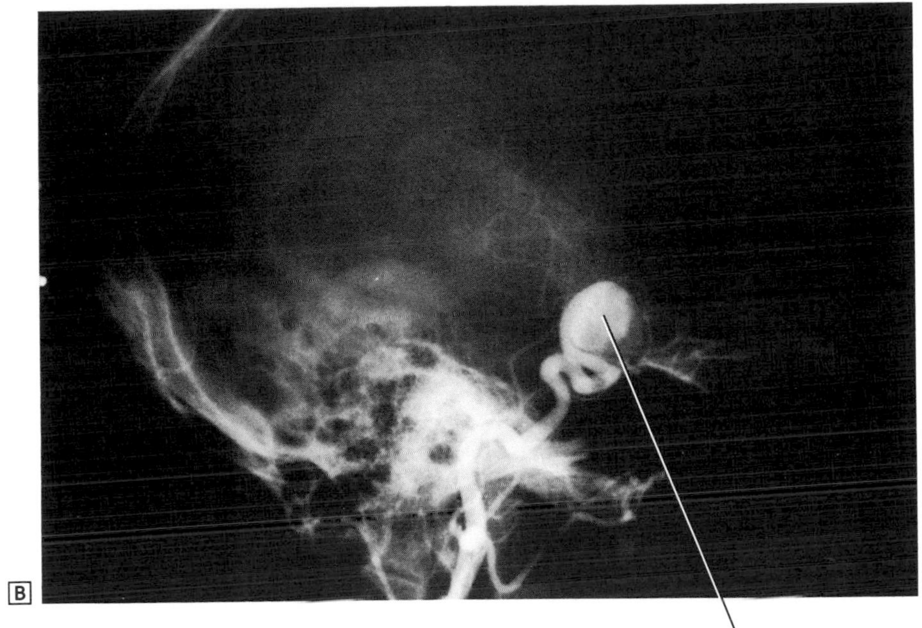

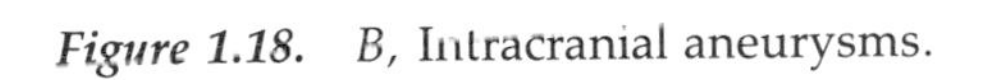

Figure 1.18. *B,* Intracranial aneurysms.

1.19 INTRACRANIAL CALCIFICATIONS

A. High attenuation (white) on CT
B. Types of calcification
  1. Physiologic
    a. Pineal gland
    b. Choroid plexus
    c. Falx cerebri and tentorium cerebelli
    d. Habenular commissure
    e. Posterior commissure
    f. Mass lesions may result in displacement of these structures.
  2. Basal ganglia
    a. Basal ganglia are composed of the caudate nucleus, putamen, globus pallidus, substantia nigra, and subthalamic nuclei.
    b. When calcification of the basal ganglia occurs, it is generally symmetric bilaterally
    c. Differential diagnosis of basal ganglia calcifications
      (1) Idiopathic
      (2) Hypoparathyroidism
      (3) Hyperparathyroidism
      (4) Pseudohypoparathyroidism
      (5) Cytomegalovirus (previous infection)
      (6) Toxoplasmosis (previous infection)
  3. Vascular calcifications
    a. Differential diagnosis
      (1) Arteriosclerosis
      (2) Arteriovenous malformation
        (a) Approximately 20% calcify
        (b) Visualized as serpiginous areas of high attenuation (white)
      (3) Aneurysm
        (a) Approximately 1% calcify
        (b) Visualized as curvilinear calcification (see Sec. 1.18)
      (4) Previous cerebral hemorrhage
        (a) Approximately 5% of subdural hematomas calcify
        (b) Visualized as an area of high attenuation located over the convexities
      (5) Sturge-Weber syndrome
        (a) One of the phakomatoses (refers to a group of diseases that have neurocutaneous manifestations)
        (b) Development of venous angiomas of the leptomeninges. Calcification appears coiled and serpiginous, usually located over the parietal region.
        (c) Ipsilateral port wine nevus of the face following the trigeminal nerve distribution
        (d) Usually associated with seizures
        (e) May have mental retardation and hemiatrophy
  4. Inflammatory diseases
    a. Differential diagnosis
      (1) Brain abscess
        (a) Most often seen in the frontal and temporal regions
        (b) Contrast-enhanced CT demonstrates ring enhancement of a low dense region.
        (c) Calcification may occur late.
      (2) Tuberculosis
        (a) Calcification may occur in involved areas.
        (b) Leptomeninges at the base of the brain are most often involved, and may undergo calcification.
        (c) May result in communicating or noncommunicating hydrocephalus
        (d) Tuberculoma (tuberculous abscess) may also calcify.

        (e) CT examination with IV contrast demonstrates enhancement of the leptomeninges, basal cisterns, and tuberculomas.
    (3) Encephalitis
5. Parasitic disease
   a. Cysticercosis
      (1) May be visualized as multiple small enhancing lesions following IV contrast
      (2) Late in the disease, a noncontrast CT may reveal multiple small calcified granulomas.
   b. Echinococcus (hydatid) disease
      (1) Forms large hydatid cysts that may calcify
      (2) Cysts occur in liver, lungs, brain, kidney, and skeleton
   c. Trichinosis
      (1) May see multiple calcified granulomas
      (2) Involves skeletal muscle, brain, heart, and any other organ
6. Congenital disease
   a. Tuberous sclerosis (Bourneville's disease)
      (1) Also one of the phakomatoses (that have neurocutaneous lesions)
      (2) Triad consists of
         (a) Mental retardation
         (b) Epilepsy
         (c) Adenoma sebaceum (facial nevi)
      (3) Inherited as autosomal dominant trait
      (4) Manifest during childhood
      (5) Angiomyolipomas of the kidney, pancreatic cysts, or rhabdomyoma of the heart may also occur.
      (6) CT or skull roentgenograms demonstrate multiple periventricular calcifications.
      (7) Hydrocephalus is present with dilatation of the ventricular system.
7. Neoplastic calcifications
   a. Between 10 and 15% of intracranial neoplasms contain calcification (see Sec. 1.17)
      (1) Meningioma
      (2) Gliomas
         (a) Oligodendroglioma
         (b) Astrocytoma, including glioblastoma multiforme
         (c) Ependymoma
         (d) Pinealoma
         (e) Medulloblastoma
      (3) Craniopharyngioma
      (4) Epidermoid
      (5) Chordoma
      (6) Chromophobe adenoma
      (7) Choroid plexus papilloma

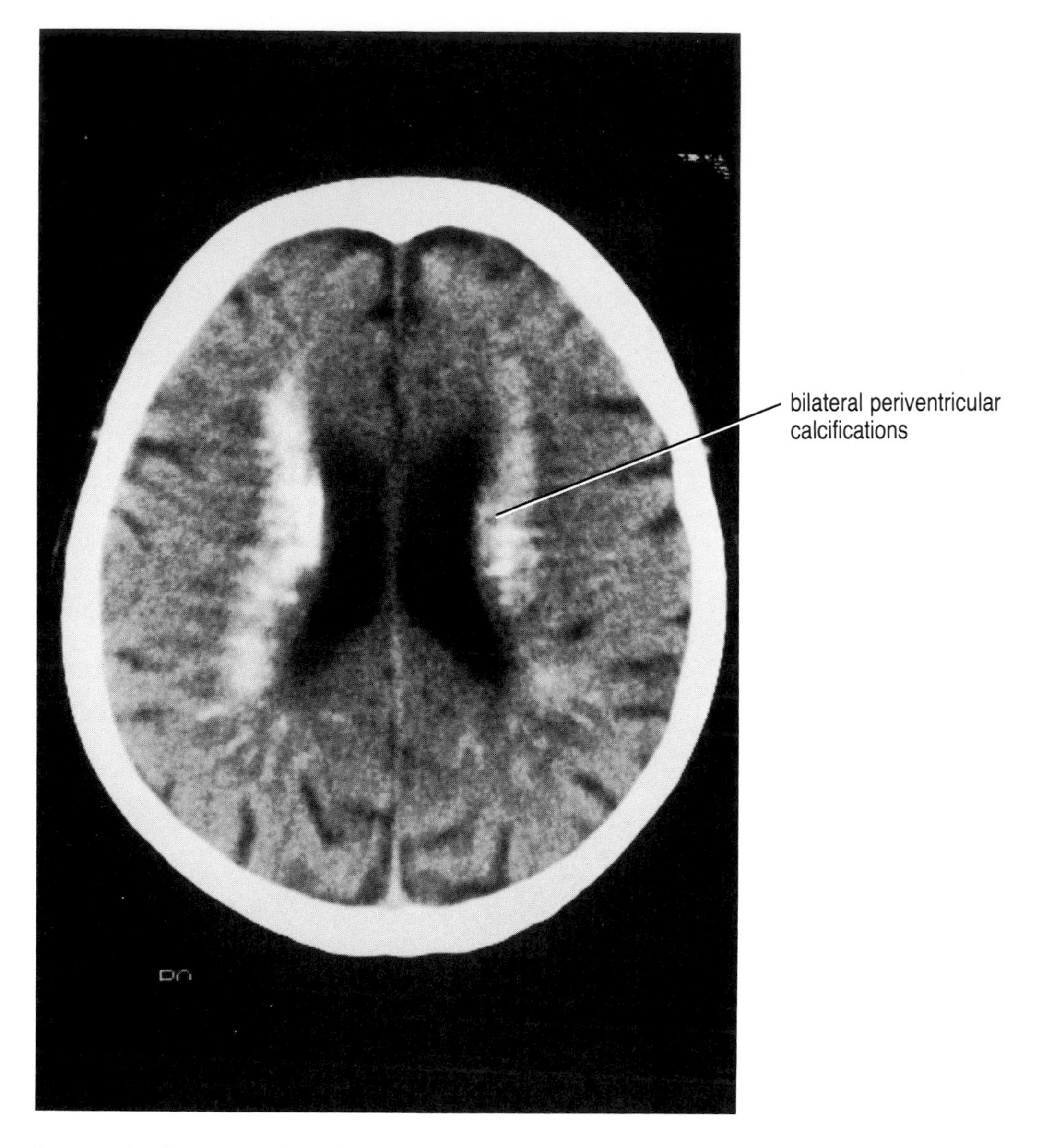

Figure 1.19. Intracranial calcifications.

References

Dorf, P.S., et al.: Harrison's Principles of Internal Medicine. 10th Ed. New York: McGraw-Hill Book Co., 1983.

Eisenberg, R.L.: Diagnostic Imaging in Internal Medicine. New York: McGraw-Hill Book Co., 1985.

Harris, J.H., and Harris, W.H.: The Radiology of Emergency Medicine. 2nd Ed. Baltimore: Williams & Wilkins, 1981.

Juhl, J.H., and Crummy, A.B.: Essentials of Radiologic Imaging. Philadelphia: J.B. Lippincott, 1987.

Levy, R.C., Hawkins, H., and Barsan, W.G.: Radiology in Emergency Medicine. St. Louis: C.V. Mosby Co., 1986.

Meschan, I., and Farrer-Meschan, R.M.: Roentgen Signs in Diagnostic Imaging, Vol. 3: Spine and Central Nervous System. Philadelphia: W.B. Saunders Co., 1985.

Taveras, J.M., and Ferrucci, J.T.: Radiology Diagnosis—Imaging—Intervention, Vol. 3: Neuroradiology and Radiology of the Head and Neck. Philadelphia: J.B. Lippincott, 1988.

2

Spine

2.01 NORMAL ANATOMY AND EVALUATION OF THE CERVICAL SPINE

A. Evaluation of the cervical spine requires attention to detail and extreme caution.
B. Routine examination of the cervical spine
   1. Lateral view
      a. This is the single most important view.
      b. A gradual smooth lordotic curve should be present. Positioning of the patient may alter the degree of the curve. The examination should be done in mild extension.
      c. The entire cervical spine along with the superior aspect of T1 should be visualized on the lateral view. If the entire cervical spine is not visualized, additional views such as the swimmer's view are required.
      d. The prevertebral soft tissues must be examined for the presence of soft tissue swelling. Anterior to the body of C3 the prevertebral space should not be greater than 5 mm. The prevertebral space anterior to the vertebral bodies below the level of C4 should not exceed 15 mm
      e. Alignment of the cervical spine should be well maintained. An imaginary line drawn along the anterior aspect of the vertebral bodies should interconnect. In this same maner, the posterior aspect of the vertebral bodies and the posterior neural arch should all maintain alignment along the same plane. If alignment is maintained, the anterior and posterior longitudinal ligaments are intact.
      f. The relationship of the posterior margin of the anterior arch of C1 to the odontoid process of C2 should be evaluated. This space should not exceed 3 mm in the adult. The maximum distance in young children is 5 mm.
      g. The amount of space between the spinous processes from level to level should be examined. Usually, each level maintains about the same distance.
      h. The facet (apophyseal) joints should be evaluated at each level.
      i. The disc interspaces should be well preserved.
      j. The volume of each vertebral body should be examined to exclude the possibility of compression. The height of the vertebral body anteriorly should be compared to the height posteriorly.
   2. AP view
      a. The spinous processes should be located in the midline and should form a straight line. Spinous processes may have a bifid appearance.
      b. The trachea should be visualized as a midline air density.
      c. The height of each level should be maintained.
      d. The lateral margins of the cervical spine should be intact.
   3. Odontoid (open-mouth) view
      a. This view allows for evaluation of the C1 to C2 articulation.
      b. The integrity of the odontoid should be evaluated.
      c. The lateral masses of C1 should have a symmetrical relationship with the odontoid and the lateral mass of C2. Improper positioning may result in some degree of asymmetry.
   4. Right and left oblique views
      a. These projections allow evaluation of the neuroforamina, facet joints, and pedicles.
C. Physiologic pseudosubluxation of C2 on C3
   1. Many young children have a normal laxity of the longitudinal ligaments. This

allows the body of C2 to appear slightly anteriorly subluxed on C3. This condition can be excluded from traumatic subluxation because the posterior neural arches of C1, C2, and C3 are in alignment.

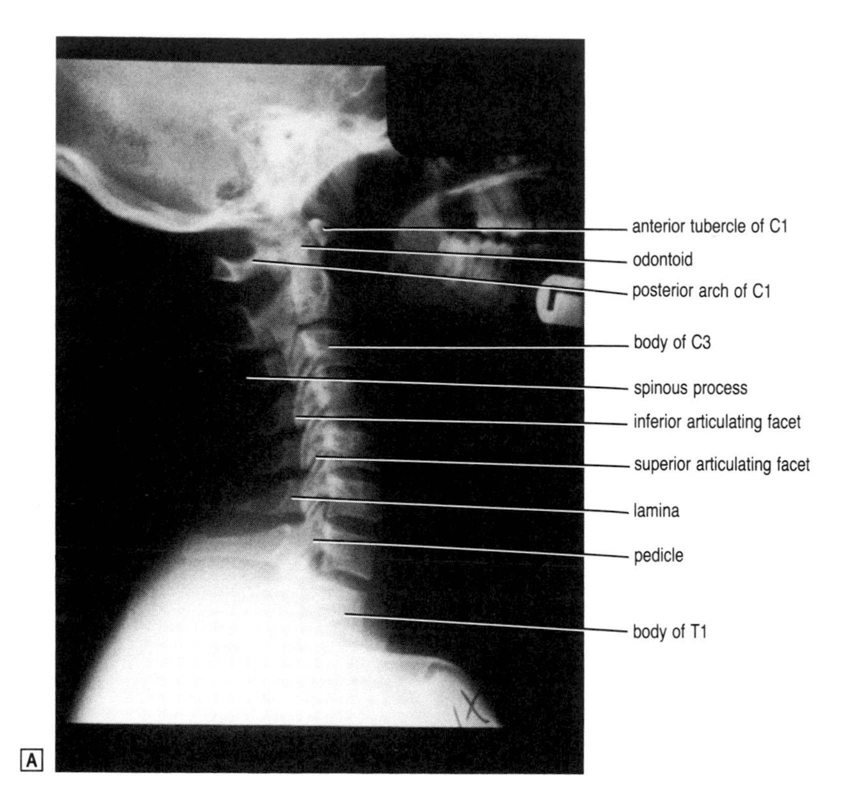

Figure 2.01. *A,* Normal anatomy and evaluation of the cervical spine.

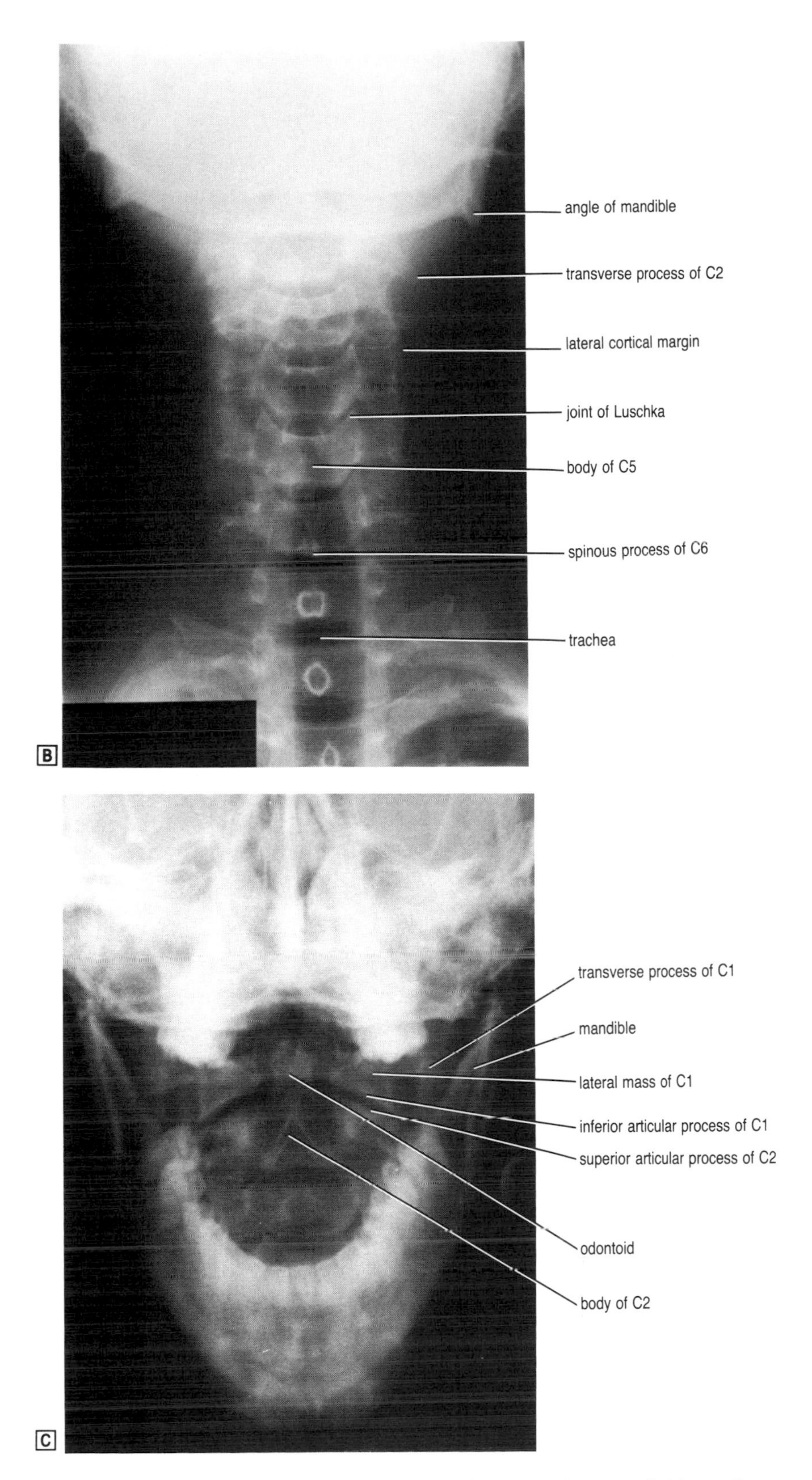

Figure 2.01. *B*, Normal anatomy and evaluation of the cervical spine. *C*, Normal anatomy and evaluation of the cervical spine.

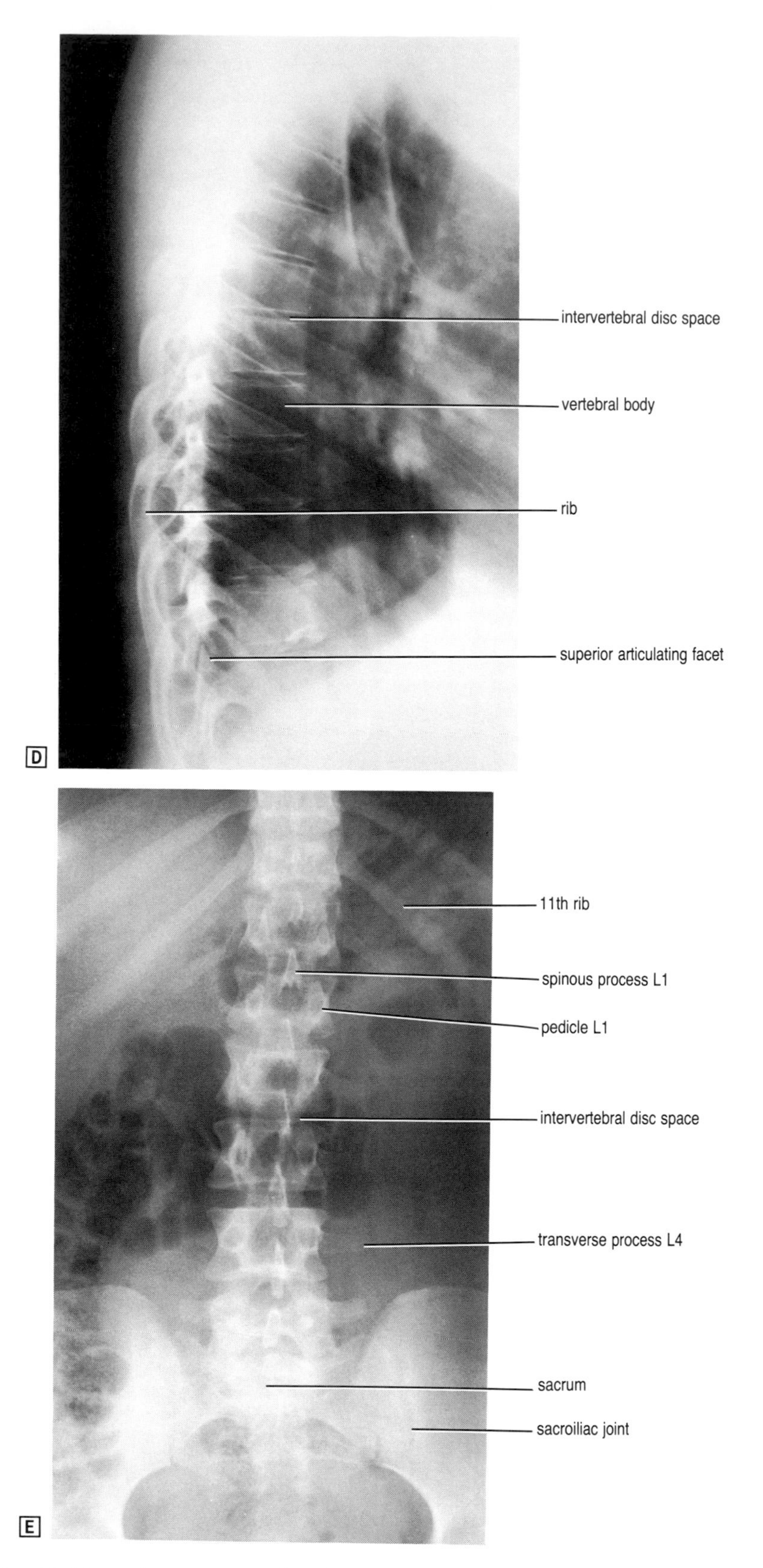

Figure 2.01. *D,* Normal anatomy and evaluation of the cervical spine. *E,* Normal anatomy and evaluation of the cervical spine.

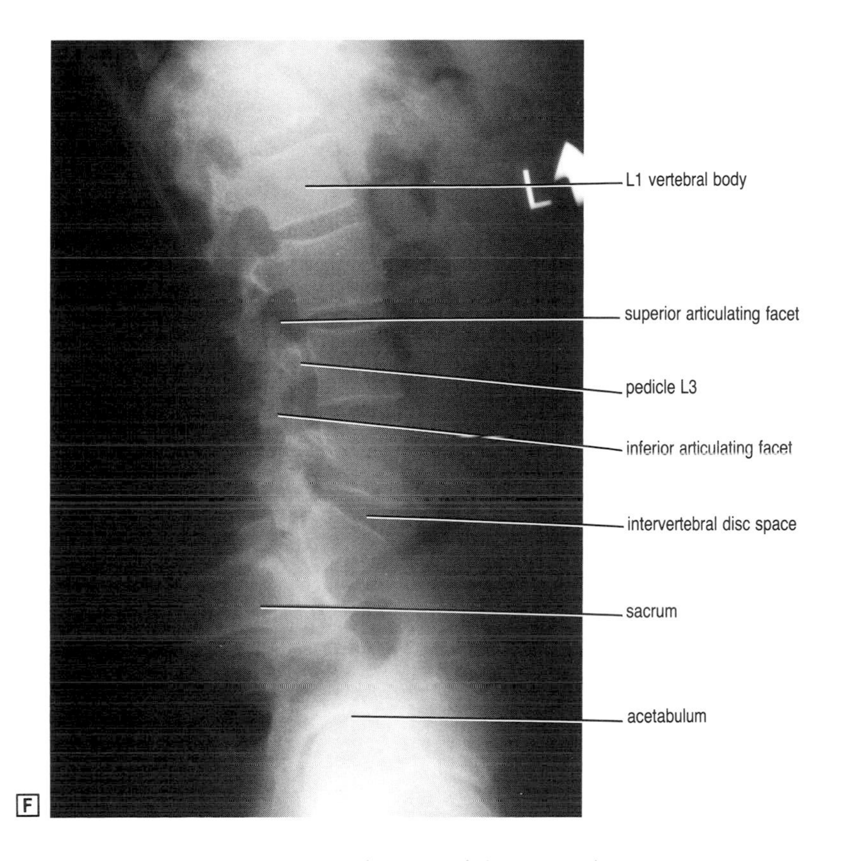

Figure 2.01. *F*, Normal anatomy and evaluation of the cervical spine.

2.02 CERVICAL SPINE: MUSCLE SPASM AND ANTERIOR SUBLUXATION

A. In the presence of cervical trauma or an unresponsive patient without an adequate history, the cross-table lateral view of the cervical spine is necessary to exclude significant cervical injury prior to complete x-ray examination (see Sec. 2.01 for evaluation of the cervical spine).
B. The entire cervical spine including C7 to T1 must be visualized because most cervical vertebrae fractures occur below the level of C4.
C. The sphenoid sinus should be evaluated on the cross-table view for a fluid level that may indicate a basilar skull fracture.
D. The normal lateral view of the cervical spine demonstrates a mild lordotic curve. In the presence of muscle spasm secondary to trauma, there is loss of the curve with straightening of the cervical spine. Improper positioning may also result in loss of the normal lordotic curve.
E. Anterior subluxation
   1. Anterior subluxation results from hyperflexion of the cervical spine.
   2. It represents a soft tissue injury that results in posterior ligament injury.
   3. The affected vertebra is displaced anteriorly.
   4. The normal lordotic curve is disrupted.
   5. There is often widening posteriorly between spinous processes at the level of involvement.
   6. It usually represents a stable injury; however, delayed instability may develop.

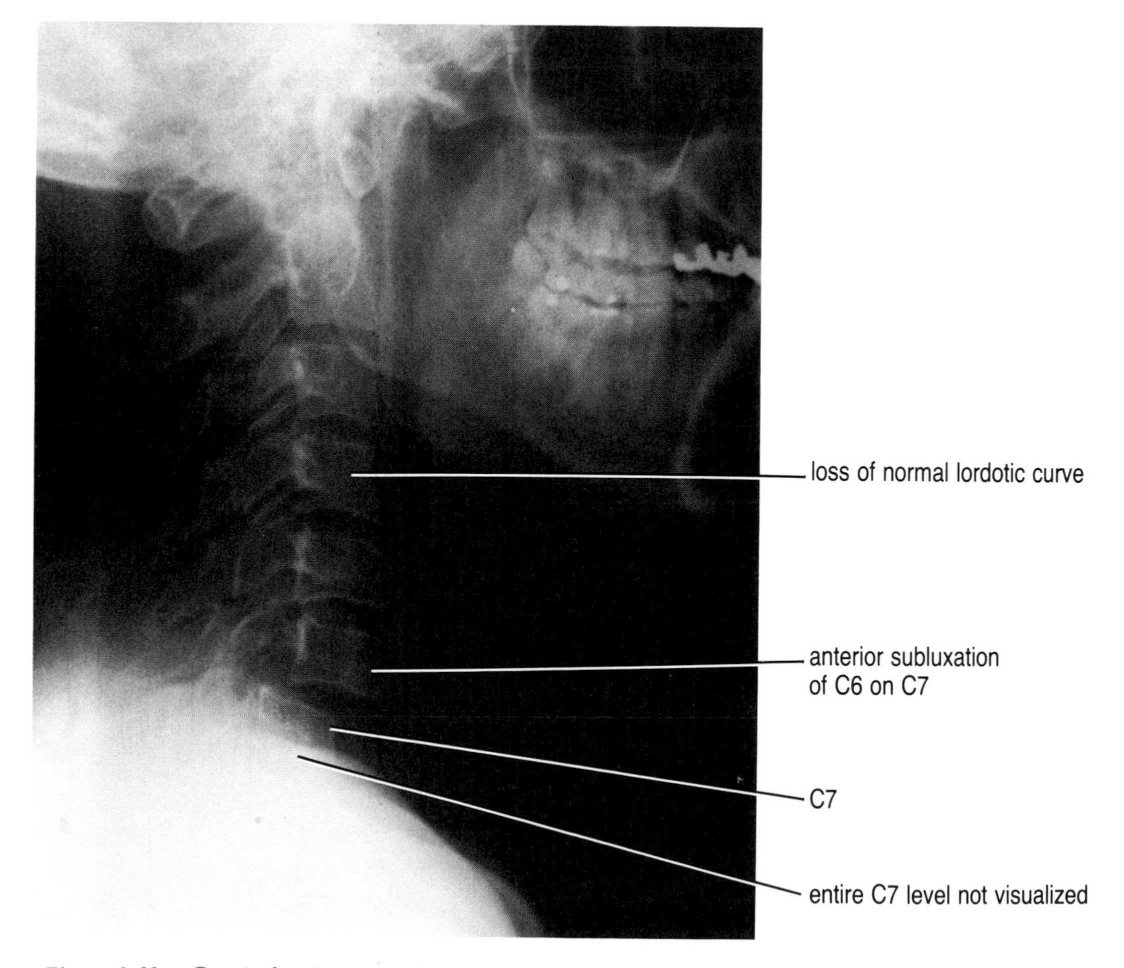

Figure 2.02. Cervical spine: muscle spasm and anterior subluxation.

2.03 CERVICAL SPINE: JEFFERSON BURST FRACTURE

A. This fracture results from axial impaction of the skull on the cervical spine while it is in a neutral position.
B. It is usually visualized on the open-mouth view of the odontoid with lateral displacement of the lateral masses of C1 with respect to C2.
C. The lateral view may demonstrate significant prevertebral soft tissue swelling.
D. This fracture results in disruption of the anterior and posterior arches of C1 and represents an unstable fracture.
E. CT evaluation provides additional valuable information.

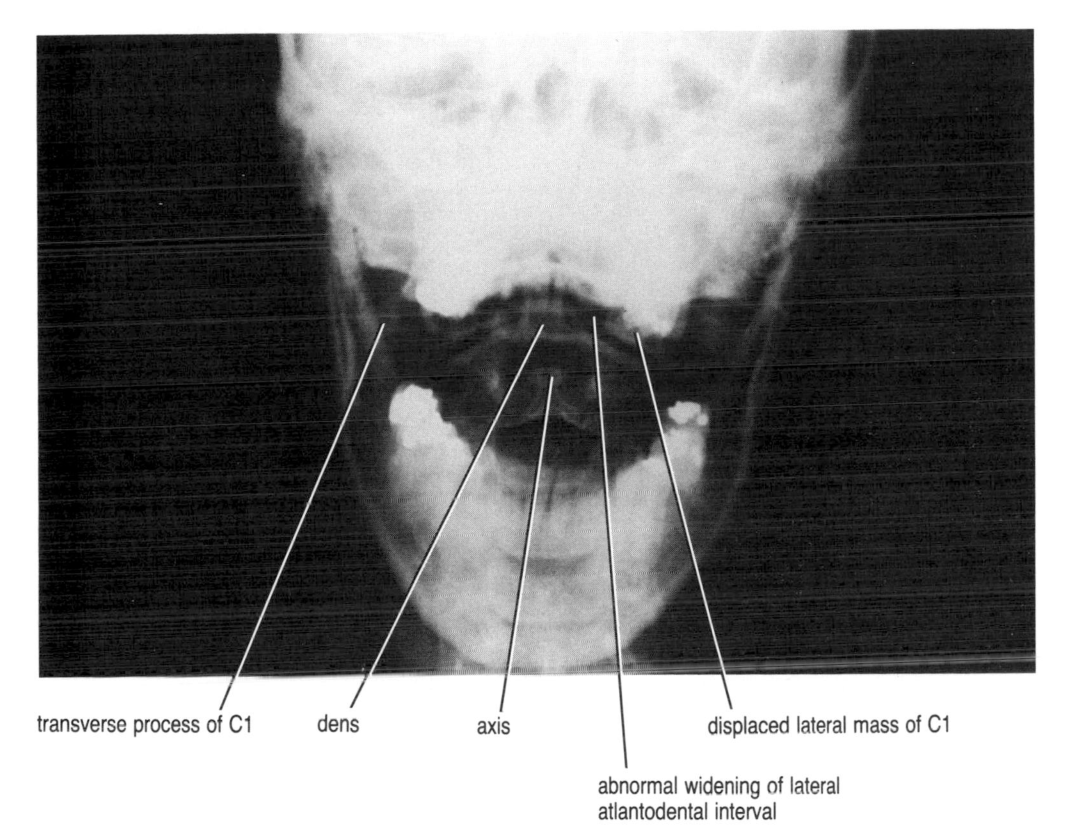

Figure 2.03. Cervical spine: Jefferson burst fracture.

2.04 CERVICAL SPINE: COMPRESSION FRACTURE

A. This injury results from hyperflexion of the cervical spine.
B. Compression of the vertebral body results in anterior compression of the involved vertebra with preservation of the normal height of the posterior aspect. Disruption of the cortical surface may be seen anteriorly, indicative of acute fracture.
C. Vertebral alignment remains intact with preservation of the disc interspace.
D. The compression is best demonstrated on the lateral view.
E. This represents a stable fracture.

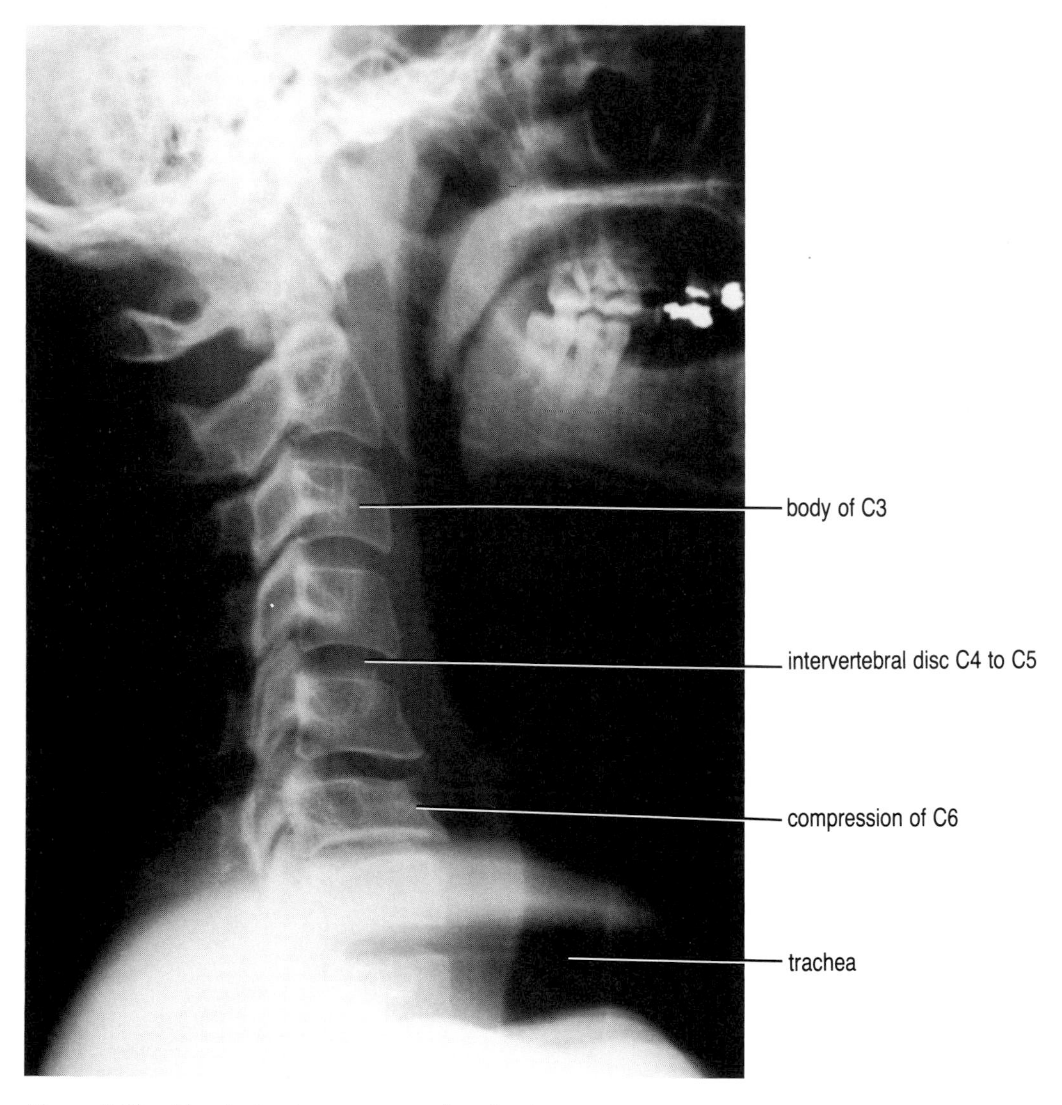

Figure 2.04. Cervical spine: compression fracture.

2.05 CERVICAL SPINE: CLAY-SHOVELER'S FRACTURE

A. This is a result of hyperflexion of the cervical spine.
B. Lateral view of the cervical spine reveals an oblique fracture through the spinous process of C6, C7, or T1.
C. C7 is the most commonly affected level.
D. This fracture is confined to the posterior elements and is considered a stable injury.

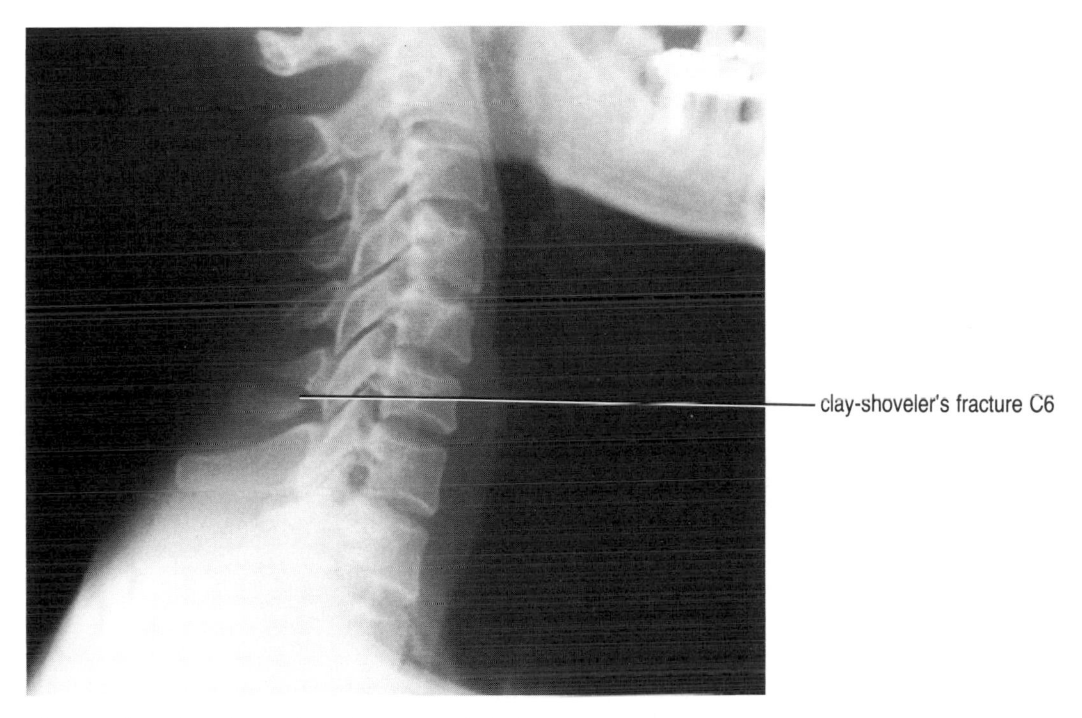

Figure 2.05. Cervical spine: clay-shoveler's fracture.

2.06 CERVICAL SPINE: UNILATERAL INTERFACETAL DISLOCATION (UID)

A. This injury results from a combination of hyperflexion and rotatory movements.
B. The lateral view demonstrates anterior subluxation at the level of involvement. The facet joints are not clearly visualized owing to rotation.
C. The AP view demonstrates abnormal alignment of the spinous processes. At the level of involvement and above the spinous process, they are displaced toward the side of dislocation. Inferior to the level of dislocation the spinous processes remain in the midline.
D. Oblique views should demonstrate the anterior dislocation of the inferior articulating facet.
E. The dislocated facet becomes locked within the neuroforamen; thus, this represents a stable injury.
F. The patient's head is turned and locked opposite to the side of dislocation.
G. Fractures may be associated with this injury. CT evaluation of the level of involvement may be used to identify the dislocated facet and any additional fractures.

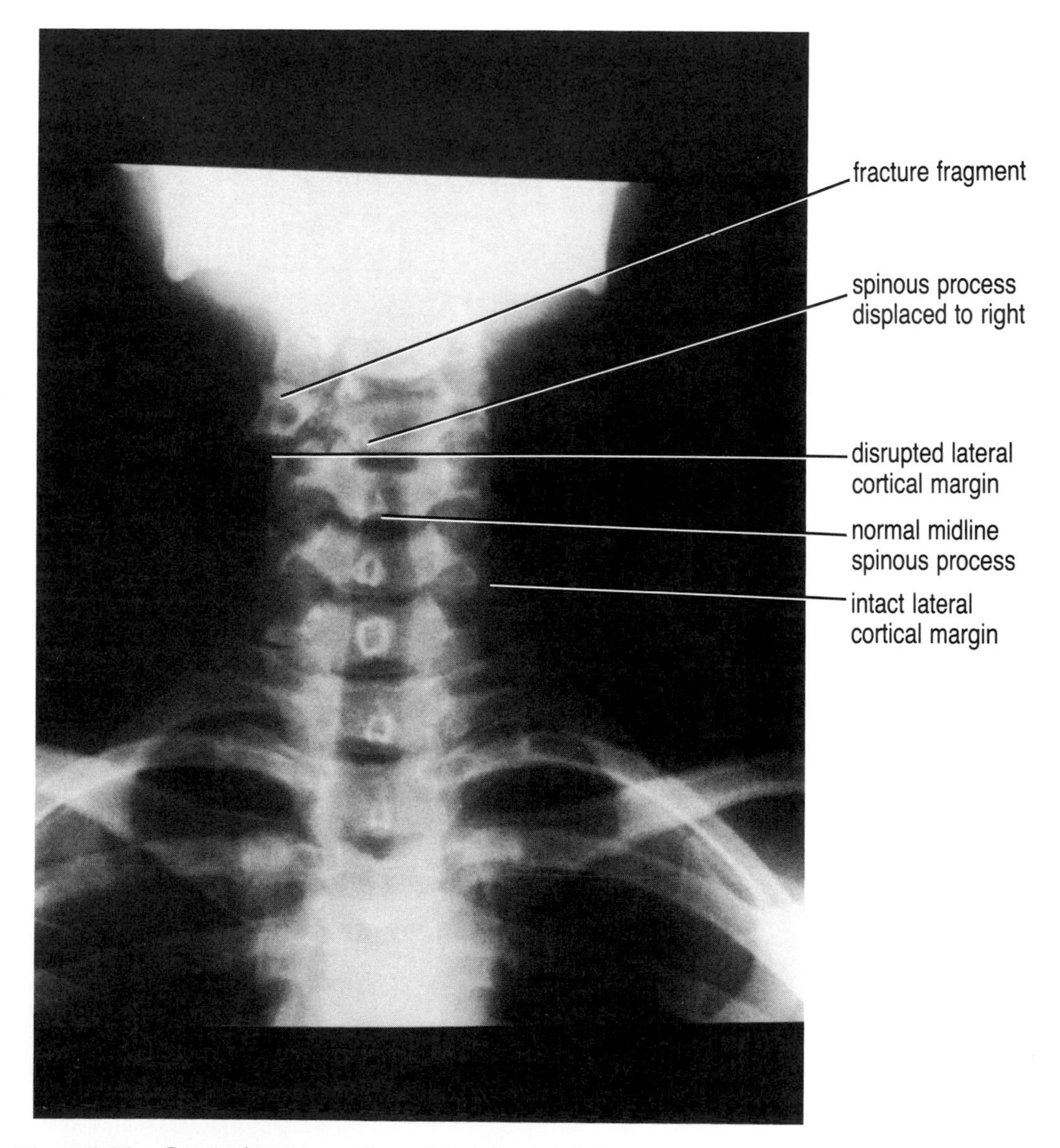

Figure 2.06. Cervical spine: unilateral interfacetal dislocation (UID).

2.07 CERVICAL SPINE: HANGMAN'S FRACTURE

A. This fracture results from hyperextension of the cervical spine.
B. There is a bilateral pedicle fracture of C2.
C. The lateral view of the cervical spine reveals disruption of the pedicles of C2, anterior subluxation of C2 on C3, and prevertebral soft tissue swelling.
D. This represents an unstable injury.

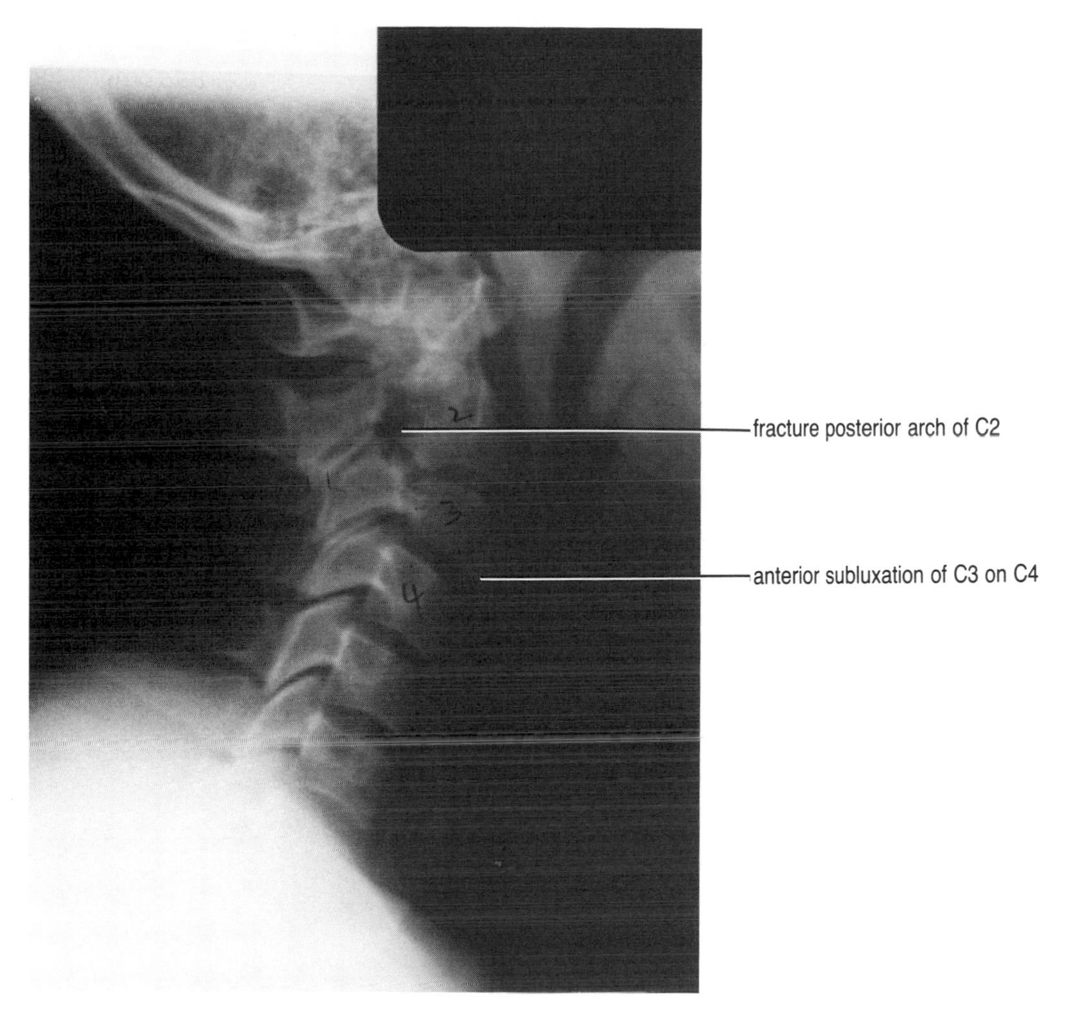

Figure 2.07. Cervical spine: hangman's fracture.

2.08 CERVICAL SPINE: FRACTURE OF THE ODONTOID PROCESS

A. Fracture of the odontoid is best visualized on the open-mouth view (see Sec. 2.01).
B. Superimposition of normal structures such as the incisor teeth or the inferior aspect of the arch of the atlas may simulate a fracture.
C. The odontoideum represents congenital nonfusion of the odontoid and the body of the axis. This entity should not be mistaken for acute fracture.
D. There are three types of odontoid fractures:
   1. Type I—an oblique fracture of the tip of the odontoid
   2. Type II—a transverse fracture of the base of the odontoid
   3. Type III—a fracture that extends through the body of C2.
E. The type II odontoid fracture is the most common.

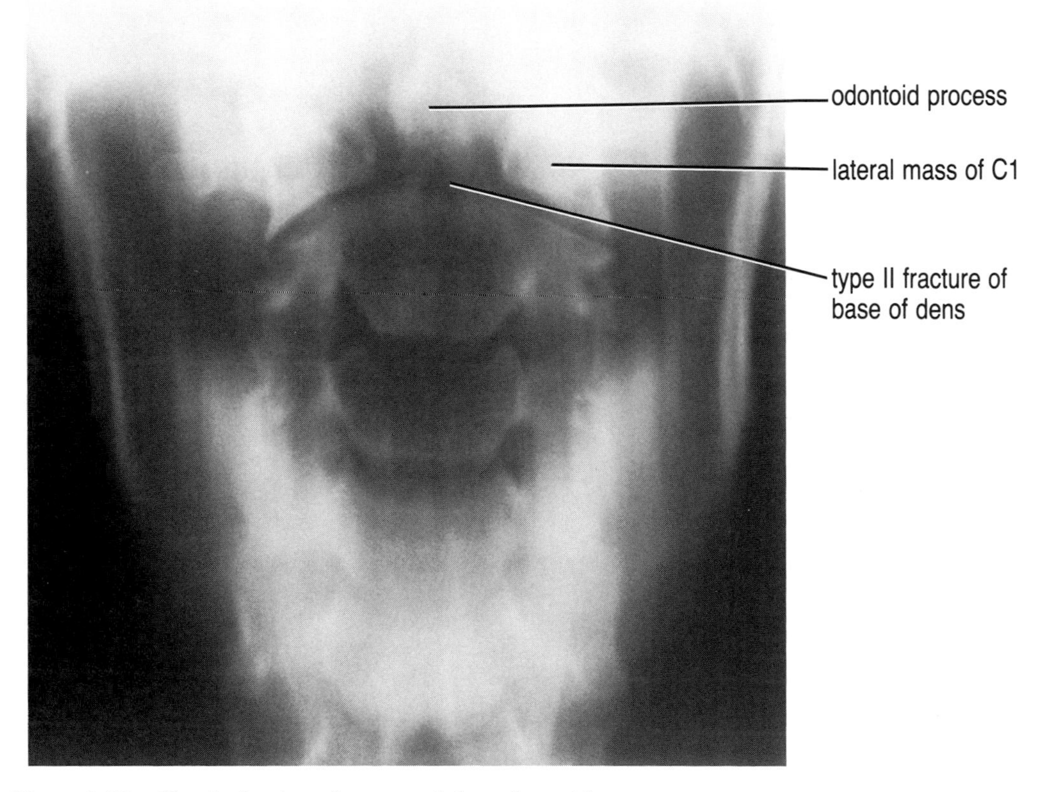

Figure 2.08. Cervical spine: fracture of the odontoid process.

2.09 CERVICAL SPINE: TEARDROP FRACTURE

A. This fracture results from forced flexion of the cervical spine.
B. The lateral view of the cervical spine reveals a displaced fracture of the anteroinferior aspect of the involved vertebra.
C. There may be associated prevertebral soft tissue swelling and kyphotic angulation at the level of involvement.
D. This represents an unstable fracture.
E. This is a severe injury associated with quadriplegia.

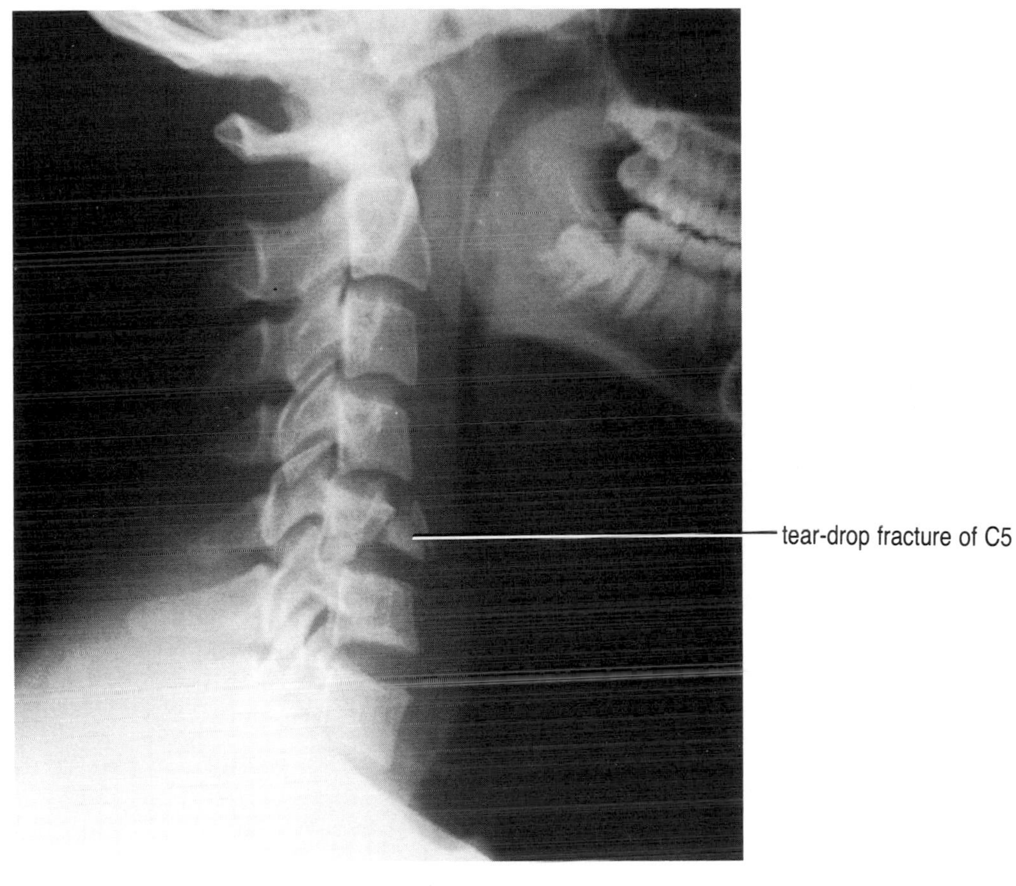

Figure 2.09. Cervical spine: teardrop fracture.

2.10 NORMAL SOFT TISSUE LATERAL VIEW OF THE NECK

A. On this examination, x-ray technique is utilized to enhance the appearance of the soft tissues.
B. Proper evaluation begins with an adequate examination. The hypopharynx should be distended with air and the cervical spine should be in mild extension.
C. Remember that the esophagus lies between the vertebral bodies and the trachea.
D. The prevertebral space should be evaluated for soft tissue swelling. The acceptable range varies with age. In the adult:
   1. The prevertebral space from the level of C1 through the majority of C4 should not exceed 5 mm.
   2. The prevertebral space located behind the trachea from the rest of C4 caudally should not exceed 15 mm.
E. The epiglottis and aryepiglottic folds should be evaluated for the presence of edema.
F. The subglottic regions should also be evaluated for the presence of edema.

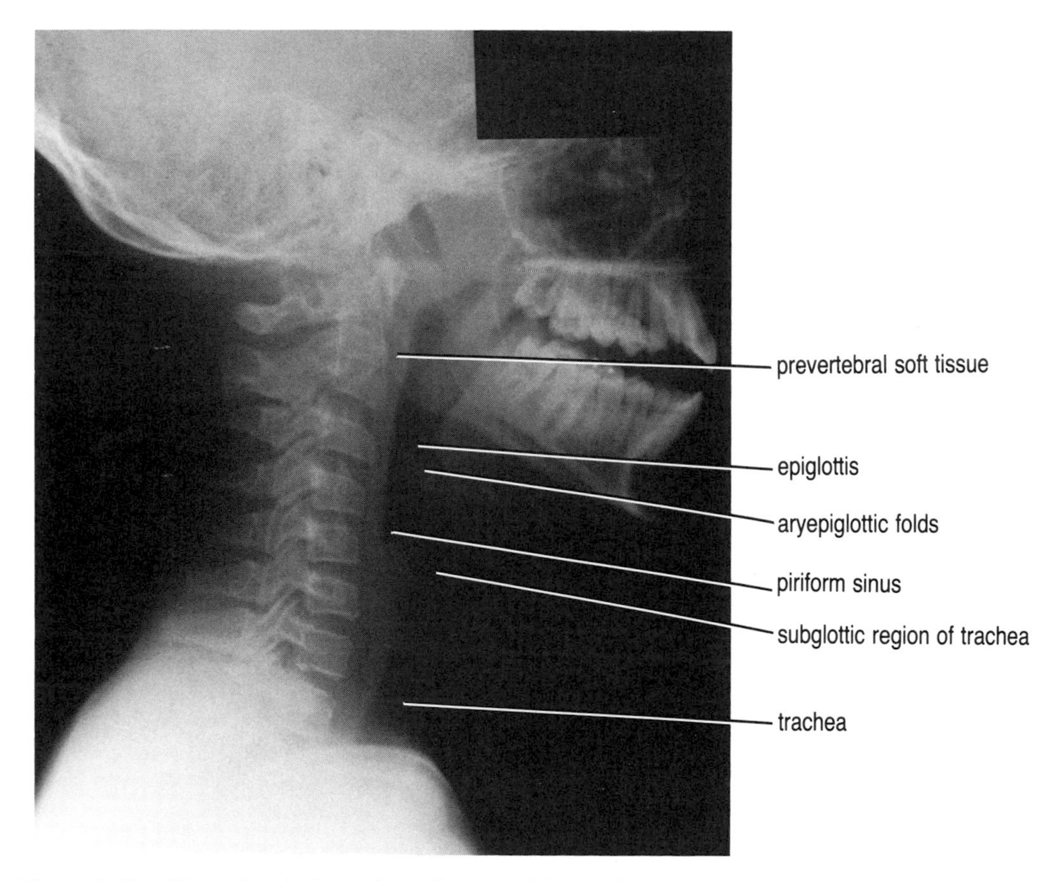

Figure 2.10. Normal soft tissue lateral view of the neck.

2.11 ACUTE OBSTRUCTION OF THE UPPER AIRWAY

A. Radiographic evaluation requires a chest roentgenogram, soft tissue lateral view of the neck, and an AP view of the neck (see Sec 2.10).

B. Infants and young children are more prone to develop acute obstruction of the upper airway because of the relative small size of the air passage.

C. Differential diagnosis
   1. Croup (laryngotracheobronchitis)
   2. Acute epiglottitis
   3. Foreign body
   4. Retropharyngeal abscess or hemorrhage
   5. Allergic angioneurotic edema

D. Croup (laryngotracheobronchitis)
   1. Radiographically, the lateral view demonstrates subglottic edema with narrowing and haziness of the airway in this region. The subglottic narrowing results in distention of the hypopharynx. The AP view demonstrates a funnel-shaped narrowing of the subglottic area.
   2. The epiglottis and aryepiglottic folds are normal in croup.
   3. Croup usually has a viral cause, most often parainfluenza.
   4. It affects young children between 6 months and 3 years of age.
   5. Presentation includes a barking cough and inspiratory stridor

E. Acute epiglottitis
   1. Radiographically, the lateral view demonstrates edematous enlargement of the epiglottis and aryepiglottic folds. There may be associated prevertebral soft tissue swelling, but the subglottic region is normal.
   2. Has a bacterial cause most often due to Haemophilus influenzae type B
   3. Affects young children between 2 and 7 years old; presentation includes fever, drooling, sore throat, inspiratory stridor, and respiratory distress

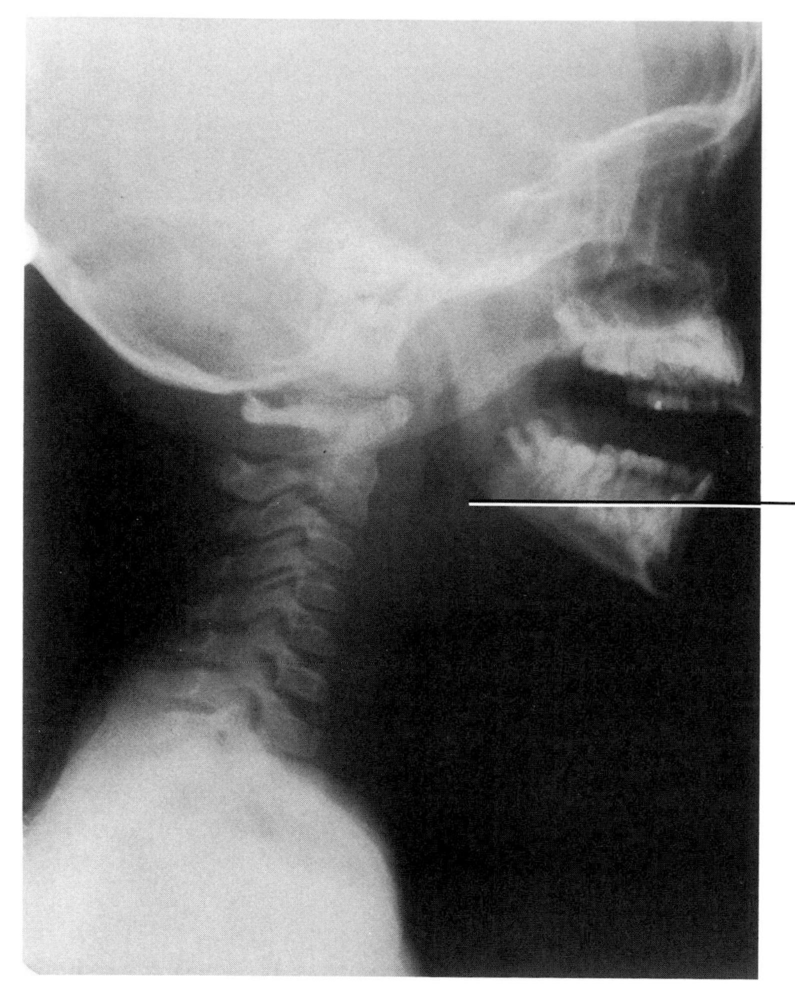

Figure 2.11. Acute obstruction of the upper airway.

2.12 THORACOLUMBAR SPINE: COMPRESSION FRACTURE AND TRANSVERSE PROCESS FRACTURE

A. Compression fractures of the thoracic and lumbar vertebrae are common traumatic lesions.
B. Compression fractures are the result of hyperflexion of the spine.
C. Usually visualized as anterior compression of the affected vertebral body with relative preservation of the posterior aspect of the involved vertebrae
D. With severe flexion, the entire superior end-plate may be depressed.
E. Paraspinous hematomas may be associated with thoracic compression fractures.
F. Alignment of the vertebrae is usually maintained, and the disc interspace is usually preserved.
G. Older females with osteoporosis are more susceptible to compression fractures. Radiographically, it can be difficult to determine the acute or chronic nature of the compression; clinical correlation is often required.
H. Chance fracture
   1. This represents a severe obliquely oriented fracture through the body, pedicles, and spinous process of a lumbar vertebra. This injury is seen in individuals who sustained severe forced flexion while in seat-belt restraint.
I. Lumbar trauma may result in fracture of the transverse processes. A retroperitoneal hematoma may be associated with transverse process fracture. The psoas margins should be examined and clearly visualized. A retroperitoneal hematoma may result in obliteration of a psoas margin or may result in an adjacent soft tissue mass.
J. Differential diagnosis of compression of a vertebra
   1. Trauma
   2. Metastatic disease; common primary tumors include lung, breast, prostate, renal, and thyroid carcinoma
   3. Osteoporosis
   4. Multiple myeloma
   5. Osteomyelitis
   6. Lymphoma
   7. Histiocytosis X
   8. Hyperparathyroidism
   9. Hemangioma

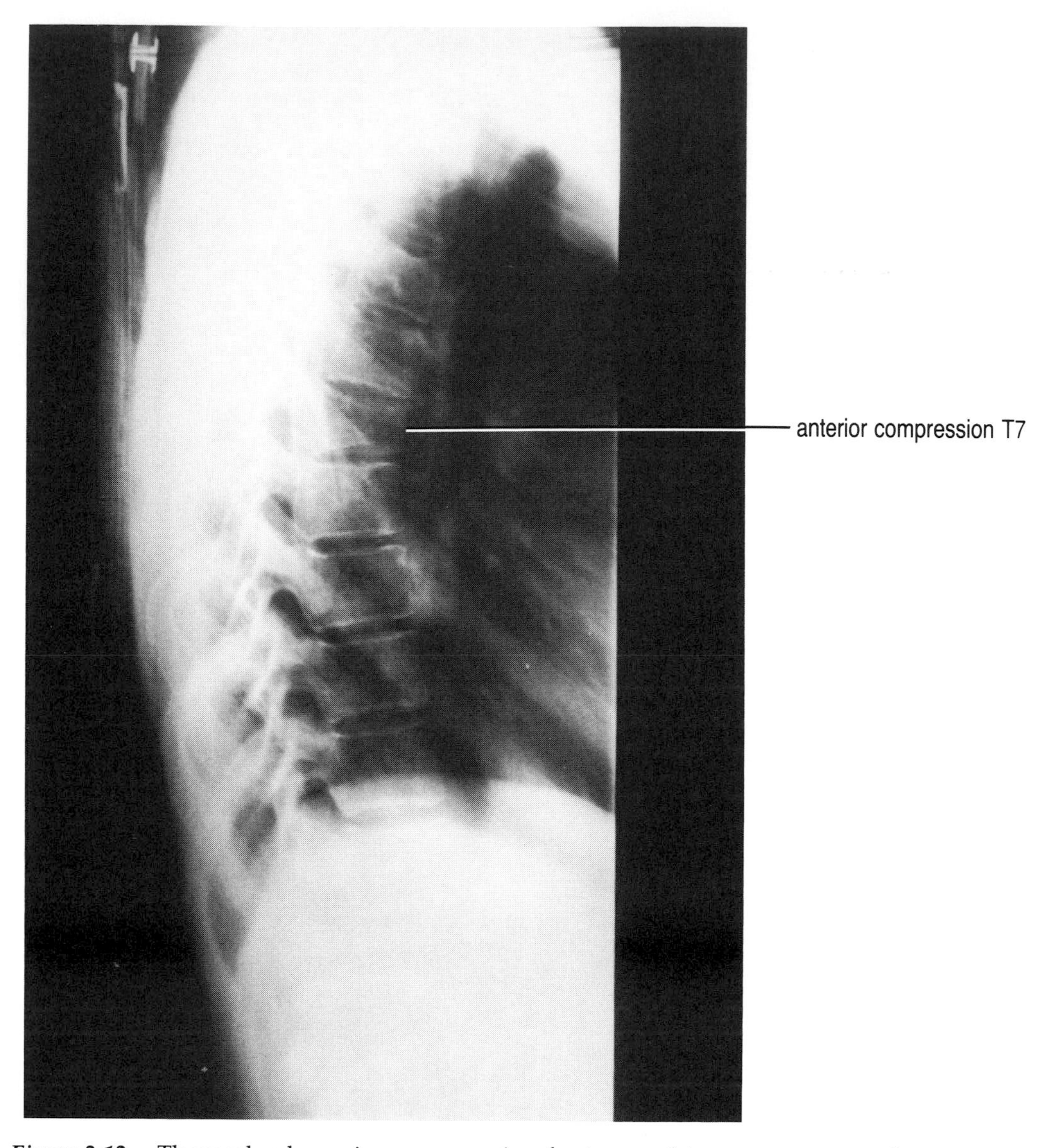

Figure 2.12. Thoracolumbar spine: compression fracture and transverse process fracture.

2.13 EVALUATION OF BACK PAIN IN THE ABSENCE OF TRAUMA

A. No radiographic abnormalities are identified in most individuals complaining of back pain. Individuals with acute back strain, herniated disc, or poor physical fitness and postural abnormalities usually have normal x-ray evaluation.
B. Following the exclusion of trauma by history, physical examination, and radiographic evaluation, other causes of back pain must be ruled out.
C. Degenerative joint disease
   1. Radiographically visualized as
      a. Irregular narrowing of the disc interspace
      b. Osteosclerosis of areas of involvement
      c. Degenerative spur formation (osteophytes) on the anterior and/or lateral aspect of the vertebral bodies and the facet joints
D. Neoplastic disease
   1. Radiographically visualized as an osteolytic process of a vertebral body that does not involve or cross the intervertebral disc
E. Inflammatory disease
   1. Osteomyelitis results in destruction of a vertebral body, but readily involves and crosses the intervertebral disc.
F. Ankylosing spondylitis
   1. A type of sacroiliitis
      a. Radiographic findings
         (1) Early changes include sacroiliac joint erosion.
         (2) Bilateral fusion of sacroiliac joints
         (3) Anterior erosions of the vertebral bodies result in a squared appearance of the vertebrae.
         (4) Osteoporosis
         (5) Syndesmophyte formation. Syndesmophytes represent calcification within the paravertebral soft tissues and ligaments parallel to the long axis of the spine.
      b. Condition is more common in males

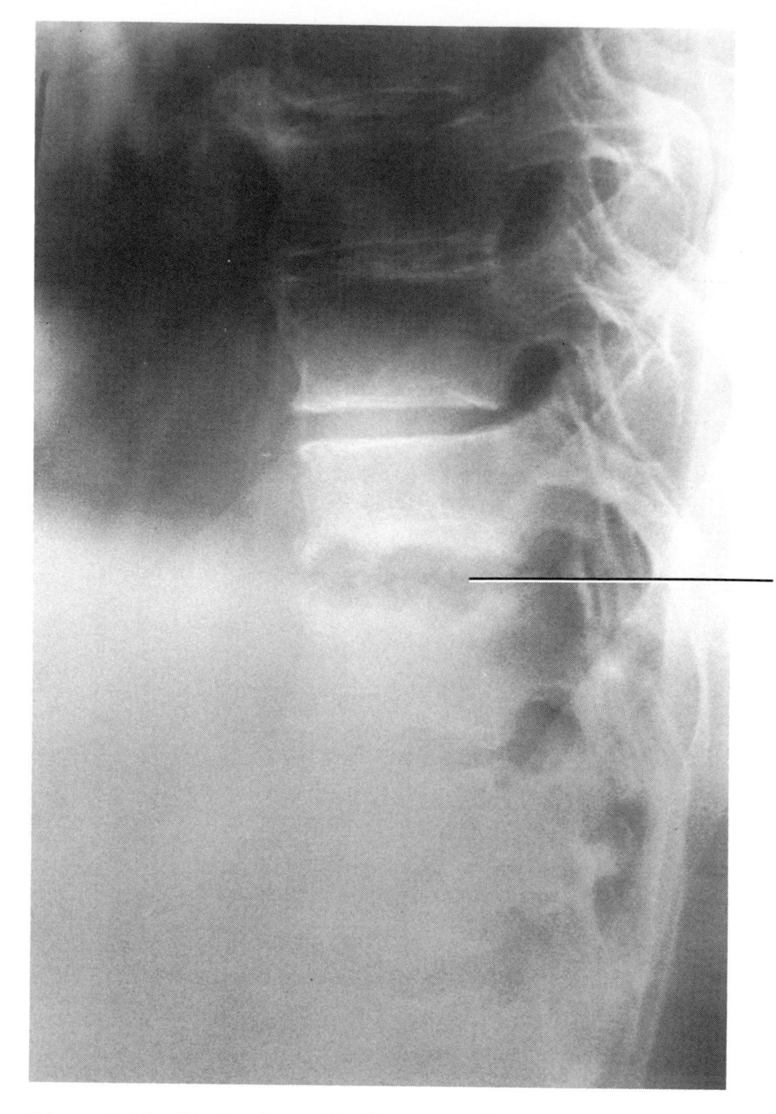

Figure 2.13. Evaluation of back pain in the absence of trauma.

2.14 DESTRUCTION OF A VERTEBRAL PEDICLE

A. On routine examination of the spine, the pedicles should be examined to look for the presence of erosion.
B. Normally, the pedicles have a symmetrical appearance unless patient rotation or scoliosis is present.
   1. Differential diagnosis
      a. Metastasis
      b. Neurofibroma
      c. Tuberculosis
      d. Multiple myeloma
      e. Aneurysmal bone cyst
      f. Giant cell tumor

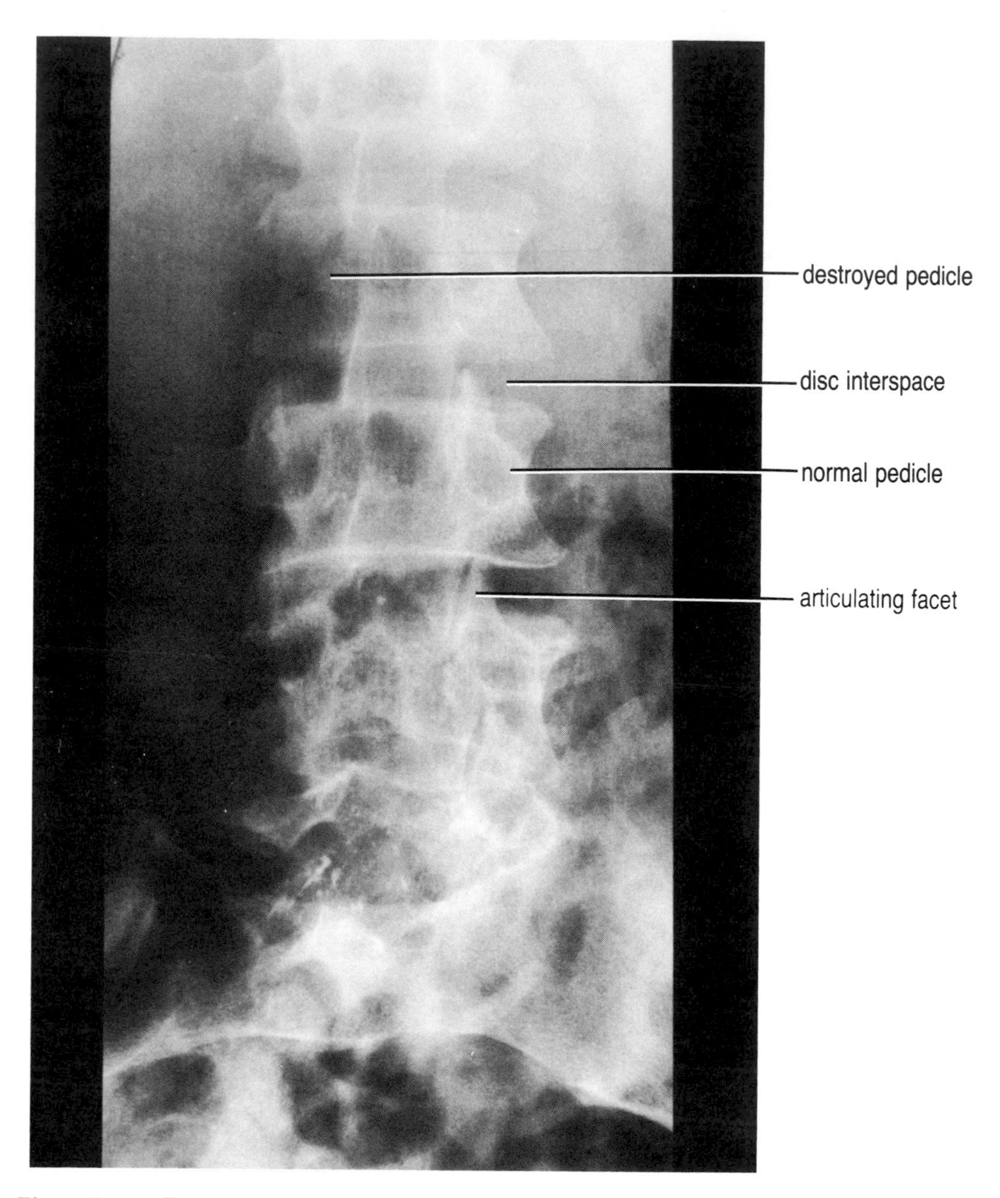

Figure 2.14. Destruction of a vertebral pedicle.

2.15 SIMULATION OF A FRACTURE BY CONGENITAL ANOMALIES

A. Spina bifida occulta is a common radiographic finding that may simulate a fracture.
B. Spondylolysis may also simulate a fracture. This represents a defect through the pars interarticularis, usually at the L5 or L4 level. This defect may be unilateral or bilateral. If the defect involves both pedicles, the involved vertebra may be anteriorly displaced forward. If this has occurred, the condition is known as spondylolisthesis.

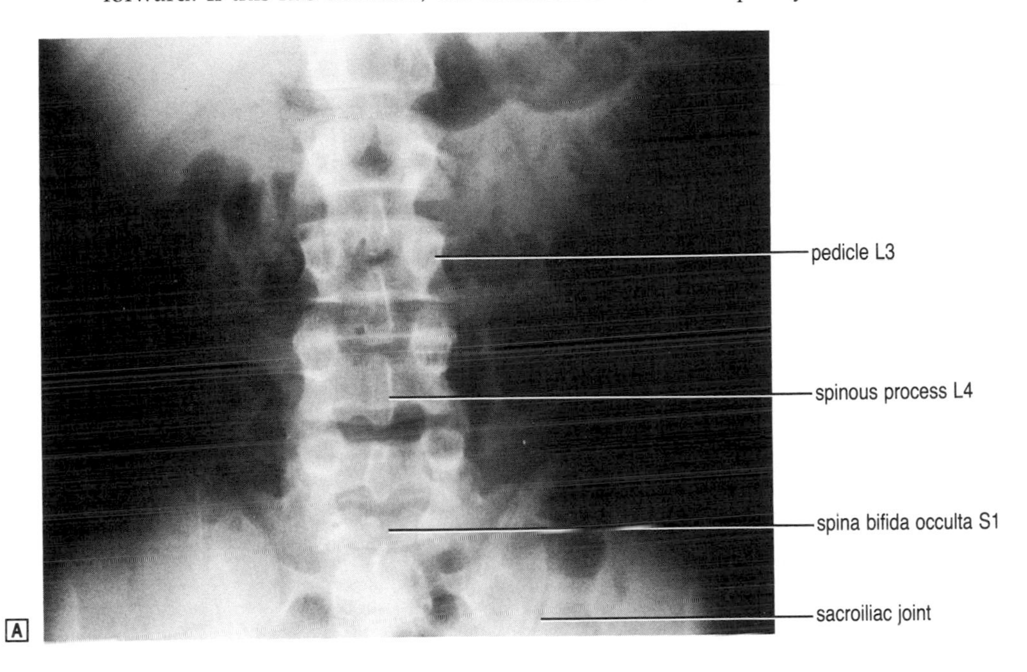

Figure 2.15. *A*, Simulation of a fracture by congenital anomalies.

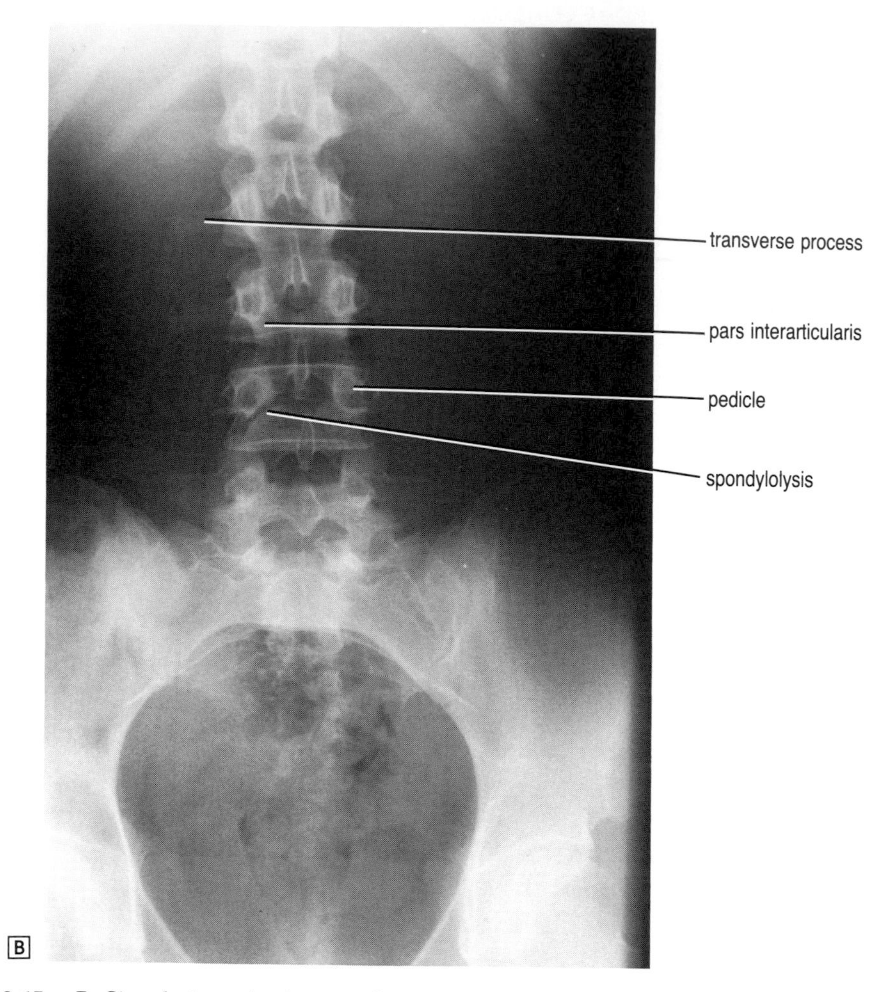

Figure 2.15. *B*, Simulation of a fracture by congenital anomalies.

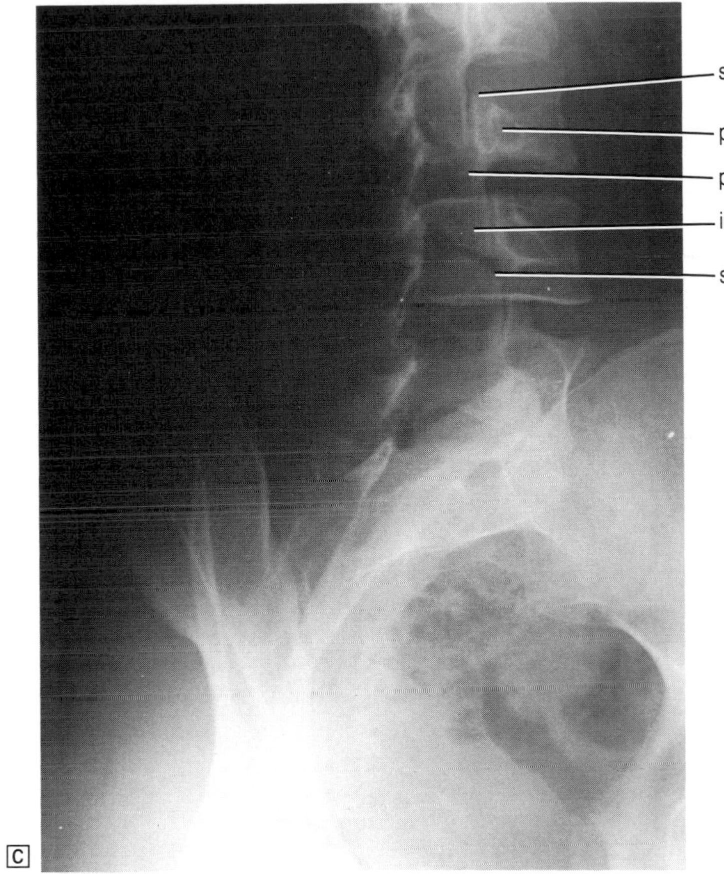

Figure 2.15. C, Simulation of a fracture by congenital anomalies.

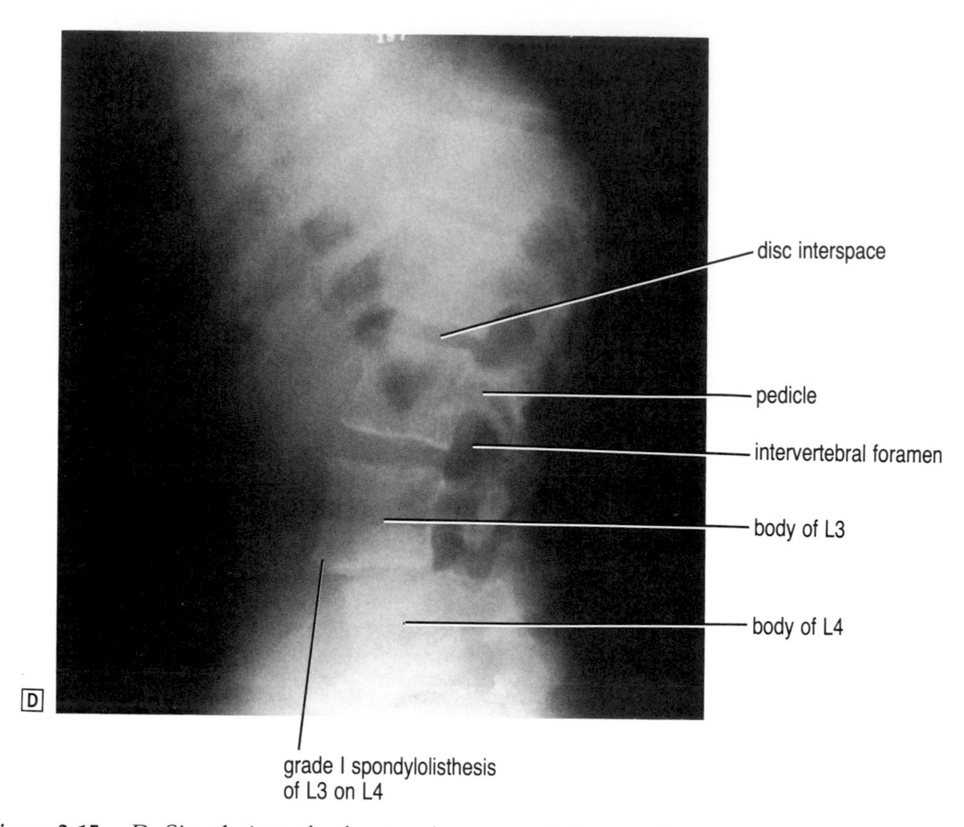

Figure 2.15. *D,* Simulation of a fracture by congenital anomalies.

References

Eisenberg, R.L.: Diagnostic Imaging in Internal Medicine. New York: McGraw-Hill Book Co., 1985.

Forrester, D.M., and Brown, J.C.: Radiographic evaluation of back pain. In: Contemporary Diagnostic Radiology, Vol. 2. Baltimore: Williams & Wilkins, 1979.

Harris, J.H., and Harris, W.H.: The Radiology of Emergency Medicine. 2nd Ed. Baltimore: Williams & Wilkins, 1981.

Juhl, J.H., and Crummy, A.B.: Essentials of Radiologic Imaging. Philadelphia: J.B. Lippincott, 1987.

Levy, R.C., Hawkins, H., and Barsan, W.G.: Radiology in Emergency Medicine. St. Louis: C.V. Mosby Co., 1986.

Meschan, I., and Farrer-Meschan, R.M.: Roentgen Signs in Diagnostic Imaging, Vol. 3: Spine and Central Nervous System. Philadelphia: W.B. Saunders Co., 1985.

Taveras, J.M., and Ferrucci, J.T.: Radiology Diagnosis—Imaging-Intervention, Vol. 3: Neuroradiology and Radiology of the Head and Neck. Philadelphia, J.B. Lippincott, 1988.

3

Chest

3.01 THE NORMAL CHEST: SYSTEMATIC SEARCH

A. The goal is to establish a logical approach to evaluation of the chest. Be thorough in your examination and repetitive in your approach. The method presented is only an example. Establish a routine that is most comfortable for you and stick with it. Repetition of your method will yield the best results. Avoid the temptation to go directly to the most visible disease. We recommend beginning at the periphery and working toward the center.

B. Remember the "ABCs" of the chest.
   1. A = Abdomen: Take advantage of all the information given to you. Looking below the diaphragm may reveal free air or abnormal calcifications.
   2. B = Bones: Examination allows you to detect fractures, destructive lesions, dislocations, degenerative changes, or demineralization.
   3. C = Cardiac/vascular structures: Evaluate cardiac size and vascular disease.
   4. S = Soft tissues and segments of the lung: Look for evidence of previous mastectomy, nipple shadows, pneumothorax, pneumonia, effusion, atelectasis, or carcinoma.

C. When evaluating a chest, you must look for disease to see it. For example, to see a pneumothorax you must be looking for it and know that it can exist.
   1. AP or PA view of the chest
      a. Systematic Search
         (1) Below diaphragm
         (2) Right humerus, shoulder, scapula, and clavicle
         (3) Left humerus, shoulder, scapula, and clavicle
         (4) Lower C-spine, T-spine, and trachea
         (5) Right hemidiaphragm and costophrenic angle
         (6) Left hemidiaphragm and costophrenic angle
         (7) Right ribs (anterior and posterior)
         (8) Left ribs (anterior and posterior)
         (9) Right lung field
         (10) Left lung field
         (11) Heart and vascular structures
         (12) Behind the heart
         (13) Apices
         (14) Overall survey; examine the entire film together
         (15) Don't forget the soft tissues
   2. Lateral view of the chest
      a. The same rules apply. Establish a systematic search and remember the ABCs.

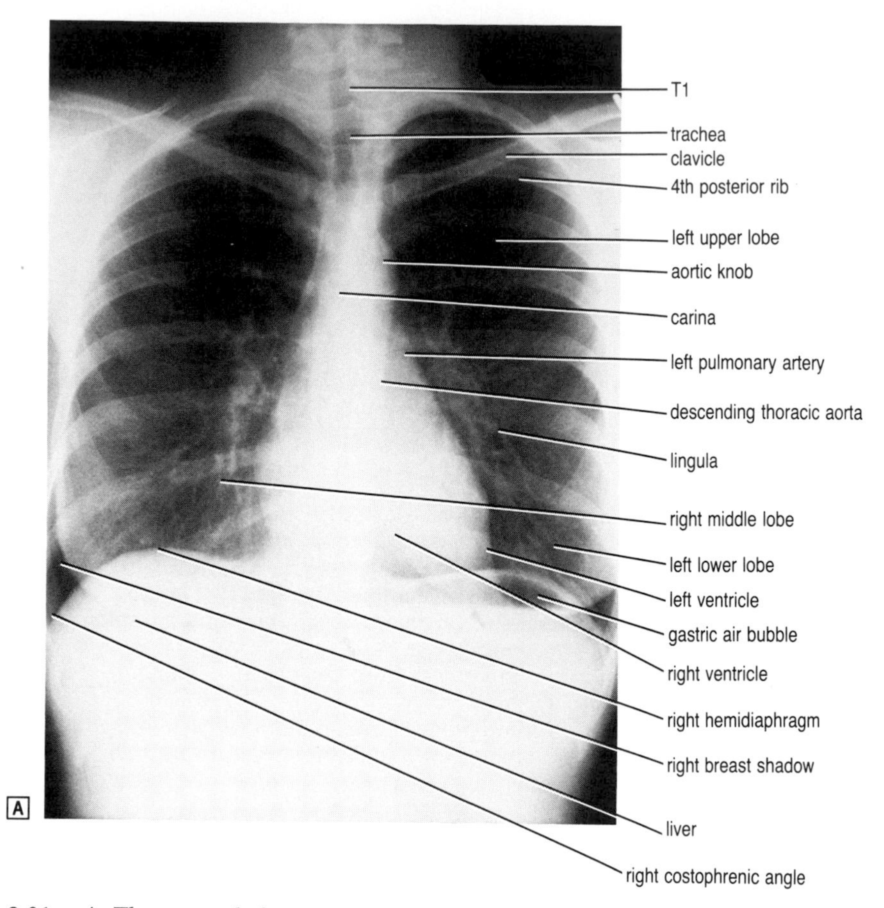

Figure 3.01. *A,* The normal chest: systematic search.

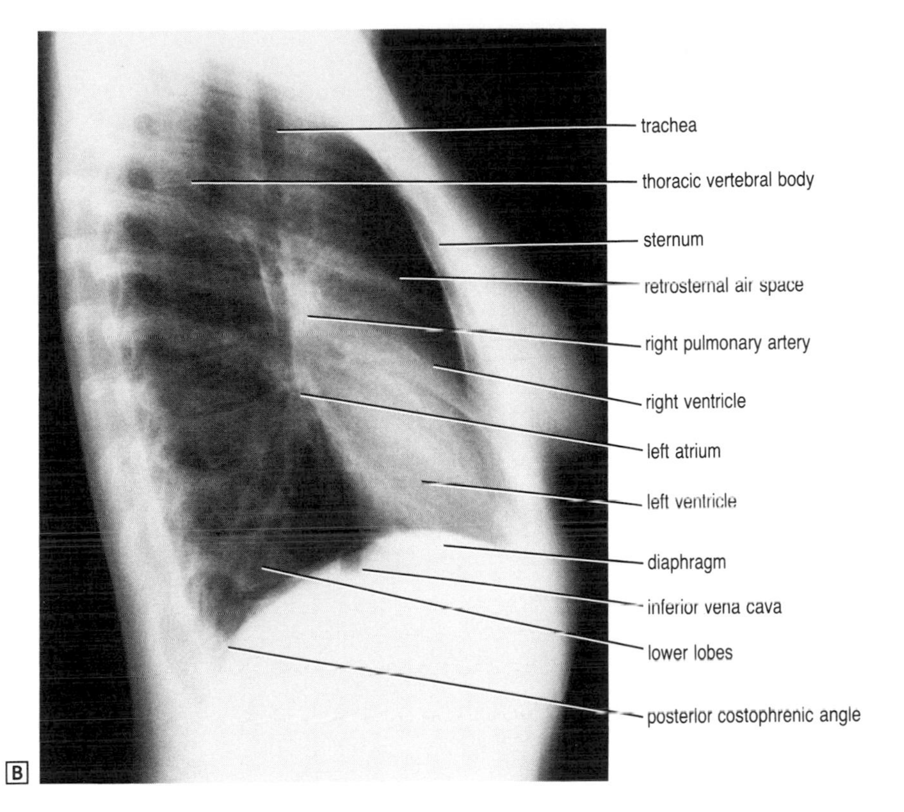

Figure 3.01. *B,* The normal chest: systematic search.

3.02 MASTECTOMY

A. Differential diagnosis: unilateral hyperlucent lung
   1. Mastectomy: removal of breast and pectoral muscles
   2. Pneumothorax: visible pleural edge with absence of peripheral lung markings
   3. Suboptimal technique: due to rotation of the patient
   4. Poland's syndrome: congenital absence of the pectorals on one side
   5. Bullous emphysema
   6. Obstructive emphysema
   7. Compensatory hyperinflation following lobectomy
   8. Swyer James syndrome
      a. History of repeated respiratory infections during childhood
      b. Acute infection causes obliteration of the small airways. The peripheral lung becomes ventilated by collateral air drift, which results in air trapping and eventual destruction. Emphysematous changes follow.
      c. May involve one or two lobes
      d. The affected lung appears hyperlucent owing to decreased lung markings and emphysematous changes.
      e. The affected lung is smaller owing to decreased volume.

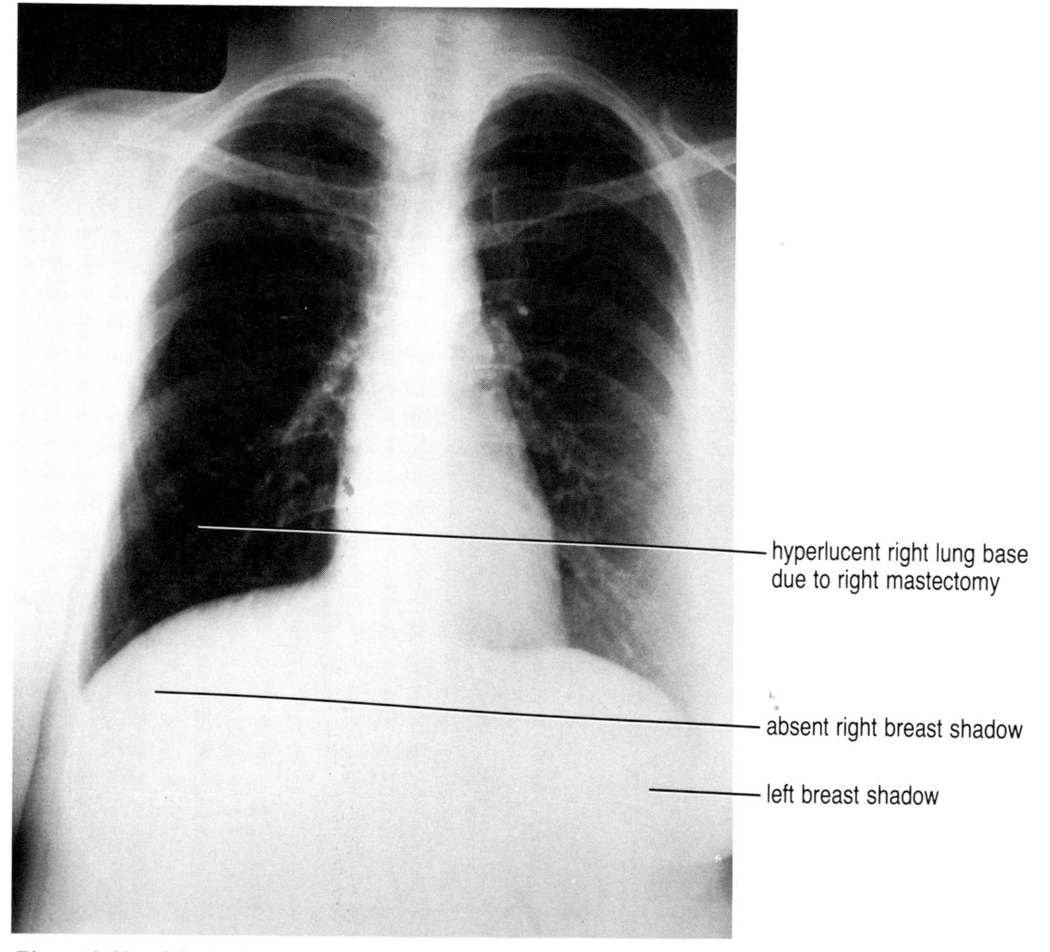

Figure 3.02. Mastectomy.

3.03 LINE PLACEMENT

A. Placement of an external apparatus within the body requires accurate localization of its position.
   1. Endotracheal tube (ETT)
      a. The level of the carina is most often between T5 and T6.
      b. If chin is in neutral position, the tip of the ETT should be approximately 5 cm above the carina.
      c. Flexion of the neck pushes the tip of the ETT 2 cm downward.
      d. Extension raises the ETT 2 cm upward.
      e. Aspiration may result if the ETT is placed too high.
      f. If placed too low, the ETT will extend into the right main-stem bronchus and may lead to collapse of the left lung.
   2. Tracheostomy tube
      a. The distal tip should be in the area of T3, approximately midway between the tracheal stoma and the carina.
   3. Central venous pressure (CVP) lines
      a. The tip should be placed within the superior vena cava proximal to any valves that may affect monitoring of right atrial pressure. The most proximal valve is located in the subclavian vein in the area of the first anterior rib.
      b. Most common ectopic locations include the internal jugular vein, right atrium, and right ventricle.
      c. Potential complications include pneumothorax (see Sec. 3.05), hemothorax, and ectopic location of the catheter tip, which may result in the infusion of fluids into the mediastinum.
   4. Nasogastric tube (NG)
      a. The tip should extend below the left hemidiaphragm and terminate within the stomach.
   5. Chest tube
      a. Placement for pneumothorax should be in the anterior superior aspect of the pleural space.
      b. Placement for hydrothorax should be in the posterior inferior aspect of the pleural space.
   6. Swan-Ganz catheter (SGC)
      a. The tip should be within the right or left main pulmonary artery.
      b. Complications include pulmonary infarction distal to catheter, arrhythmia, or rupture of the pulmonary artery and pneumothorax (see Sec. 3.05).
   7. Intra-aortic counterpulsation balloon pump (IACB)
      a. The tip should be at the level of the aortic knob.
      b. Inflation of the balloon occurs during diastole producing an elevation of diastolic pressure, which increases coronary blood flow.
      c. Also decreases afterload on the heart
      d. Deflation occurs during systole.
      e. Potential complications include aortic dissection and obstruction of blood flow to the abdomen if placement is too distal.
   8. Pacemaker
      a. The tip should be in the area of the apex of the right ventricle.
      b. Ectopic locations include right atrium, pulmonary artery, and coronary sinus. If the pacemaker is placed within the coronary sinus, the anterior view appears nearly normal, but the lateral view shows that the lead is directed posteriorly rather than anteriorly.

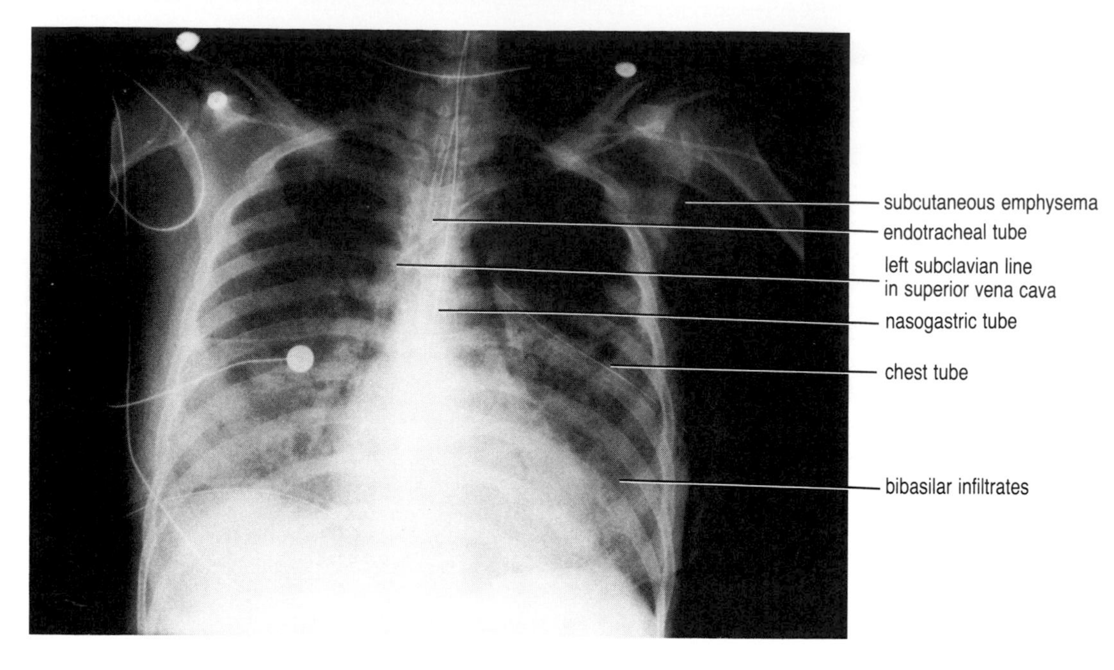

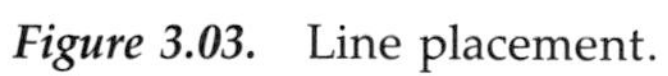

Figure 3.03. Line placement.

3.04 PNEUMONIA

A. Pneumonia represents an inflammatory process of the lung.

B. Pneumonic infiltrates are radiographically visualized as alveolar infiltrates, interstitial infiltrates, or a combination of both. Alveolar infiltrates represent air space consolidation of the alveoli and are visualized as patchy, fluffy densities that become confluent. Interstitial infiltrates represent an inflammatory process within the interstitium of the air passages. They are visualized as linear streaks of increased density with sparing of the alveoli.

C. Air bronchograms
   1. Following consolidation of an area of the lung, sections of air within the passageways become visible and are known as air bronchograms. These are visualized as linear streaks of air density within areas of air space consolidation.

D. Silhouette sign
   1. The silhouette sign allows localization of a pneumonic infiltrate to the involved segment of the lung.
   2. An area of infiltrate in contact with the border of the heart or diaphragm results in obliteration of its visible margin.
   3. If an infiltrate in the right lung obscures the right cardiac margin, a right middle lobe infiltrate is suspected and can be confirmed on a lateral view.
   4. If the right cardiac margin is clearly visualized despite adjacent infiltrate, a right lower lobe infiltrate is suspected. Once again a lateral view will confirm the location of the infiltrate.
   5. Infiltrates within the lingular segment of the left upper lobe obscure the left cardiac margin while left lower lobe infiltrate does not. The left hemidiaphragm may become obscured with a left lower lobe infiltrate.
   6. If an infiltrate is in contact with the diaphragm, it will obliterate its appearance.
   7. This same principle applies for mass lesions in the chest.

E. A few examples of pneumonia
   1. Streptococcal pneumonia
      a. Is a common community-acquired pneumonia
      b. May occur in debilitated individuals, such as alcoholics, or may occur in relatively healthy individuals
      c. Produces air space consolidation
      d. Gram-positive organism
   2. Staphylococcal pneumonia
      a. Is a common hospital-acquired pneumonia
      b. Often seen in debilitated patients
      c. Occurs in children
      d. Empyema and pneumatoceles may form in young children
      e. Pleural effusion may occur
      f. Gram-positive organism
   3. Klebsiella pneumoniae
      a. Most often seen in debilitated patients such as chronic alcoholics
      b. Typically, an entire segment consolidates with bulging of the adjacent fissure.
   4. Aspiration pneumonia
      a. Aspiration of foreign substances usually involves the right middle lobe or right lower lobe. The left lower lobe is less frequently affected.
      b. Represents a mixed bacterial infection
      c. Usually appears as a patchy infiltrate with a rapid onset.
   5. Mycoplasmal pneumonia
      a. Most common cause of nonbacterial pneumonia
      b. Usually affects teenagers and young adults
      c. Radiographic appearance consists of linear interstitial infiltrates, which may gradually result in air space consolidation.
      d. Viral pneumonias in general produce interstitial infiltrates.

F. There are numerous different types of pneumonia. The diagnosis depends upon the combination of bacteriologic sputum evaluation, clinical presentation, and radiographic findings.

G. Differential diagnosis of alveolar infiltration
   1. Pneumonia
   2. Pulmonary edema, CHF
   3. Hemorrhage, trauma, Goodpasture's syndrome
   4. Metastatic disease
   5. Neoplasm
   6. Fat emboli

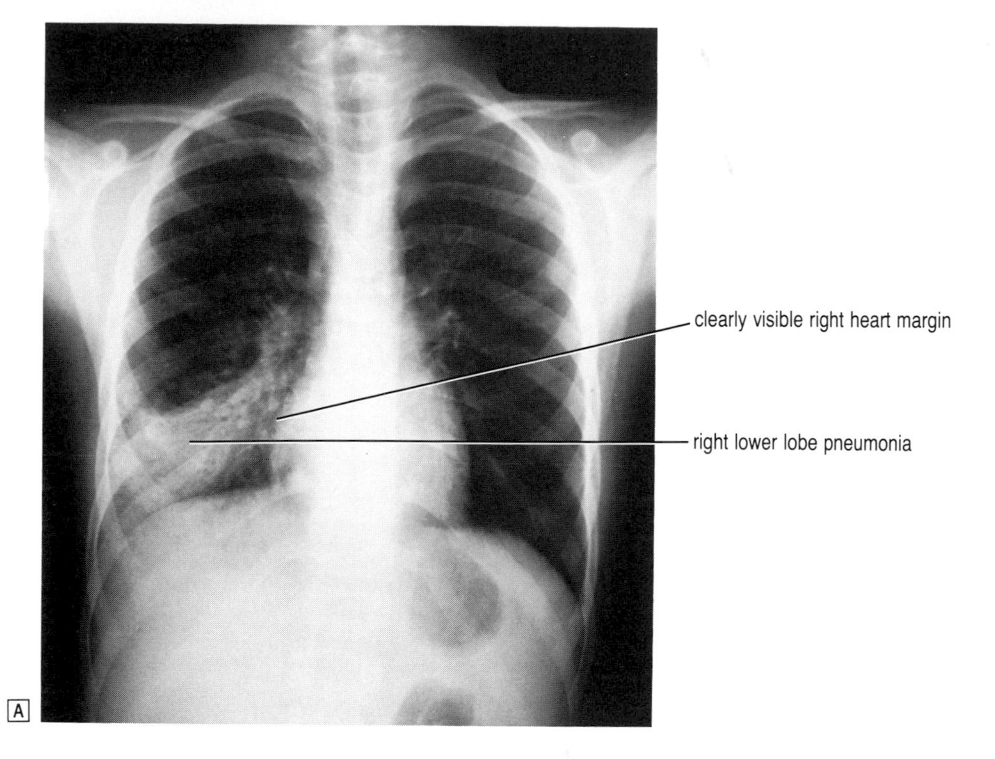

Figure 3.04. *A,* Pneumonia.

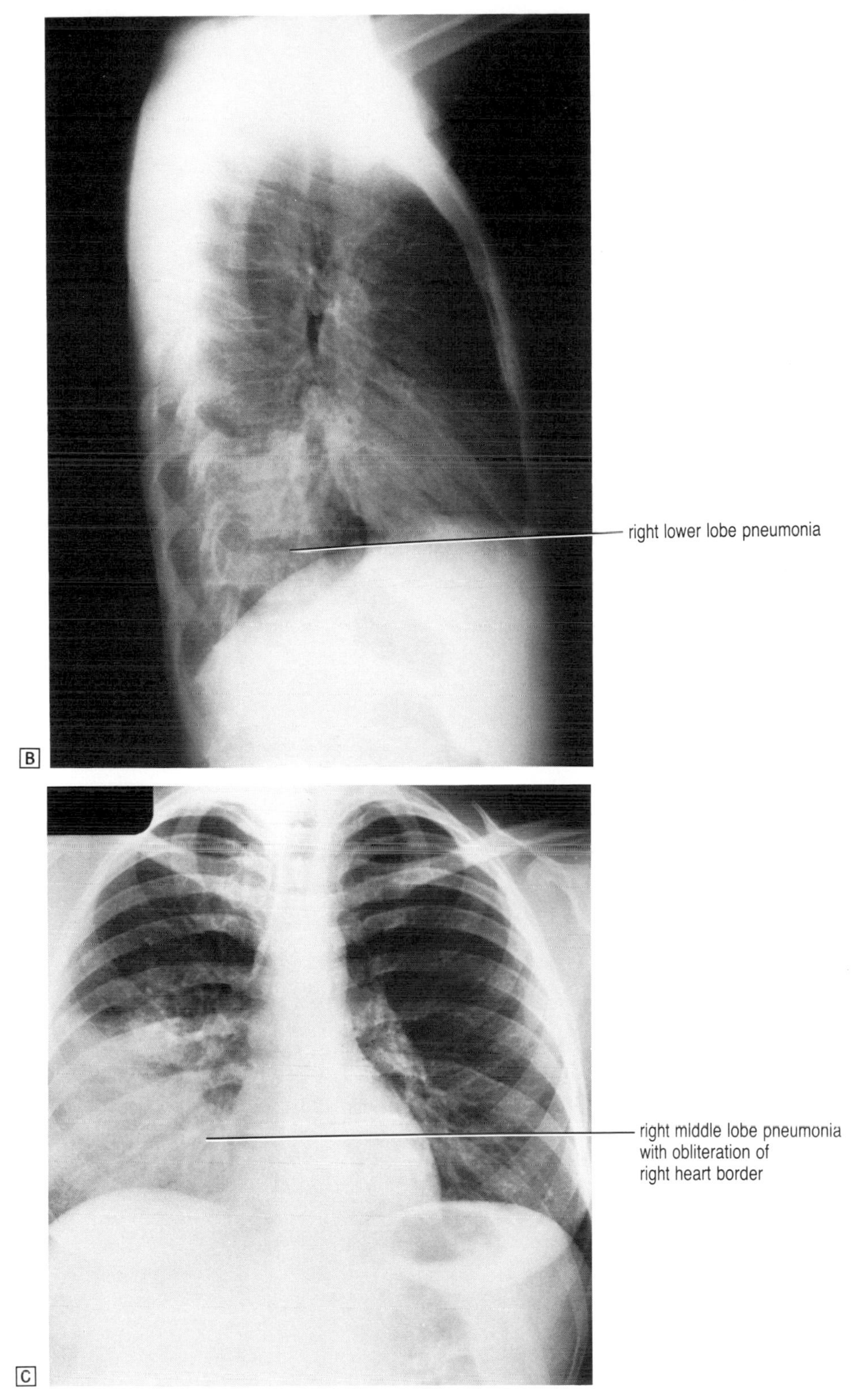

Figure 3.04. *B*, Pneumonia. *C*, Pneumonia.

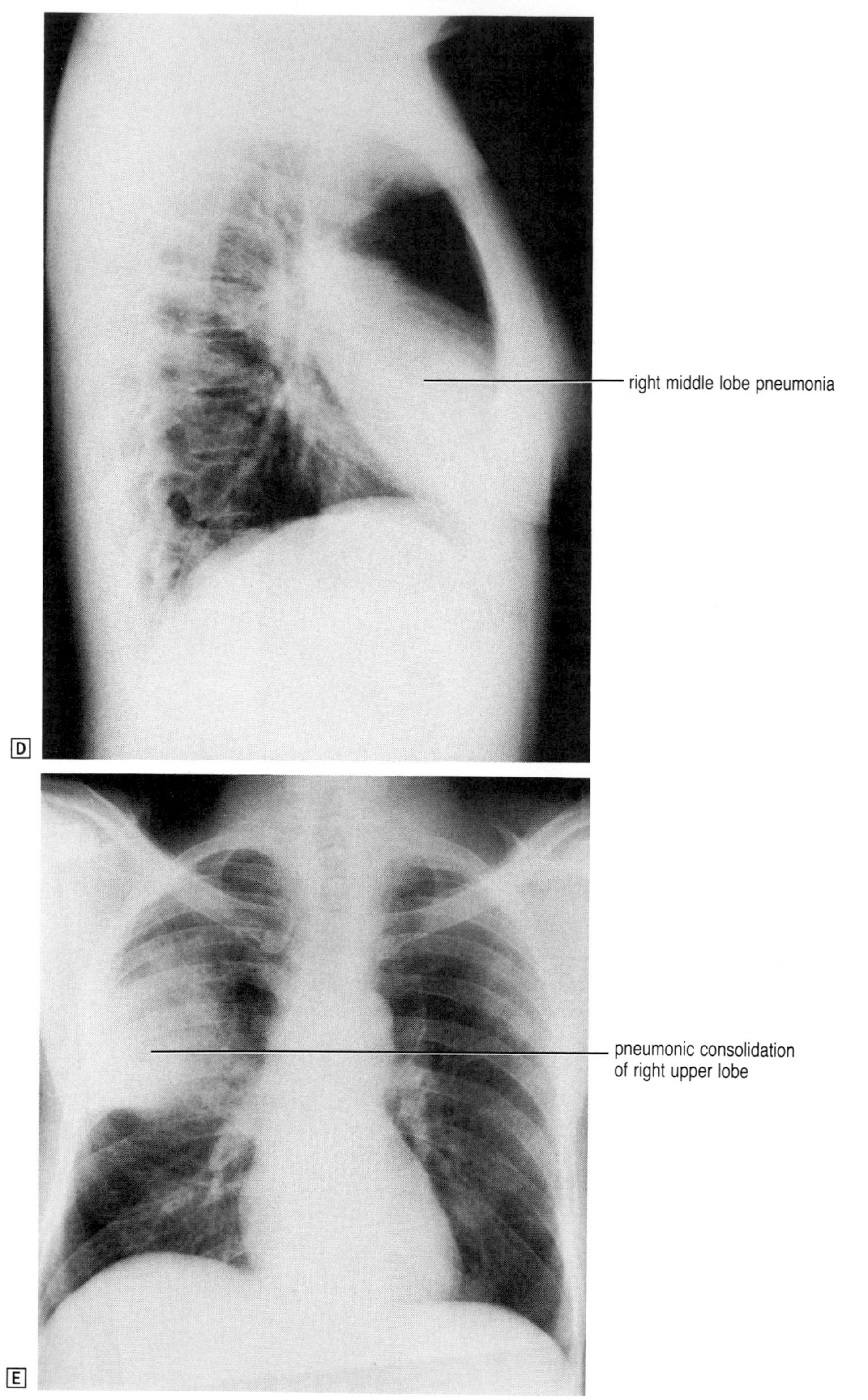

Figure 3.04. *D*, Pneumonia. *E*, Pneumonia.

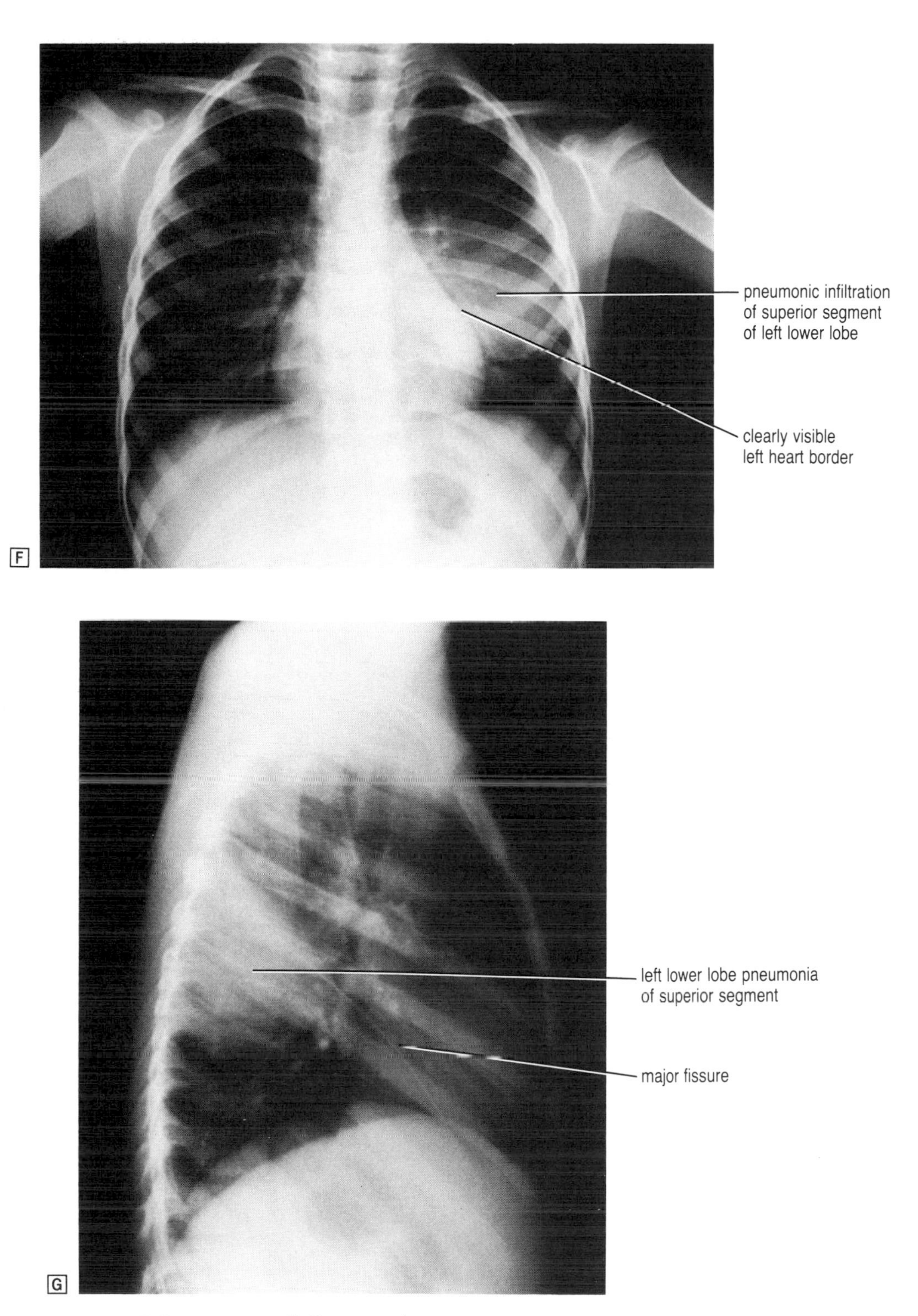

Figure 3.04. *F,* Pneumonia. *G,* Pneumonia.

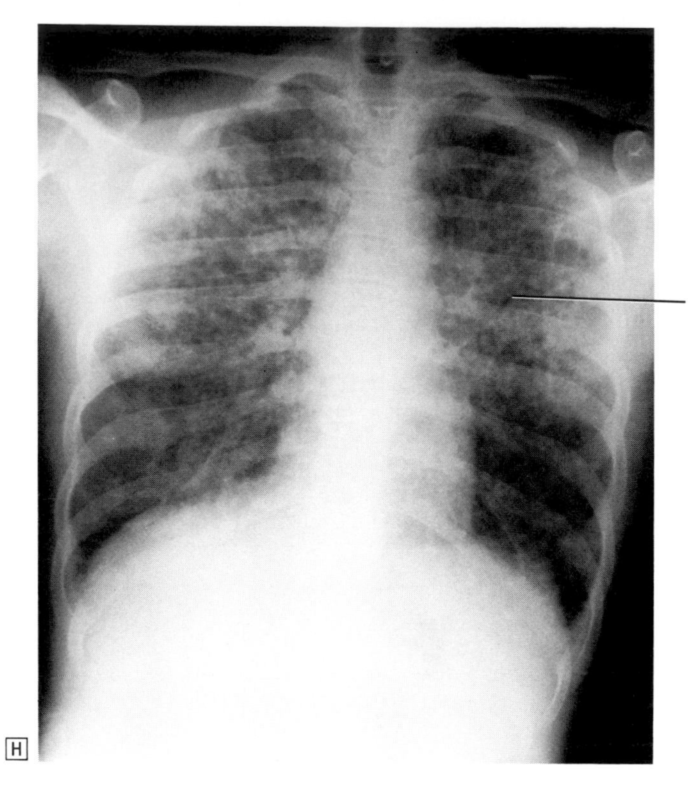

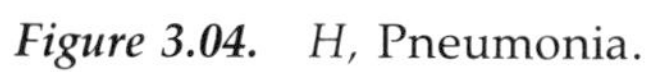
Figure 3.04. *H,* Pneumonia.

3.05 PNEUMOTHORAX

A. Major diagnostic finding: unilateral hyperlucent lung (see Sec. 3.02)
   1. An abnormal collection of air located between the visceral and parietal pleura
   2. In the erect position is a visible pleural edge with an absence of peripheral lung markings, usually near the apex.
   3. In the supine position, abnormal air collections seen at the bases indicate possibility of a pneumothorax.
   4. Normal variants that simulate pneumothorax
      a. Skin folds; peripheral lung markings cross this line
      b. Companion rib shadows; seen as a symmetrical linear density along the inferior border of a rib

B. Differential diagnosis
   1. Iatrogenic: following insertion of a CVP line or following a lung biopsy
   2. Spontaneous: affects males more than females 8:1, typically a tall, thin male
   3. Trauma: look for rib fractures or pleural fluid accumulation.
   4. Secondary to neoplasm
   5. Secondary to COPD or asthma
   6. Secondary to many other types of intrinsic lung disease.
   7. Unilateral hyperlucent lung (see Sec. 3.02)

C. Clinical signs
   1. Chest pain, dyspnea, decreased breath sounds
   2. Hyperresonant to percussion

D. Tension pneumothorax
   1. An opening allows air to enter the pleural space during inspiration, and a flap prevents its escape during expiration. Accumulation of air forces the mediastinal structures to the contralateral side resulting in compression of the opposite lung and venous circulation. This is a life-threatening condition that must be identified quickly.

E. Remember, if the chest film is equivocal for pneumothorax, get a follow-up erect chest roentgenogram with forced expiration.

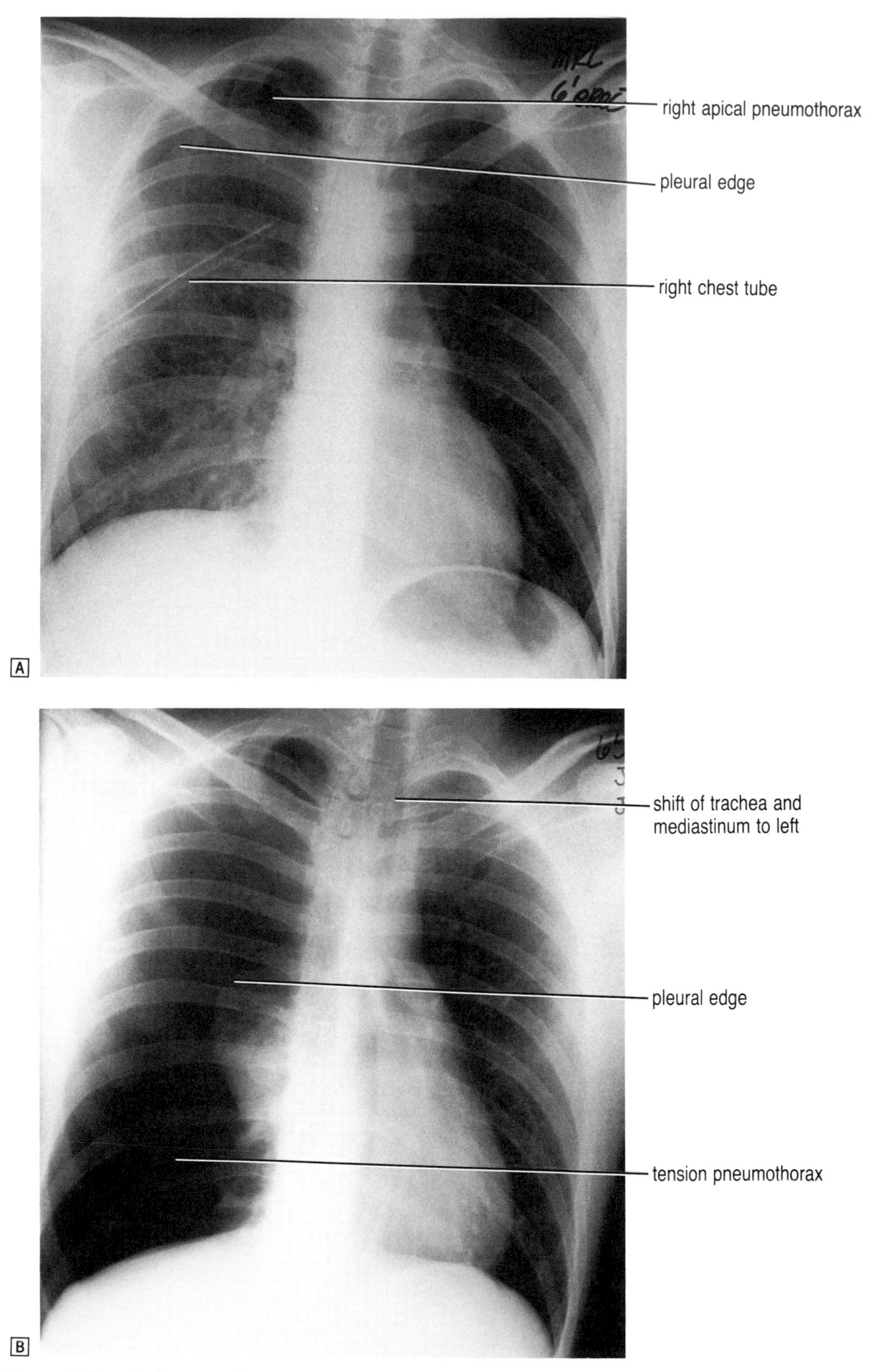

Figure 3.05. *A,* Pneumothorax. *B,* Pneumothorax.

3.06 CONGESTIVE HEART FAILURE (CHF)

A. Radiographic manifestations result from elevated pulmonary venous pressures.
   1. 6 to 12 mm Hg: normal left atrial pressure
   2. 12 to 20 mm Hg: redistribution of pulmonary blood flow known as cephalization of flow. In the erect position, blood flow becomes greater to the upper lung fields than to the lower fields.
   3. 20 to 30 mm Hg: there is transudation of fluid into the interstitium. Fluid accumulates in the perihilar regions and produces perihilar haziness. Pleural effusions of the right side are greater than those of the left. Visualization of Kerley B lines represents transudation of fluid from interlobular septal lymphatics into the surrounding space.
   4. 30 to 40 mm Hg: fluid moves into the alveolar spaces producing alveolar pulmonary edema, predominantly perihilar in distribution, and fluffy alveolar infiltrates.

B. Differential diagnosis for pulmonary edema
   1. Heart disease: left ventricular failure
   2. Iatrogenic: fluid overload
   3. Cerebral: head injury, stroke
   4. Drugs: heroin overdose, morphine, nitrofurantoin
   5. Mendelson's syndrome: aspiration of gastric contents
   6. Renal failure
   7. Near drowning
   8. High altitude
   9. Radiation therapy

C. Clinical presentation of CHF
   1. Dyspnea
   2. Orthopnea
   3. Tachypnea and tachycardia
   4. Cardiomegaly
   5. Auscultation of S3 gallop
   6. Jugular venous distention
   7. Peripheral edema
   8. Weakness and fatigue

D. Left ventricular enlargement
   1. PA view
      a. The left heart border is prominent with displacement of the apex inferiorly. The cardiothoracic ratio is greater than 50%.
   2. Lateral view
      a. The posterior inferior aspect of the cardiac silhouette is prominent.
   3. Differential diagnosis for left ventricular enlargement
      a. CHF
      b. Arteriosclerotic coronary heart disease
      c. Aortic stenosis (pressure overload)
      d. Aortic insufficiency (volume overload)
      e. Ventricular septal defect (VSD)
      f. Cardiomyopathy
      g. Patent ductus arteriosus
      h. Coarctation of the aorta (see Sec. 3.19)

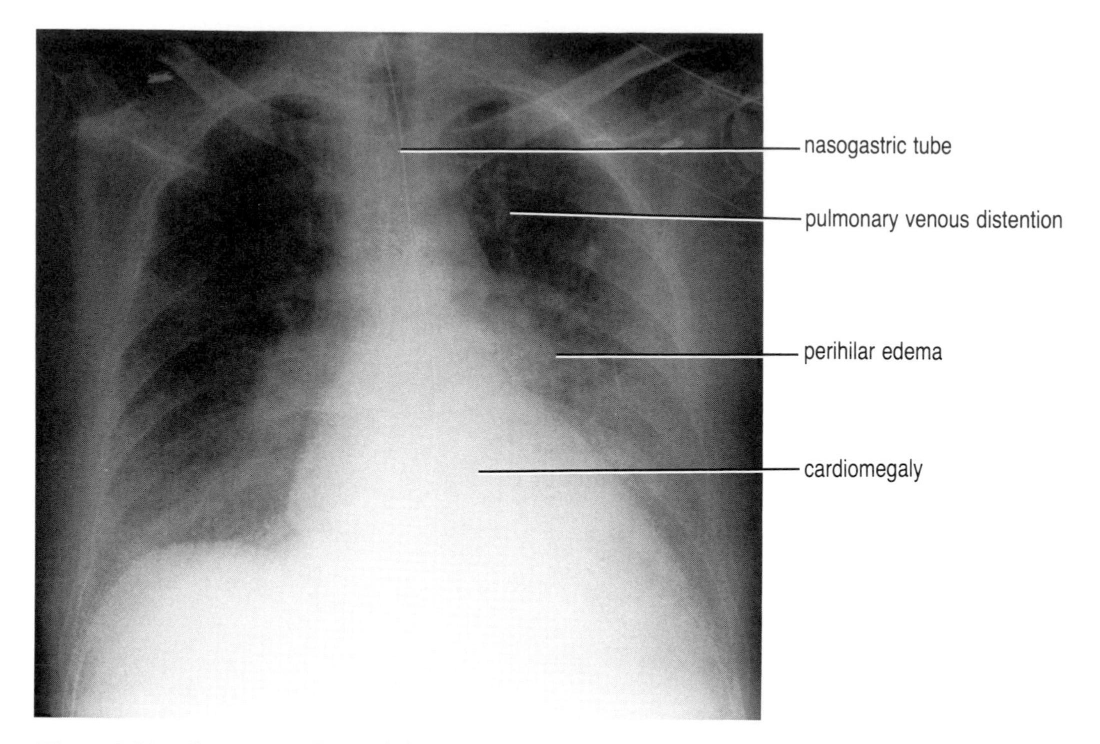

Figure 3.06. Congestive heart failure (CHF).

3.07 ATELECTASIS

A. Atelectasis is a loss of lung volume.

B. There are different forms of atelectasis. Most types result in visible air bronchograms. In the presence of an obstructing endobronchial lesion, atelectasis will occur without evidence of air bronchograms.

C. Loss of lung volume may result in small linear plate-like areas of increased density or may result in complete lobar collapse.

D. Radiographic signs of atelectasis
  1. Focal, linear areas of opacity
  2. Elevation of hemidiaphragm
  3. Shift of the mediastinum to the side of involvement
  4. Shift of interlobar fissures
  5. Possible hyperinflation of contralateral lung
  6. Rib approximation

E. Lobar collapse
  1. Left lower lobe and right lower lobe
     a. Seen on the anterior view as an obliquely oriented density located behind the cardiac silhouette. Right lower lobe collapse has a similar appearance at the right base.
  2. Left upper lobe
     a. Anterior view demonstrates haziness in the upper lung field while the lateral view reveals an area of increased density located behind the sternum.
  3. Right upper lobe
     a. Visualized on the anterior view as haziness of the right upper lobe with elevation of the minor fissure.
  4. Right middle lobe
     a. Best visualized on the lateral view, which demonstrates a triangular density superimposed on the cardiac silhouette.

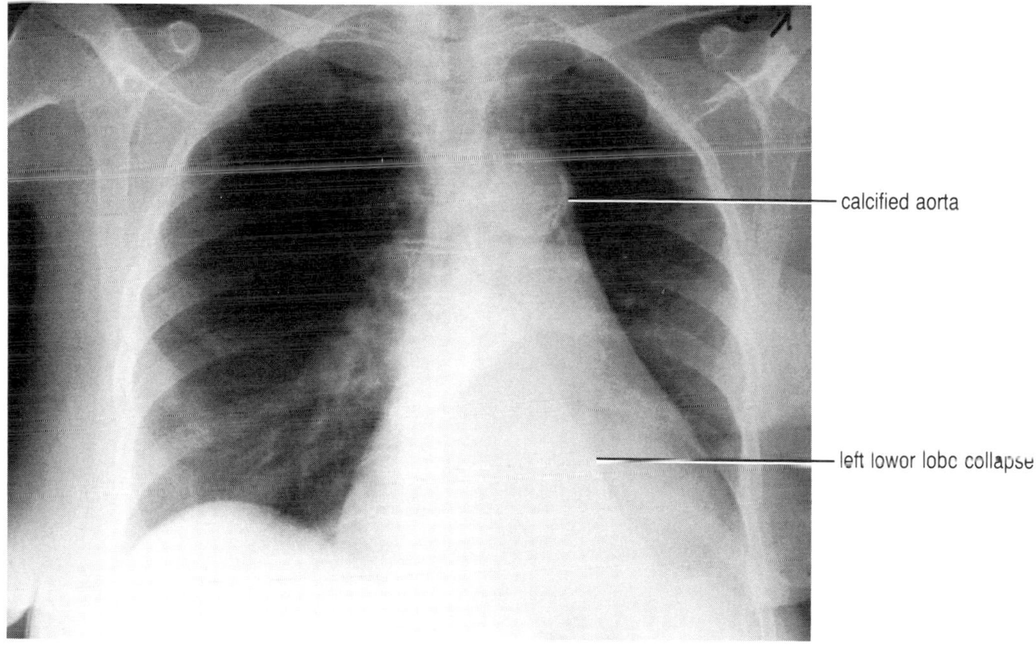

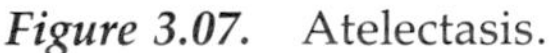

Figure 3.07. Atelectasis.

3.08 CHRONIC OBSTRUCTIVE PULMONARY DISEASE (COPD)

A. Major diagnostic finding: bilateral hyperlucent lung fields
B. Chronic lung disease produces enlargement of the air space distal to the terminal bronchiole, which leads to air trapping.
C. Characterized by air flow obstruction during expiration.
D. The two most important types of COPD
  1. Centrilobular: The respiratory bronchiole is enlarged while the alveolar ducts, alveolar sacs, and alveoli are uninvolved, i.e., the periphery of the acinus is spared. This type occurs in smokers and has upper lobe predominance.
  2. Panlobular: There is diffuse involvement of the acinus with lower lobe predominance.
E. Alpha-1 antitrypsin deficiency is an inherited disorder that results in emphysematous changes predominantly involving the lower lobes.
F. Radiographic findings
  1. Hyperinflation of the lungs characterized by low flattened hemidiaphragms and enlargement of the retrosternal air space. There is limited movement of the diaphragm with inspiration and expiration.
  2. Hyperluceny of both lung fields
  3. Cardiac silhouette appears elongated and narrowed.
  4. Pulmonary oligemia (diminished vascular markings most visible at the lung periphery)
  5. Development of interstitial fibrosis
  6. Bullae formation represents a localized area of emphysema. It is a cystic air space greater than 1 cm that is formed by alveolar destruction.
  7. Blebs are smaller than bullae and represent small areas of interstitial emphysema surrounded by visceral pleura.
G. Differential diagnosis: bilateral hyperlucent lungs
  1. COPD
  2. Asthma
  3. Obstruction of trachea or larynx due to foreign body or mass lesion.
  4. Acute bronchiolitis
  5. Hyperventilation
  6. Multiple, bilateral pulmonary emboli
  7. Cyanotic form of congenital heart disease (right-to-left shunt)

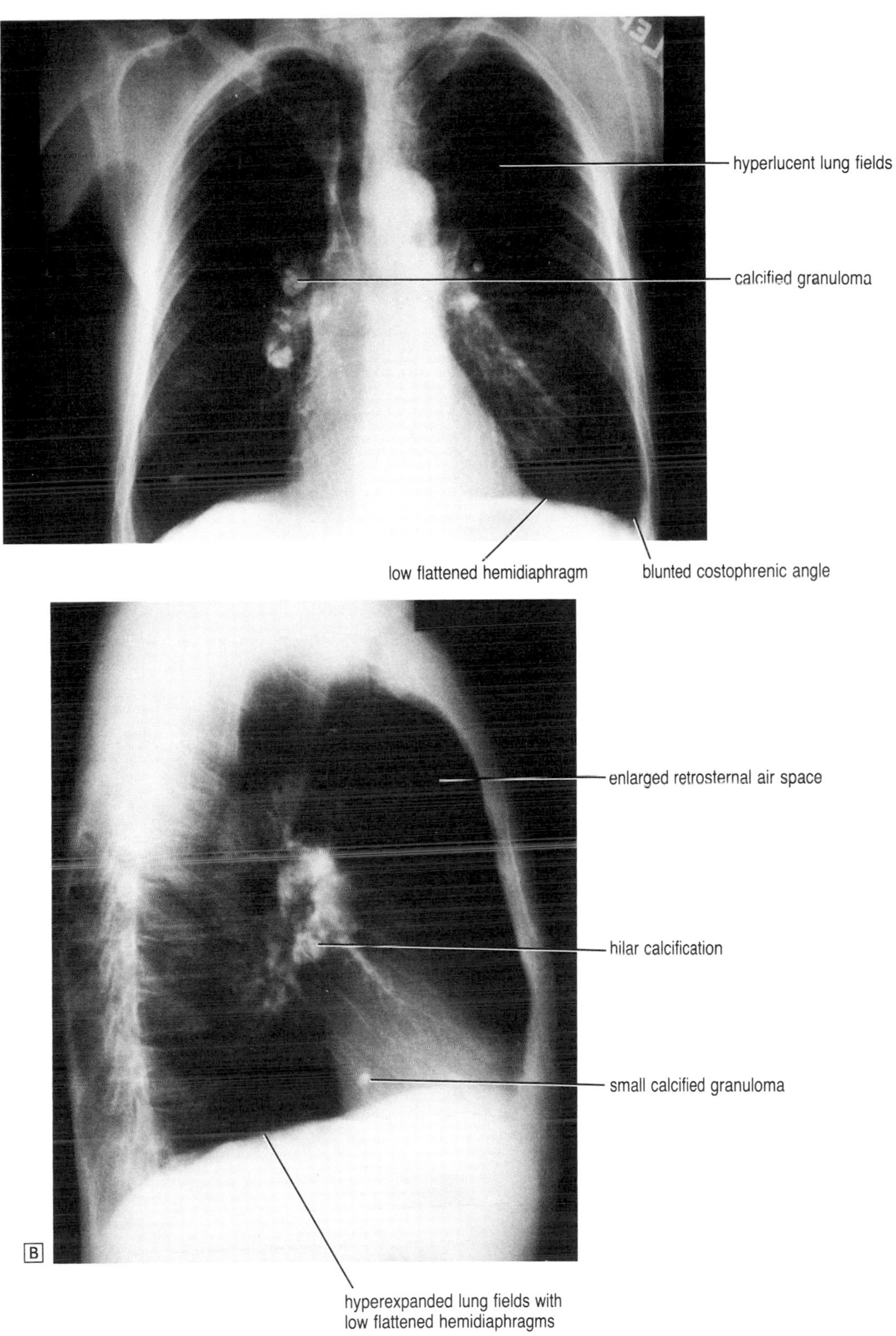

Figure 3.08. *A*, Chronic obstructive pulmonary disease (COPD). *B*, Chronic obstructive pulmonary disease (COPD).

3.09 PLEURAL-BASED MASS

A. Pleural-based masses appear as soft tissue densities located laterally with smooth margins and obtuse angles with the chest wall.
B. If a pleural mass is identified, look for additional lesions, overlying rib destruction, and pleural fluid.
C. Differential diagnosis
   1. Trauma resulting in a localized hematoma
   2. Multiple myeloma
   3. Metastasis
   4. Loculated pleural fluid
   5. Mesothelioma
   6. Bronchogenic carcinoma
   7. Callus formation from previous rib fracture
   8. Fibrin ball

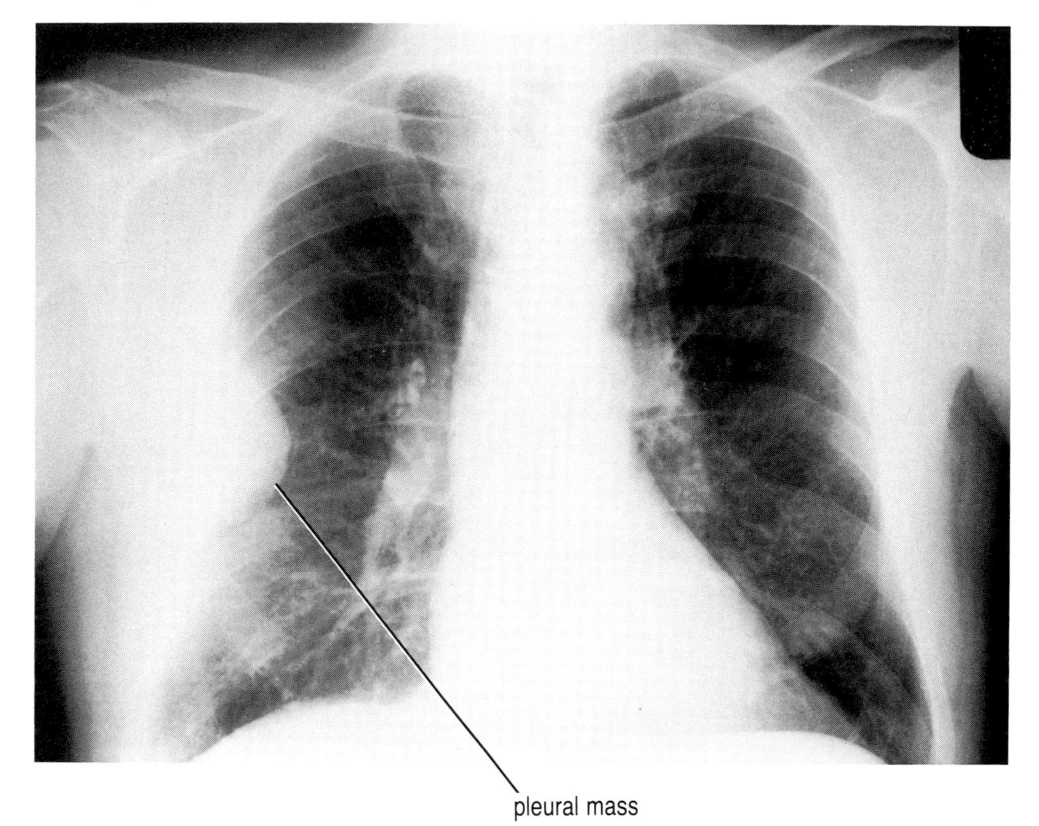

Figure 3.09. Pleural-based mass.

3.10 PNEUMOMEDIASTINUM

A. An accumulation of air within the mediastinum
B. Visualized as linear streaks of air density within the mediastinum
C. The accumulation of air forces the mediastinal pleura laterally, producing a visible pleural edge adjacent to the mediastinal structures.
D. More common in infants than adults
E. Always look for the presence of a pneumothorax or subcutaneous emphysema
F. Differential diagnosis
   1. Spontaneous: most common
   2. Trauma: bronchial or tracheal tear
   3. Asthma: bronchial obstruction results in alveolar rupture with dissection of air through the interstitium into the mediastinum
   4. Rupture of the esophagus (Boerhaave's esophagus): may be secondary to violent vomiting in an alcoholic
   5. Hyaline membrane disease
   6. Intra-abdominal free air due to perforated viscus or diagnostic procedure: air enters the mediastinum from below
   7. During childbirth: due to repeated episodes of increased abdominal pressure during delivery

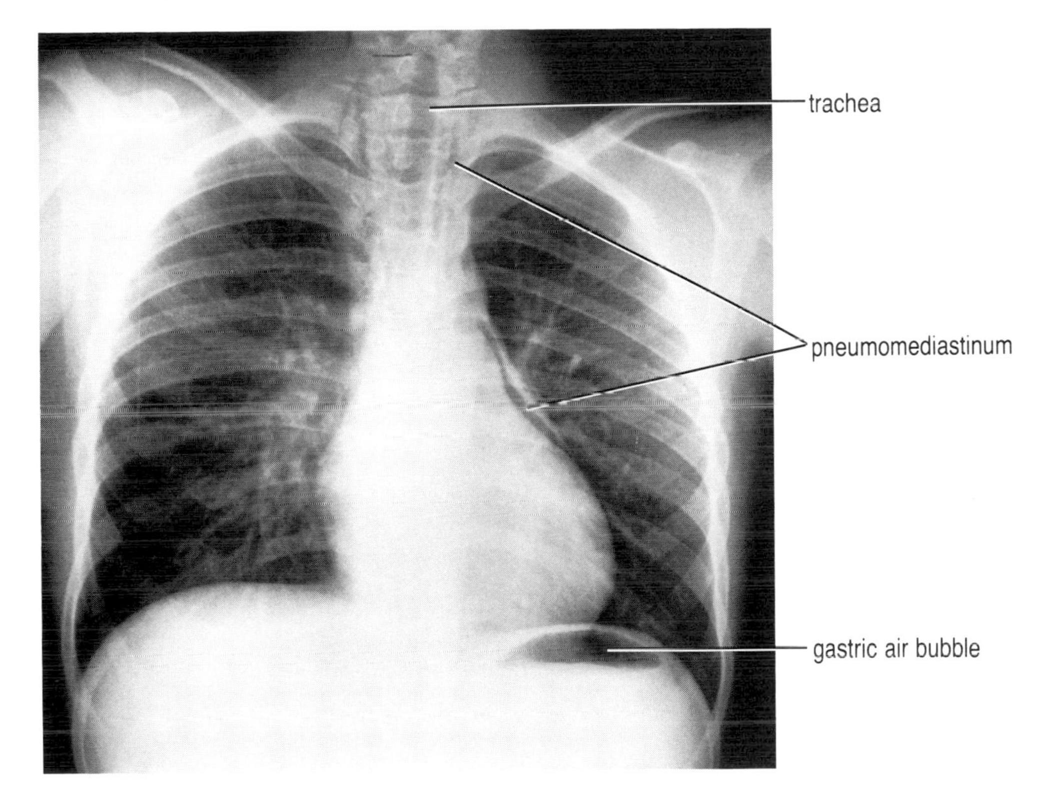

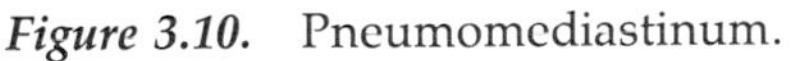

Figure 3.10. Pneumomediastinum.

3.11 LUNG METASTASES

A. Pulmonary metastases are often identified on routine chest roentgenograms.
B. Patient is usually asymptomatic from pulmonary involvement.
C. Approximately 30% of all cancer demonstrates lung metastases.
D. Pulmonary metastases may occur via direct extension, hematogenous spread, or lymphangitic spread.
E. Carcinomas of the breast, musculoskeletal system, urogenital system, thyroid, and colon tend to metastasize to the lung.
F. Carcinomas of the breast, stomach, pancreas, and esophagus metastasize by direct extension.
G. Carcinomas of the breast, thyroid, pancreas, and stomach undergo lymphatic spread.
H. Solitary metastases occur approximately 25% of the time.
I. Multiple metastases occur approximately 75% of the time.
J. Lung metastases are usually nodular, well defined, and variable in size and are most often located in the lower lobes.
K. Lymphangitic involvement produces an interstitial pattern.
L. A diffuse miliary pattern occurs with vascular tumors such as carcinoma of the thyroid, renal cell carcinoma, and trophoblastic disease (see Sec. 3.12).

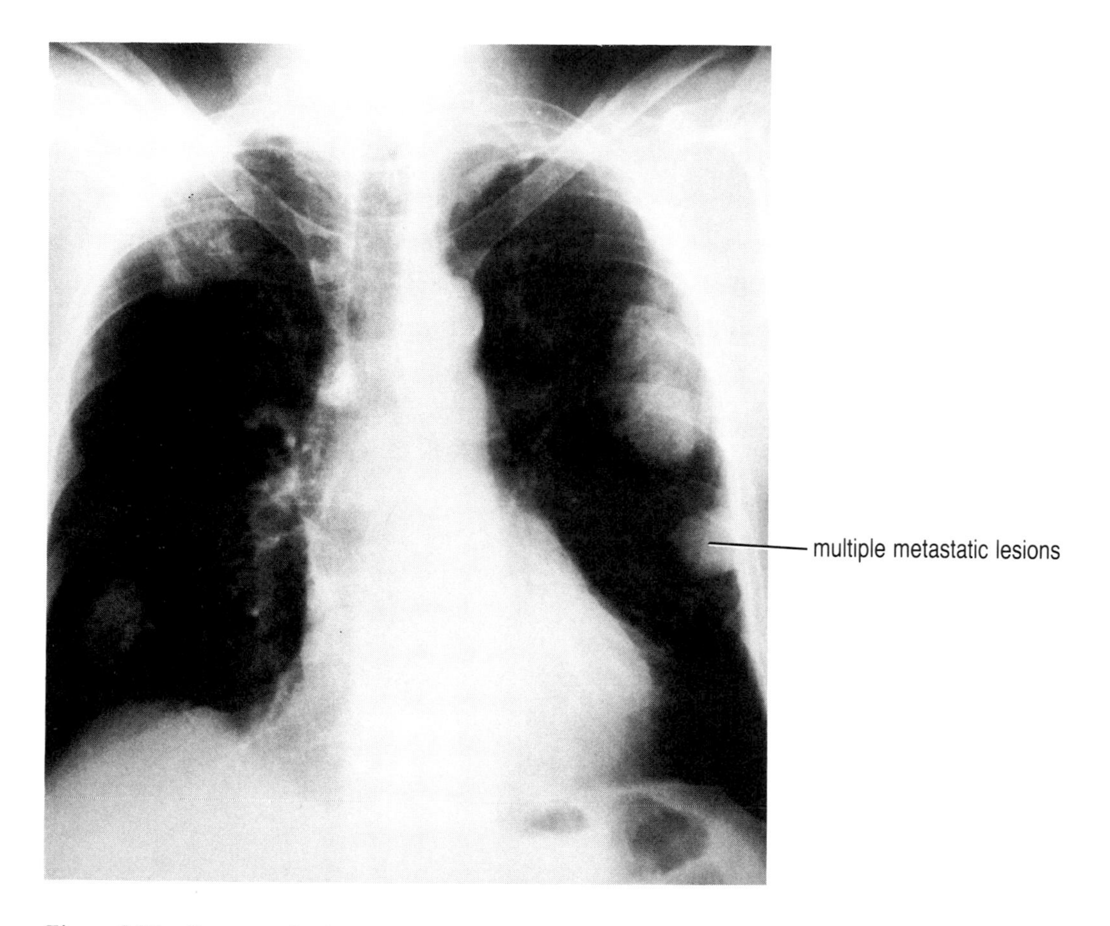

Figure 3.11. Lung metastases.

3.12 Solitary Pulmonary Nodule

A. Identification of a solitary pulmonary nodule requires a comparison with any previous chest roentgenograms.
B. Benign characteristics
   1. Well defined with smooth borders
   2. Complete calcification of the lesion
   3. Central core of calcification
   4. Does not change in appearance over time
C. Malignant characteristics
   1. Irregular shape with ill-defined borders
   2. Growth of nodule over time
   3. Eccentric calcification (rare) seen with scar carcinoma
D. Serial examinations are helpful in further evaluation.
E. Chest tomography can be used for identification of calcification.
F. CT of the chest is helpful in evaluating a solitary pulmonary nodule.
G. Differential diagnosis
   1. Inflammatory
      a. Granuloma
         (1) Histoplasmosis
         (2) Tuberculoma: more often in upper lobes
         (3) Sarcoidosis (see Sec. 3.16)
         (4) Cryptococcosis
         (5) Coccidioidomycosis
         (6) Pneumonia (see Sec. 3.04)
         (7) Abscess
         (8) Hydatid cyst: more often in lower lobes
   2. Neoplastic
      a. Benign
         (1) Bronchial adenoma: 80 to 90% centrally located near the hilum. Location within a bronchus often results in obstruction, which leads to atelectasis and obstructive pneumonitis (no visible air bronchograms). Almost all bronchial adenomas are carcinoids (90%)
         (2) Hamartoma: located peripherally, irregular "popcorn" type of calcification
         (3) Lipoma: composed of adipose tissue, 80% arise in tracheobronchial tree
         (4) Hemangioma: composed of a mass of thin-walled vessels, usually in the periphery, hemoptysis is common
         (5) Leiomyoma: arises from smooth muscle of the lung periphery or tracheobronchial walls
      b. Malignant
         (1) Bronchogenic carcinoma: has malignant characteristics and is generally larger in size than benign neoplasms. Lesion may also obstruct involved bronchus producing atelectasis and obstructive pneumonitis (no visible air bronchograms).
            (a) Unilateral hilar enlargement may occur secondary to tumor and adenopathy.
            (b) There may be cavitation and local lytic destruction of ribs or vertebrae.
         (2) Alveolar cell carcinoma: peripheral solitary lesion
         (3) Metastasis: carcinoma of breast, thyroid, stomach, colon, testis, kidney, myeloma, sarcoma
         (4) Lymphoma
   3. Other densities that mimic a solitary pulmonary nodule
      a. Nipple shadows: usually small round symmetrical densities projected over the fourth or fifth anterior rib space. Repeat chest roentgenogram with placement of nipple markers to exclude the presence of nipple shadows
      b. Rib lesions
      c. Skin lesions: neurofibromatosis, lipoma, mole
      d. Artifacts: buttons or other items
   4. Vascular

   a. Arteriovenous malformation: lobulated with efferent and afferent vessels
   b. Pulmonary infarct
   c. Hematoma
5. Immunologic
   a. Rheumatoid nodule: usually multiple; pleural effusion may be present
   b. Wegener's granulomatosis
6. Congenital
   a. Bronchogenic cyst: 30 to 40 years old, usually lower lobes
   b. Bronchopulmonary sequestrations: usually lower lobes

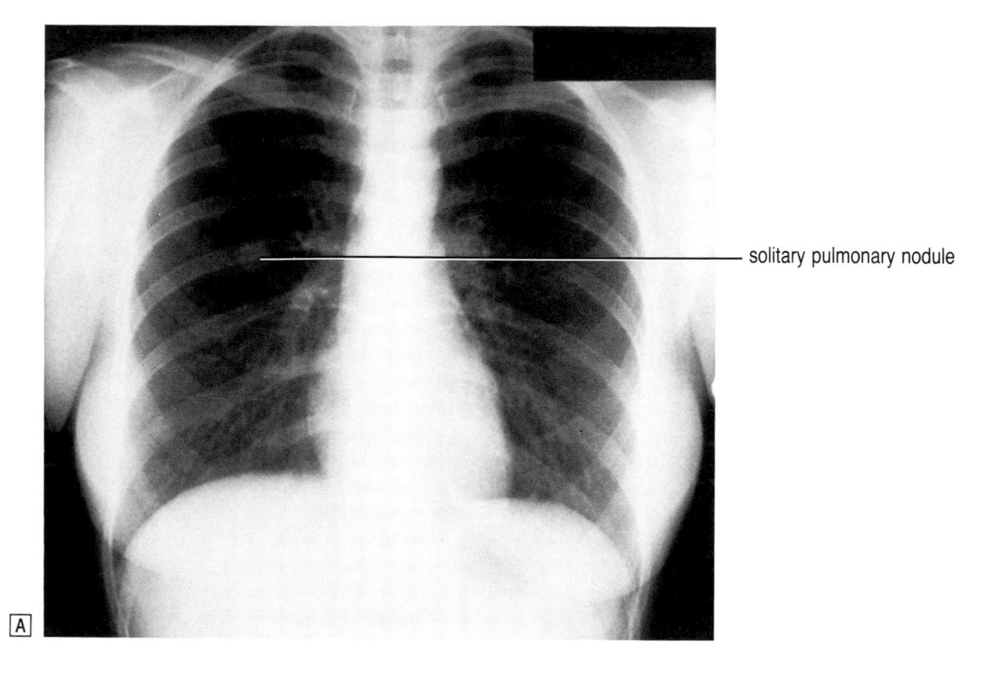

Figure 3.12. *A,* Solitary pulmonary nodule.

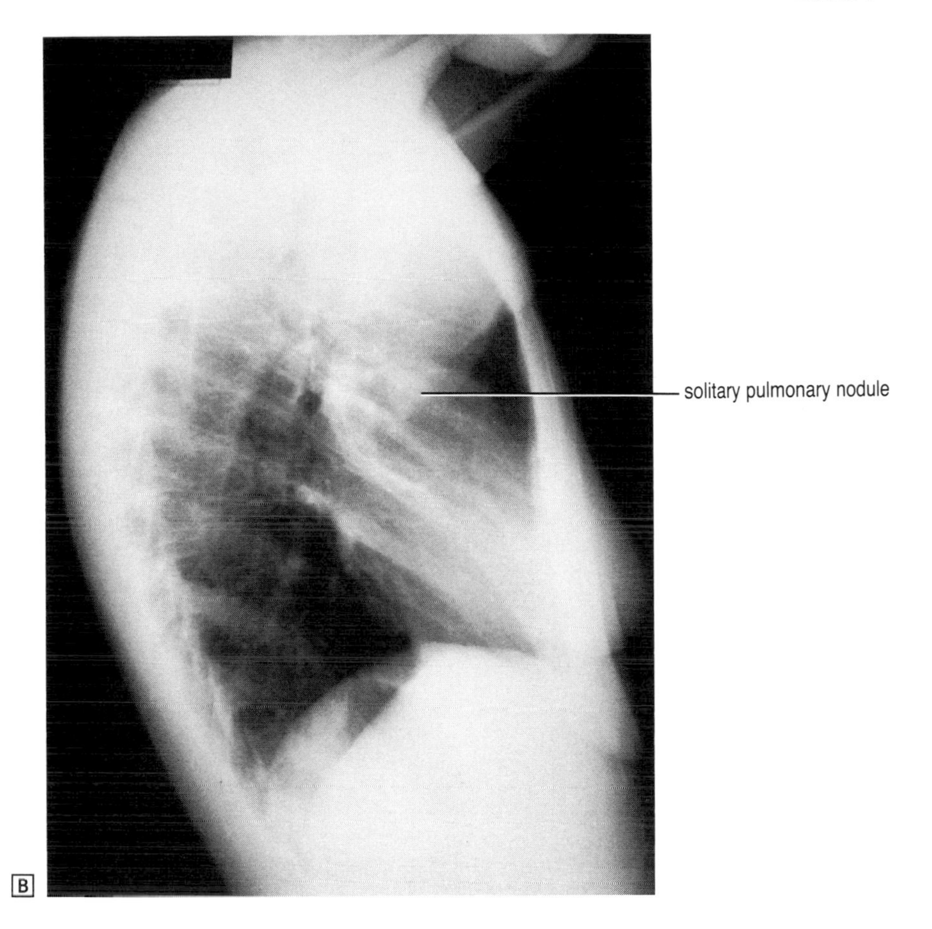

Figure 3.12. *B*, Solitary pulmonary nodule.

3.13 MEDIASTINAL MASSES

A. Anterior mediastinal masses
   1. Involves the retrosternal air space
   2. Differential diagnosis
      a. Thymoma: present in 15 to 20% of patients with myasthenia gravis
      b. Thyroid: may displace trachea posteriorly and laterally. Focal calcification is common
      c. Teratoma: contains tissue derived from ectoderm, mesoderm, and endoderm Calcification may be present in the form of a tooth or bone fragment; remainder of germ cell neoplasms are also included
      d. Lymph node enlargement
      e. Lipoma
      f. Parathyroid mass
   3. Remember the four Ts of anterior mediastinal masses: thymoma, thyroid, teratoma, and "terrible" lymphoma.

B. Middle mediastinal masses
   1. Involves the heart, major vessels, and trachea
   2. Differential diagnosis
      a. Lymph node enlargement: involves paratracheal and tracheobronchial nodes secondary to neoplasm or infection
      b. Aneurysm of the thoracic aorta: if traumatic, most common site is distal to the origin of the left subclavian artery
      c. Bronchogenic cyst
      d. Pericardial fat pad and pericardial cyst
      e. Hernia of Morgagni: congenital defect within the diaphragm. Herniation of abdominal contents usually seen to the right of midline

C. Posterior mediastinal masses
   1. Involves the area between the posterior pericardium and the vertebral column Involves esophagus and descending thoracic aorta
   2. Differential diagnosis
      a. Neurogenic tumors: neurofibroma, ganglioneuroma, paraganglioma
      b. Achalasia: dilatation of esophagus with air fluid level
      c. Hiatal hernia
      d. Hernia of Bochdalek
      e. Meningocele
      f. Paravertebral mass: secondary to abscess or extramedullary hematopoiesis
      g. Neuroenteric cyst

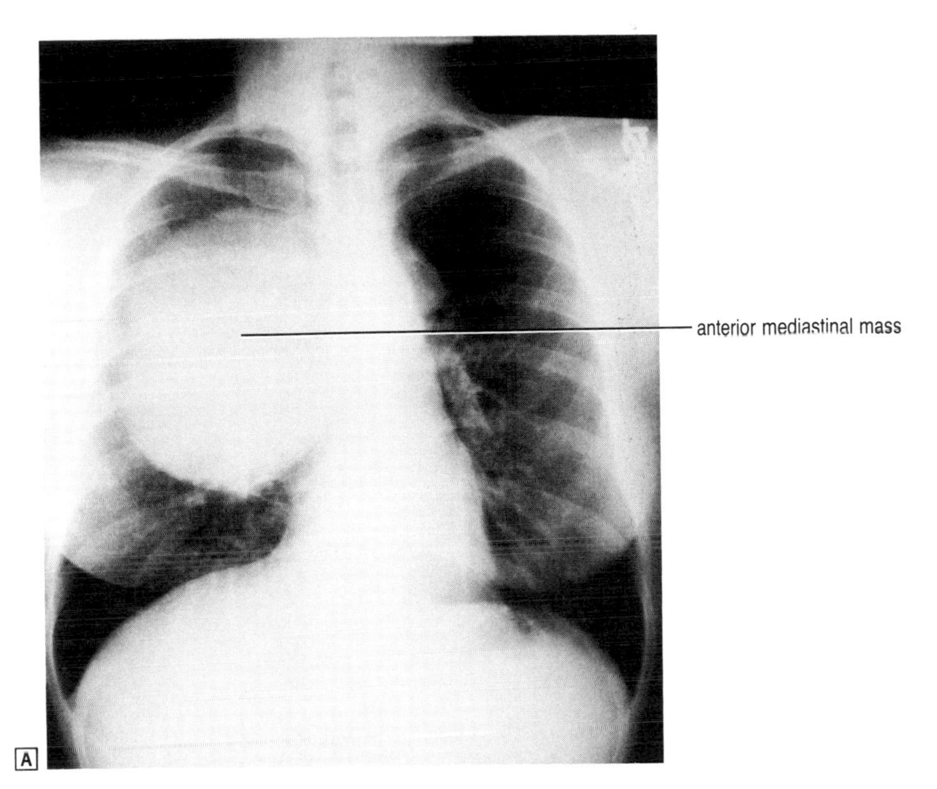

Figure 3.13. *A*, Mediastinal masses.

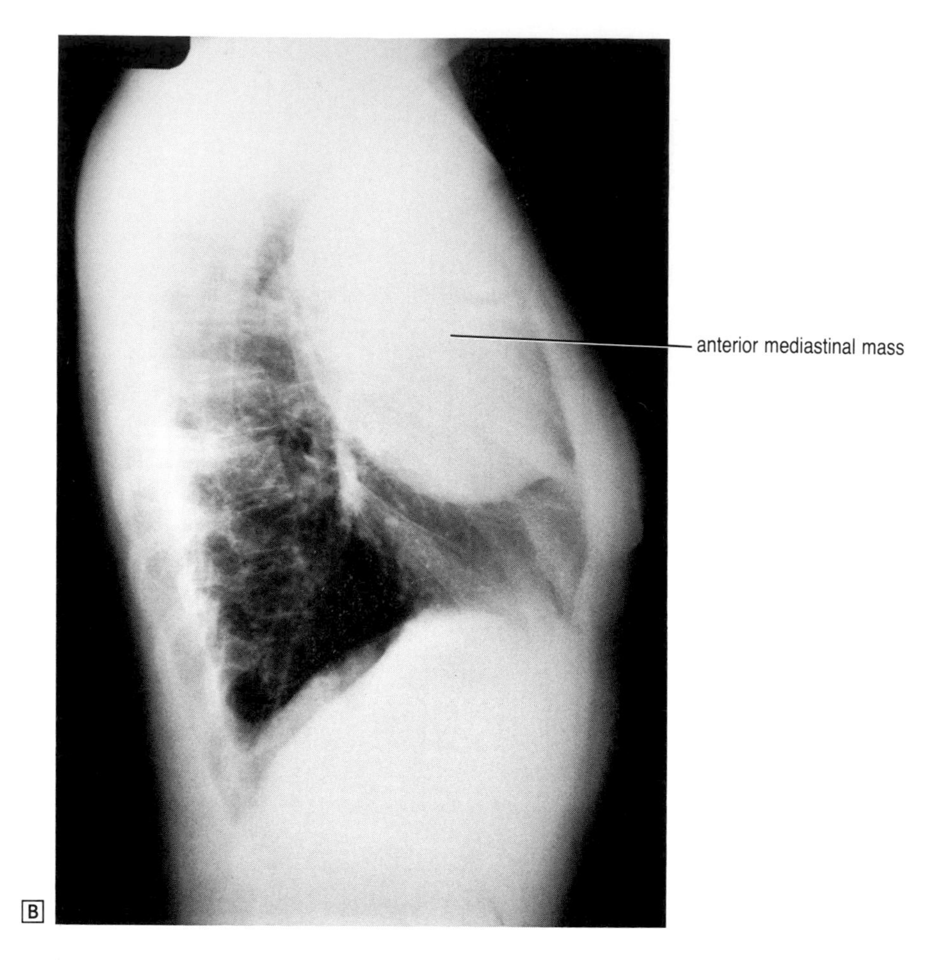

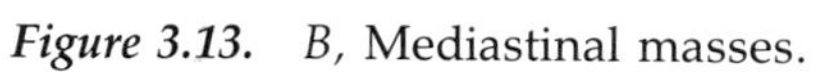
Figure 3.13. *B,* Mediastinal masses.

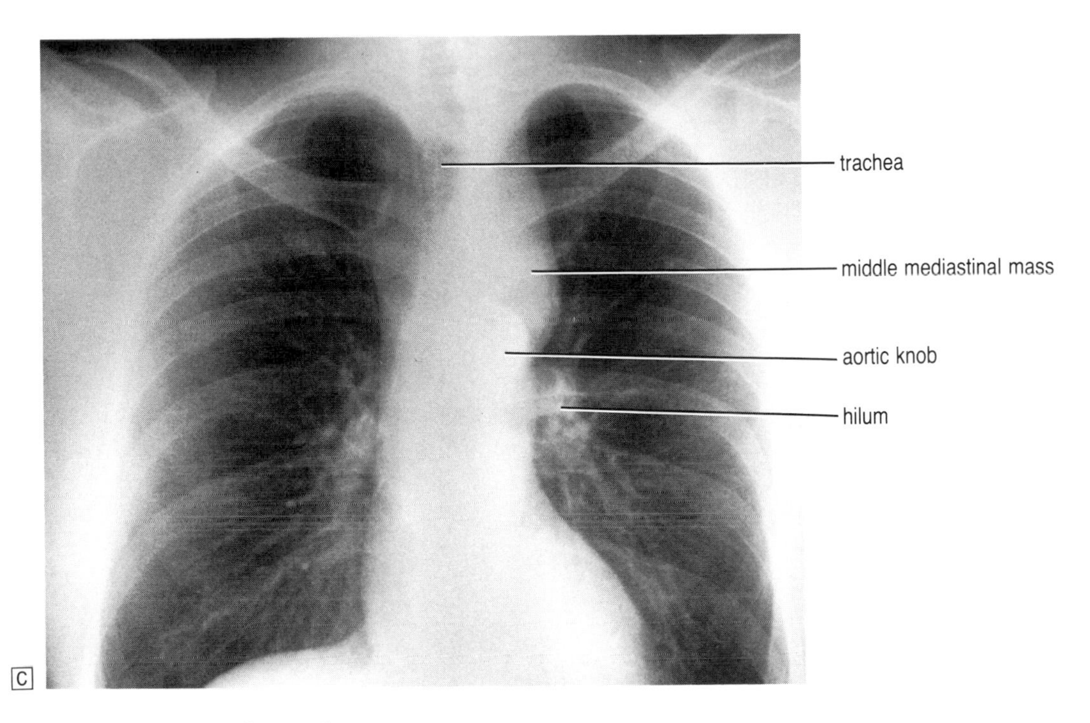

Figure 3.13. C, Mediastinal masses.

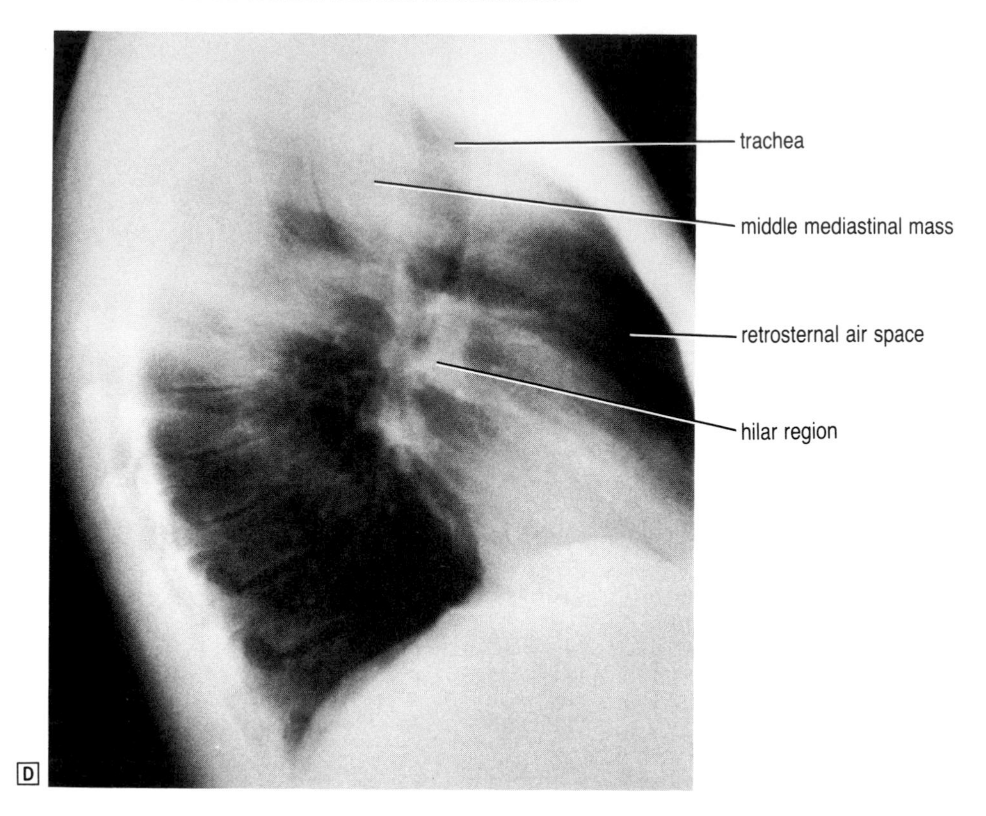

Figure 3.13. *D,* Mediastinal masses.

3.14 PLEURAL EFFUSION

A. An accumulation of fluid between the visceral and parietal pleura
* B. In the erect position, causes blunting of the costophrenic angle (CPA)
C. In the supine position, causes a generalized haziness over the affected hemithorax due to layering of fluid into the dependent portion of the pleural space. Degree of haziness is relative to the amount of pleural fluid.
D. Differential diagnosis
   1. Heart failure
   2. Liver failure
   3. Nephrotic syndrome
   4. Inflammatory
      a. Bacterial: Staphylococcus aureus, Streptococcus pneumoniae, gram-negative bacilli, Klebsiella, and Mycobacterium tuberculosis
      b. Viral
      c. Mycoplasma
      d. Fungal: Actinomyces and Nocardia
   5. Neoplastic
      a. Bronchogenic carcinoma
      b. Lymphoma
      c. Metastatic disease
      d. Mesothelioma
   6. Pulmonary embolus
   7. Trauma
   8. Iatrogenic fluid overload
   9. Subphrenic abscess
   10. Pancreatitis
   11. Immunologic
      a. Rheumatoid arthritis (RA)
      b. Systemic lupus erythematosus (SLE)
   12. Asbestosis
   13. Meigs' syndrome
      a. Pleural effusion, ascites, and pelvic mass
   14. Chylothorax: obstruction of thoracic duct due to trauma or tumor

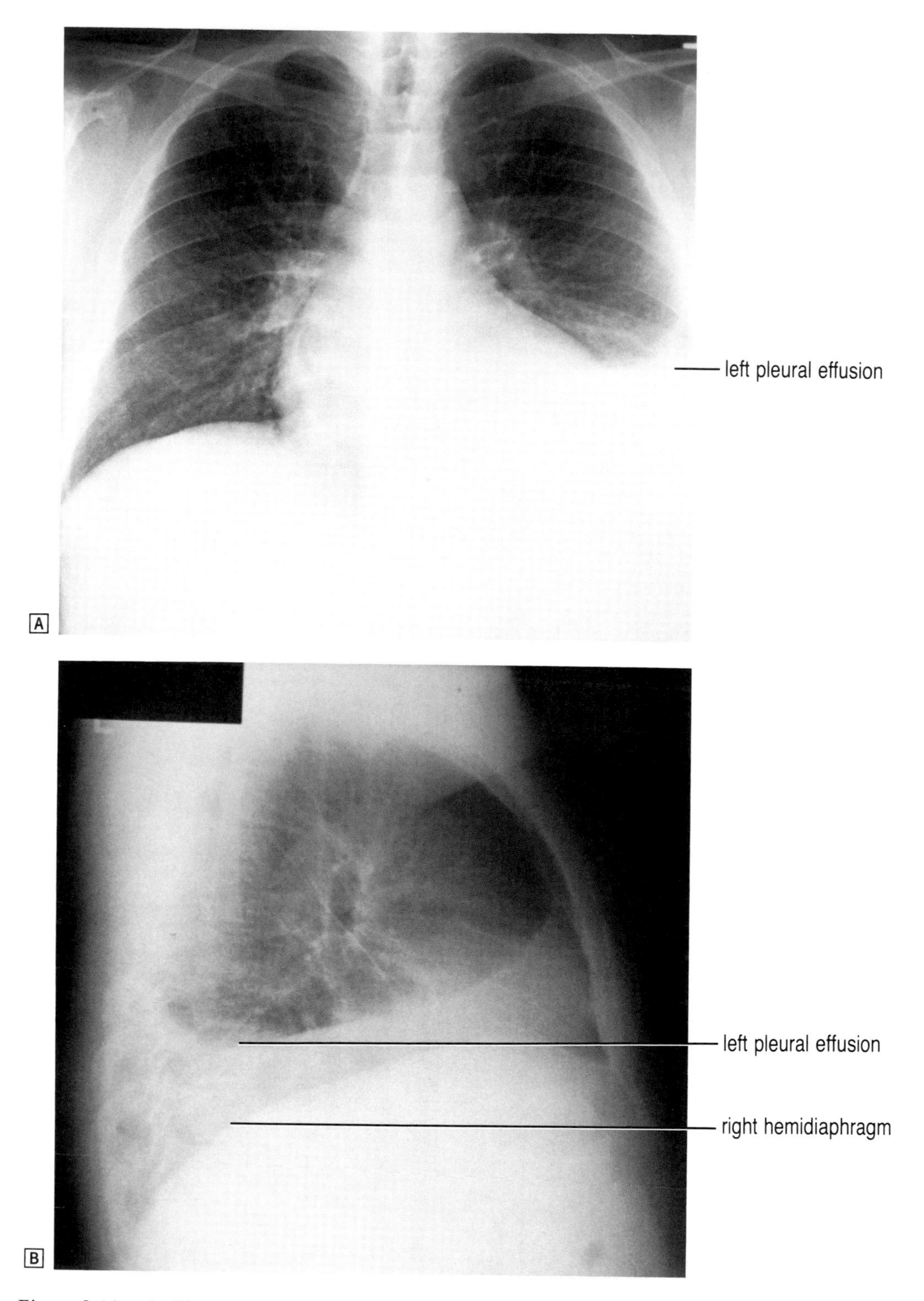

Figure 3.14. *A*, Pleural effusion. *B*, Pleural effusion.

3.15 TUBERCULOSIS

A. Caused by Mycobacterium tuberculosis, which is an acid-fast aerobic organism
B. Infants, children, and the elderly are more susceptible to infection
C. Blacks more often affected than whites. Incidence is related to overcrowding and poverty.
D. Infection has been well controlled, but with recent influx of Asian immigrants, more TB infections are likely.
E. Primary tuberculosis
   1. Seen most often in children
   2. Affects upper lobes of the lungs more often than lower lobes
   3. The presence of hilar or paratracheal lymphadenopathy differentiates primary from reactivation tuberculosis.
   4. Most patients are asymptomatic, but may experience fever, cough, weight loss, anorexia.
F. Reactivation tuberculosis
   1. Occurs mainly in adults who have developed acquired hypersensitivity from previous exposure
   2. Affects the apical and posterior segments of the upper lobes predominantly. About 10% involve the superior segment of the lower lobes.
   3. Absence of lymphadenopathy
   4. Fibrocavitary lesions form secondary to caseous necrosis followed by fibrosis.
   5. Tuberculoma is a small round density most often in the upper lobes.
   6. Clinically, most patients are asymptomatic; may present with nonspecific symptoms of weakness, fever, weight loss, anorexia, or cough.
   7. Hematogenous spread of the bacilli may result in miliary tuberculosis, visualized as multiple small foci of increased density bilaterally.

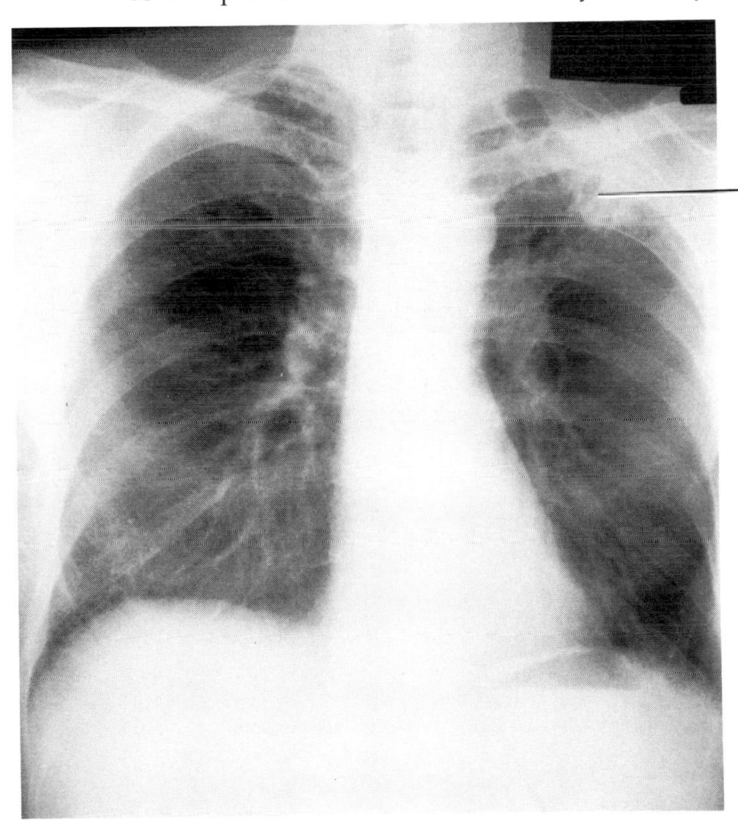

Figure 3.15. Tuberculosis.

3.16 SARCOIDOSIS

A. A multisystem disease of unknown cause characterized by noncaseating granuloma formation
B. May involve lung, lymph node, liver, spleen, bone, and skin
C. Usually identified on a routine chest roentgenogram in an asymptomatic individual
D. Blacks more commonly affected than whites
E. Commonly, bilateral hilar adenopathy involving the paratracheal and tracheobronchial groups
F. Involvement is generally symmetrical.
G. Sites of involvement
   1. Lymphadenopathy: usually asymptomatic with hilar adenopathy
   2. Pulmonary involvement: diffuse reticulonodular pattern present within both lungs. May present with shortness of breath and nonproductive cough
   3. Ocular sarcoidosis: presents as an acute uveitis
   4. Cutaneous sarcoidosis: presents as multiple small raised nodules
   5. Bone sarcoidosis: primarily involves the small bones of the hands and feet. Coarsely trabeculated pattern, well defined, punched out lucent defects. Approximately 15% present as an acute polyarthritis involving the knees, ankles, wrists, and interphalangeal joints.
H. Lab
   1. Hypercalcemia (5 to 10%)
   2. Elevated serum alkaline phosphatase
   3. Elevated angiotensin I-converting enzymes
I. Clinically
   1. Usually asymptomatic
   2. May manifest fever, weight loss, fatigue, and malaise

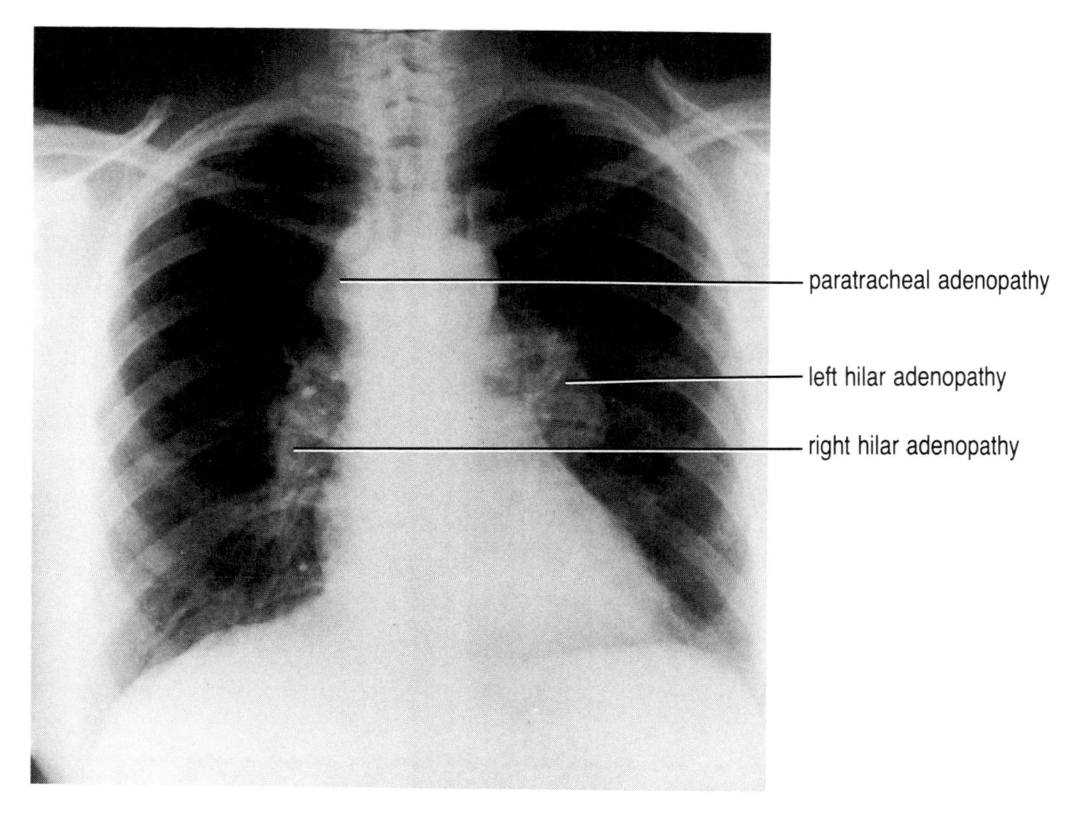

Figure 3.16. Sarcoidosis.

3.17 ELEVATION OF HEMIDIAPHRAGM

A. The right hemidiaphragm is usually slightly higher than the left.
B. There is an adequate level of inspiration on a chest roentgenogram if nine posterior ribs are visualized overlying the lung fields.
C. On an erect chest, examine below the diaphragm for the presence of free intraperitoneal air. A gas bubble within the stomach is often seen below the left hemidiaphragm. Interposition of the colon between the liver and the right hemidiaphragm may occur and simulate free air (Chilidite's syndrome). The presence of haustral markings excludes free air. If the chest film is equivocal, obtain a left lateral decubitus view of the abdomen to rule out free air.
D. Unilateral elevation: differential diagnosis
   1. Eventration of diaphragm: more common on left
   2. Phrenic nerve damage: tumor or trauma
   3. Pulmonary collapse
   4. Gaseous distention of the stomach or splenic flexure
   5. Splinting secondary to rib fractures
   6. Pulmonary infarction
   7. Pleural disease; acute or chronic process
   8. Trauma: ruptured spleen or liver
   9. Subphrenic abscess
   10. Scoliosis: elevation on side of concavity
   11. Pseudoelevation: rupture of diaphragm
   12. Organomegaly: hepatomegaly, splenomegaly, or pancreatitis
E. Bilateral elevation: differential diagnosis
   1. Poor level of inspiration (see Sec. 3.01)
   2. Ascites
   3. Large abdominal neoplasm, e.g., ovarian carcinoma
   4. Obesity
   5. Hepatosplenomegaly
   6. Pregnancy
   7. Pneumoperitoneum
   8. Bilateral lobar collapse

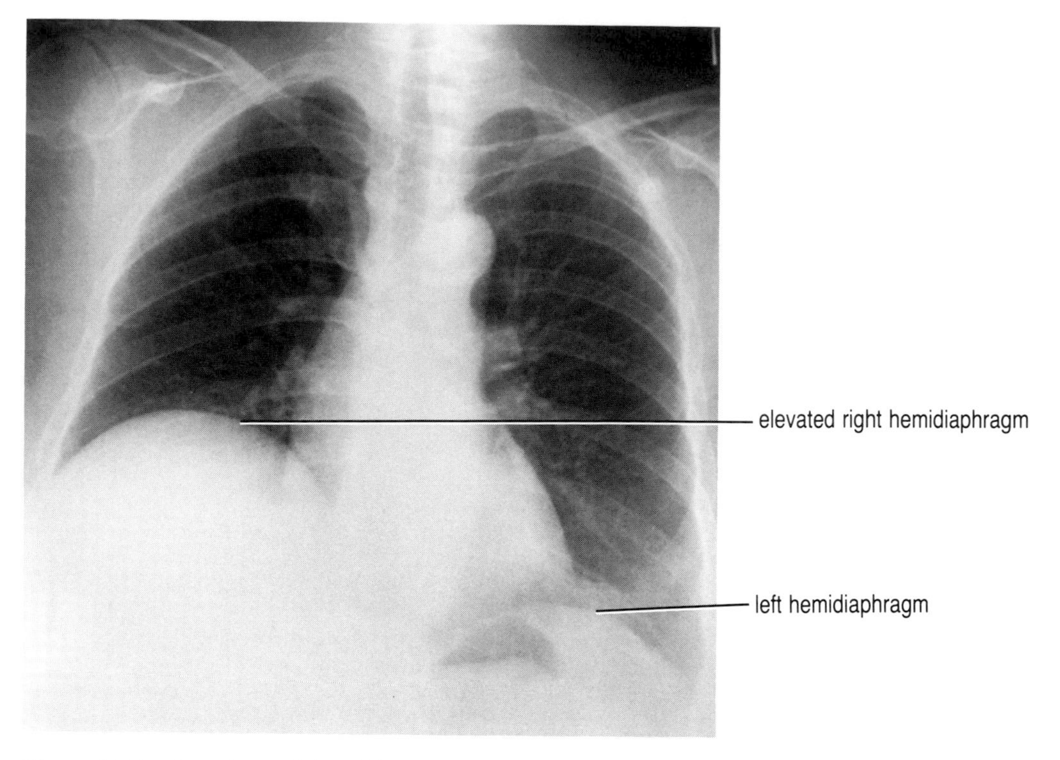

Figure 3.17. Elevation of hemidiaphragm.

3.18 ADULT RESPIRATORY DISTRESS SYNDROME (ARDS)

A. Refers to a clinical syndrome of respiratory distress secondary to pulmonary injury
B. Synonyms of ARDS
   1. Shock lung, post-traumatic pulmonary insufficiency, "stiff lung" syndrome
   2. Hemorrhagic lung syndrome, respiratory lung, congestive lung, "Da Nang" lung
   3. Pump lung, oxygen toxicity, adult hyaline membrane disease, fat embolism
   4. Disseminated intravascular coagulation
C. Predisposing conditions
   1. Hemorrhagic shock, septic shock, major trauma, cardiac arrest
   2. Aspiration of gastric contents (Mendelson's syndrome), extensive viral pneumonia
   3. Near drowning, fat embolism, drug overdose, cardiopulmonary bypass
   4. Smoke inhalation, burns, oxygen toxicity, disseminated intravascular coagulation, pancreatitis, high altitude
   5. Transfusion reaction, allergic reaction, prolonged ventilatory support
D. Endothelial damage occurs within the microvasculature resulting in increased permeability and pulmonary edema.
E. Radiographic presentation
   1. Latent period up to 12 hours with no radiographic abnormality
   2. During the first 24 hours, patchy alveolar infiltrates occur bilaterally similar to CHF with pulmonary edema.
   3. During the first two days, massive air space consolidation that resembles severe pulmonary edema occurs.
   4. Gradual resolution of alveolar infiltrates during the first week with patchy infiltrates remaining
   5. Development of interstitial infiltrates associated with patchy infiltrates
F. Radiographically a picture of pulmonary edema following the latent period; however, there is no cardiomegaly or cephalization of flow.
G. The presence of pleural fluid usually indicates another diagnosis, i.e., CHF, PE, fluid overload.
H. Clinical signs
   1. Dyspnea, hypoxia, tachypnea, and cyanosis
   2. Differential diagnosis early in the course with onset of symptoms and unremarkable chest roentgenogram should include pulmonary embolus.
   3. Ventilatory support with positive end-expiratory pressure (PEEP) is necessary.
   4. High mortality rate—at least 50%

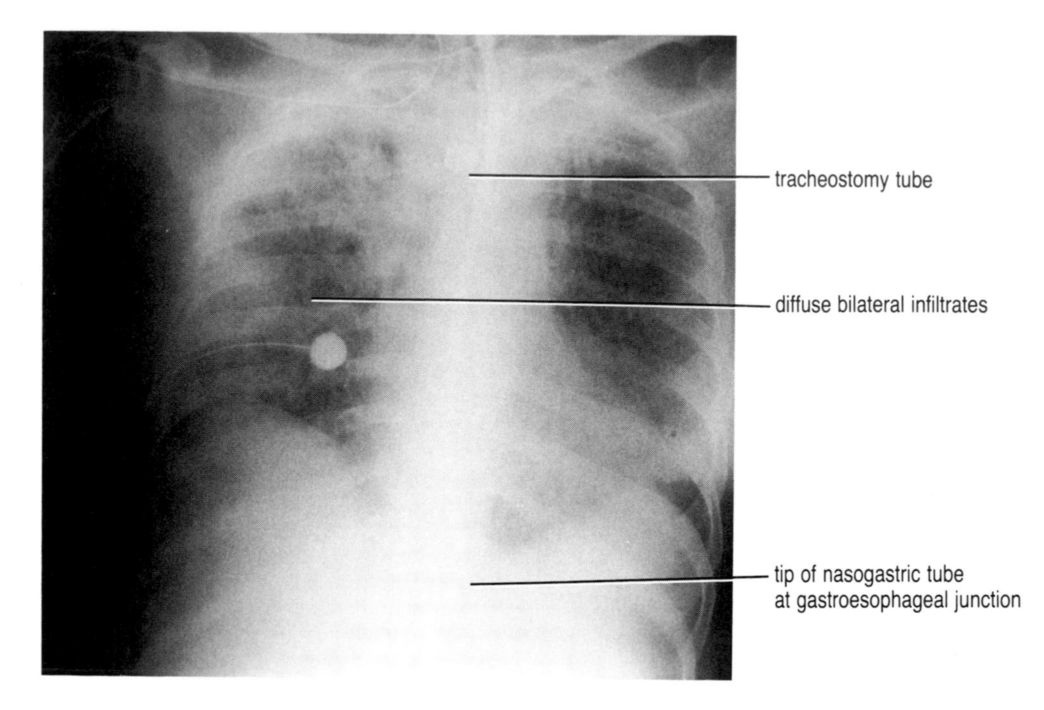

Figure 3.18. Adult respiratory distress syndrome (ARDS).

3.19 COARCTATION OF THE AORTA

A. Major diagnostic finding: Rib notching of the inferior rib surface
B. Congenital malformation resulting in constriction of a focal area of the aorta
C. Most commonly occurs in utero distal to ductus arteriosus with establishment of collateral blood flow
D. Rib notching occurs as a result of dilatation of intercostal arteries involving the fourth to the eighth ribs.
E. Ascending aorta is dilated, while the aortic knob is small, followed by poststenotic dilatation; the "3" sign
F. Heart may be enlarged
G. Differential diagnosis of inferior rib notching
   1. Coarctation of the aorta
   2. Obstruction of subclavian artery
      a. Postoperative (Blalock procedure for repair of tetralogy of Fallot)
      b. Affects the ipsilateral side
   3. Thrombosis within the aorta
      a. Generally involves lower ribs
   4. Obstruction of superior vena cava
   5. AV malformation within the lung
   6. Neurofibromatosis
H. Clinically: elevated blood pressure in upper extremities
   1. Decreased or absent femoral pulse
   2. Majority are asymptomatic
I. Most common associated cardiac anomaly is a bicuspid aortic valve.
J. Differential diagnosis of superior rib notching
   1. Rheumatoid arthritis
   2. Hyperparathyroidism
   3. Systemic lupus erythematosus
   4. Neurofibromatosis
   5. Scleroderma

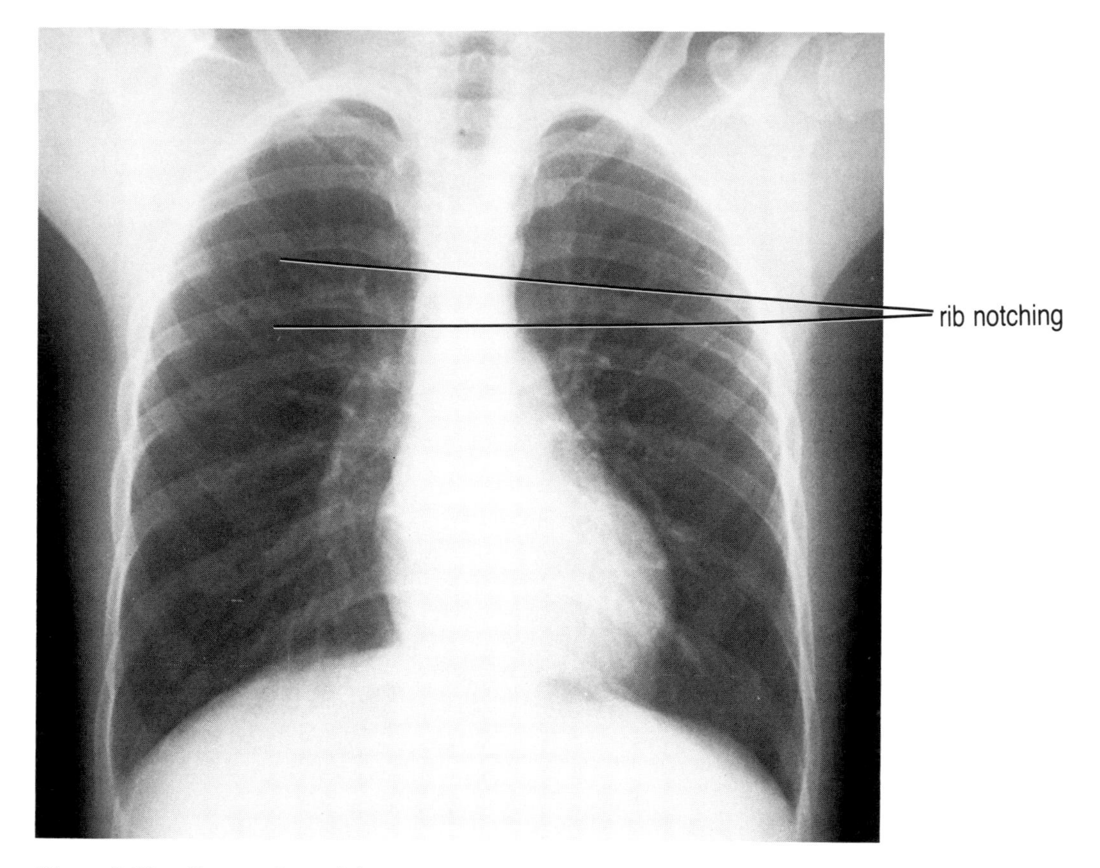

Figure 3.19. Coarctation of the aorta.

3.20 UNILATERAL OPACIFICATION OF A LUNG

A. If complete opacification of a hemithorax is present, the volume status of the affected lung should be determined.
B. If volume loss is present, i.e., shifting of the mediastinal structures toward the ipsilateral side or elevation of ipsilateral hemidiaphragm, lung collapse is suspected.
C. If volume loss is not evident or the mediastinal structures have shifted to the contralateral side, the presence of pleural fluid or consolidation of the lung should be considered.
D. Look for postoperative changes that may indicate previous pneumonectomy.
E. Differential diagnosis
   1. Lung collapse
   2. Large pleural effusion
   3. Pneumonic consolidation
   4. Previous pneumonectomy
   5. Agenesis of a lung
   6. Large mass (pulmonary or mediastinal in origin)
   7. Large hematoma of the chest wall

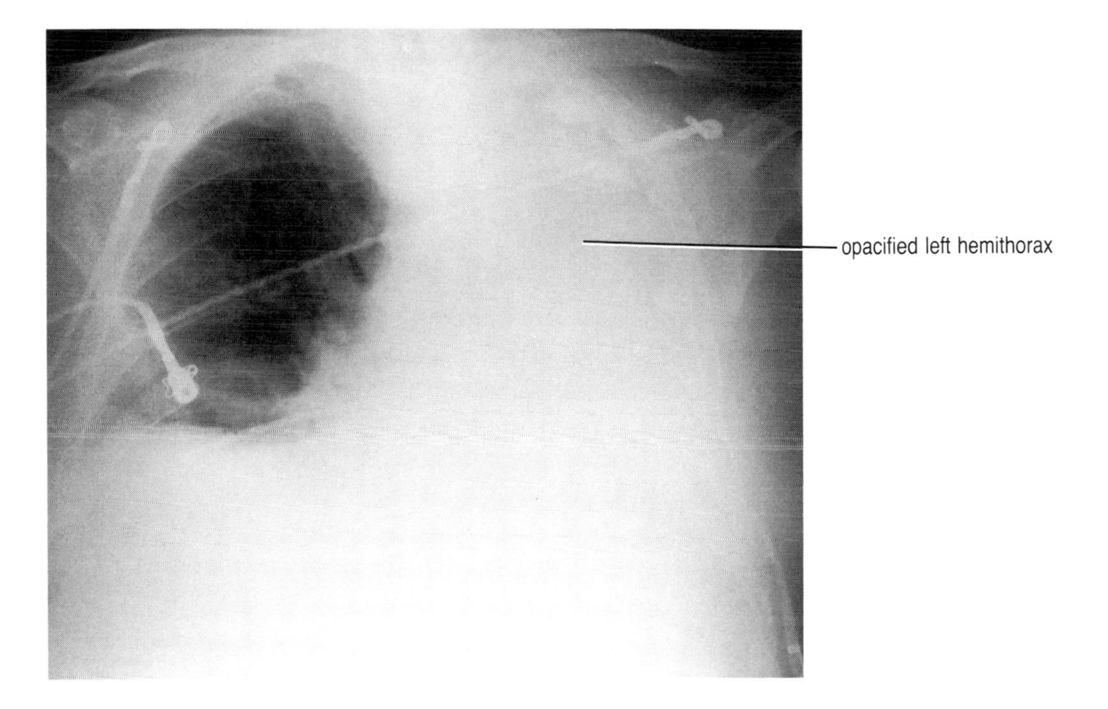

Figure 3.20. Unilateral opacification of a lung.

3.21 ASBESTOSIS

A. Long-term exposure to asbestos may result in interstitial lung disease, pleural abnormalities, and malignant neoplasms.
B. Asbestos is composed of a group of silicate salts; silicic acid is combined with magnesium, calcium, and iron.
C. Occupational and environmental exposure occurs as a result of the widespread use of asbestos in manufacturing and construction industries.
D. Increased risk of bronchogenic carcinoma with exposure to asbestos. If the person is a smoker, the risk increases sevenfold.
E. There is an association between asbestos exposure and malignant pleural mesothelioma as well as peritoneal mesothelioma.
F. Radiographic findings
   1. Pleural involvement is the most common.
   2. Pleural thickening occurs in the form of linear pleural plaques that are faintly seen along the lower lateral chest wall and along the diaphragm.
   3. Calcification of pleural plaques frequently occurs. Curvilinear calcifications are often seen along both diaphragms.
   4. Pleural effusion may occur, which may be unilateral or bilateral.
   5. Interstitial fibrosis may produce a reticulonodular pattern. Usually involves the lower lobes and produces the "shaggy heart border."

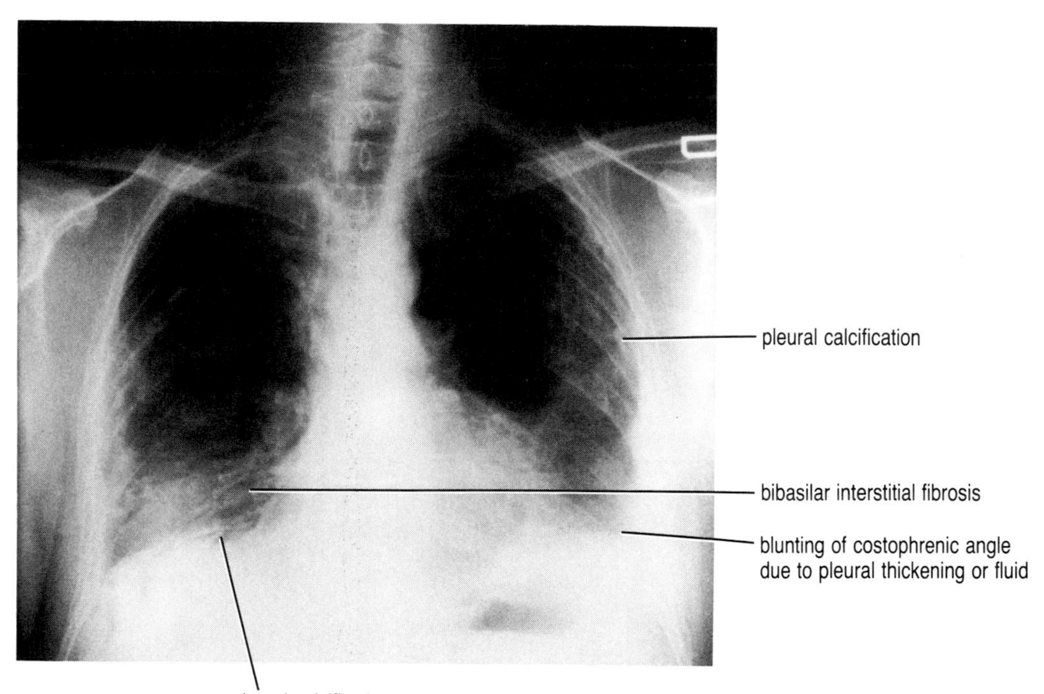

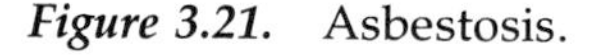

Figure 3.21. Asbestosis.

3.22 TETRALOGY OF FALLOT

A. Is a cyanotic form of congenital heart disease
B. Consists of four main components
   1. High interventricular septal defect
   2. Pulmonic stenosis
   3. Right ventricular hypertrophy
   4. Aorta overrides the septal defect.
C. Cyanosis occurs as a result of right-to-left shunt.
D. A patent foramen ovale may be an associated anomaly.
E. Radiographic findings
   1. Diminished pulmonary vascularity (pulmonary oligemia)
   2. Hypertrophy of the right ventricle produces elevation and rounding off of the apex, known as "coeur en sabot." Lateral view demonstrates filling of retrosternal air space.
   3. Overall heart size is usually within normal limits.
F. It is the most common congenital heart disease that causes decreased pulmonary blood flow following the immediate neonatal period.

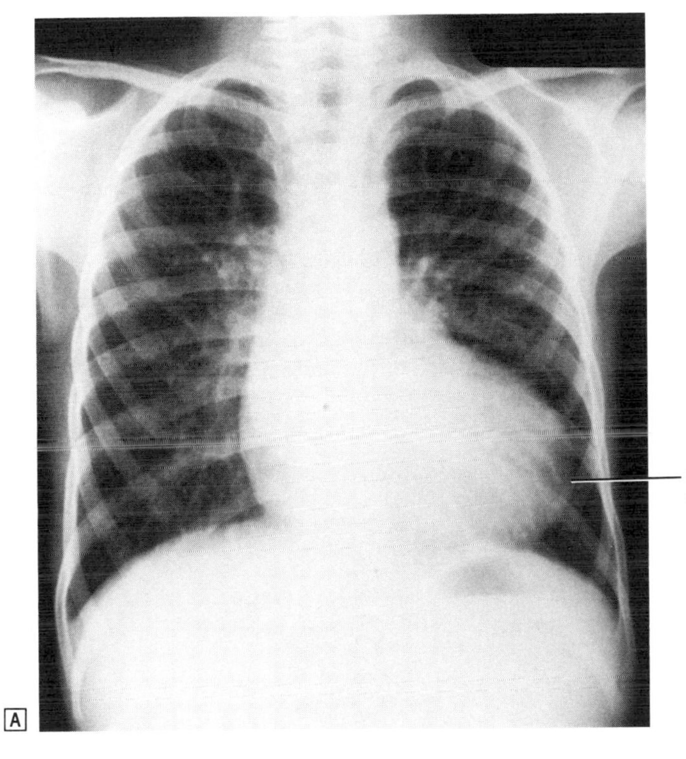

Figure 3.22. *A,* Tetralogy of Fallot.

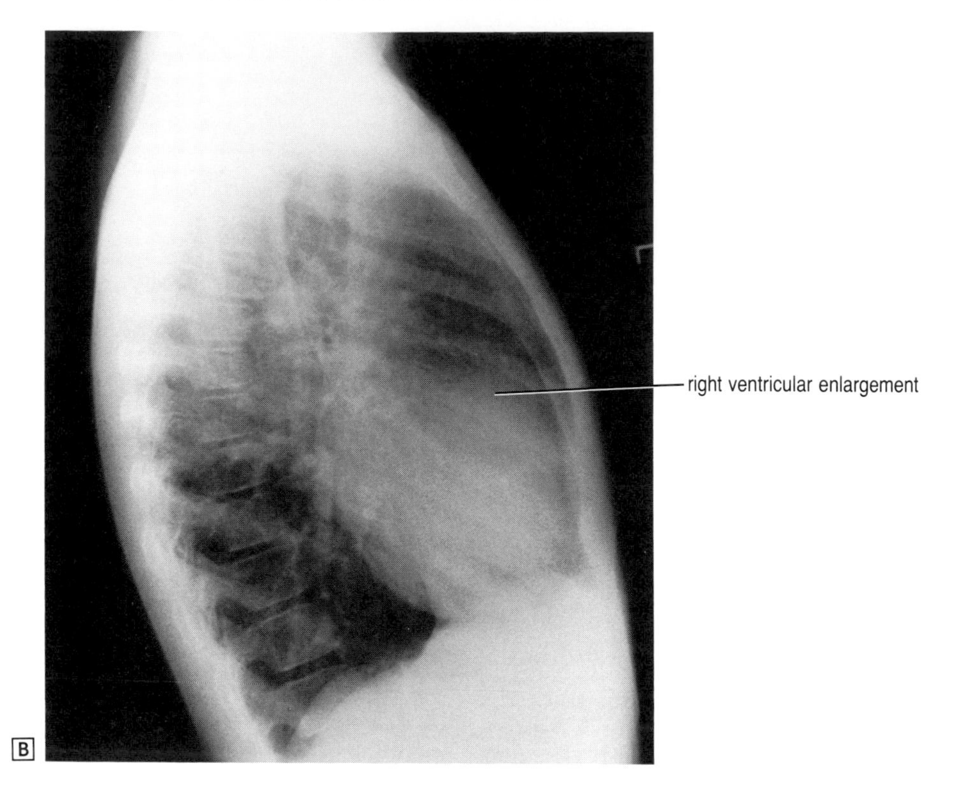

Figure 3.22. *B,* Tetralogy of Fallot.

3.23 PERICARDIAL EFFUSION

A. An accumulation of fluid within the pericardial sac
B. Seen as a generalized enlargement of the cardiac silhouette with a globular ("water bottle") configuration
C. Approximately 200 ml of fluid required in the acute setting to be radiographically visible
D. Development of an acute angle between the right heart border and the right hemidiaphragm (at the costophrenic angle)
E. Differential diagnosis
   1. Trauma
   2. Pericarditis: viral, bacterial, tuberculous
   3. Postoperative coronary artery bypass
   4. Immunologic: rheumatoid arthritis, systemic lupus erythematosus
   5. Dressler's syndrome (postmyocardial infarction syndrome)
   6. Renal failure
   7. Neoplastic disease
   8. Must exclude CHF, cardiac enlargement, but no other signs of decompensation, i.e., pulmonary venous congestion, pulmonary edema (see CHF)
   9. The differential diagnosis includes other causes of cardiac enlargement.
      a. Left ventricular hypertrophy
      b. Right ventricular hypertrophy
      c. Cardiomyopathy
      d. Valvular heart disease
F. Clinical signs
   1. Heart sounds are muffled
   2. Pulsus paradoxus
   3. EKG shows low voltage
G. Diagnosis is confirmed by echocardiography.
H. CT examination of the heart can also establish the diagnosis.

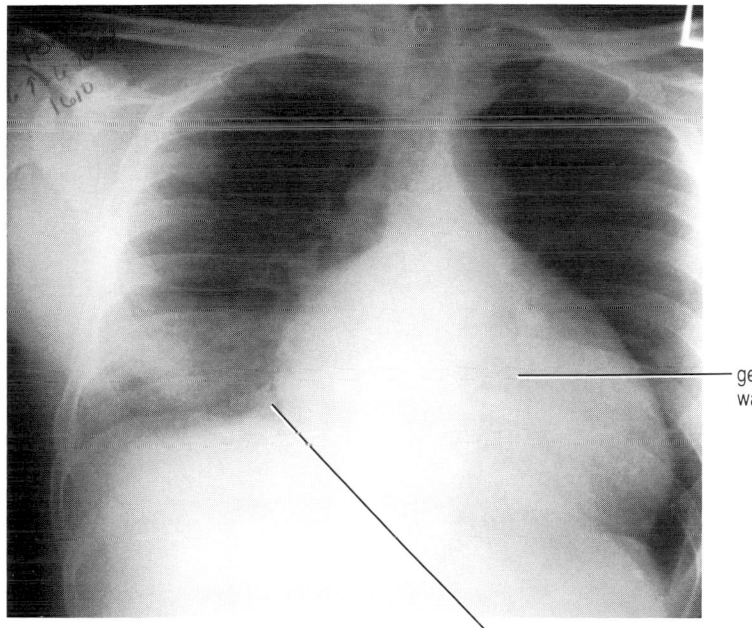

Figure 3.23. Pericardial effusion.

3.24 LEFT ATRIAL ENLARGEMENT

A. PA view
   1. Straightening of the left heart border
   2. Prominence of left atrial appendage
   3. Double density superimposed on the right heart border
   4. Elevation of left main stem bronchus

B. Lateral view
   1. There is prominence of the posterior superior aspect of the cardiac silhouette, which may result in posterior displacement of the esophagus.

C. Differential diagnosis
   1. Mitral stenosis: (pressure overload), valve may be calcified
   2. Mitral insufficiency (volume overload)
   3. Patent ductus arteriosus (PDA)
   4. Ventricular septal defect (VSD)
   5. Left atrial myxoma

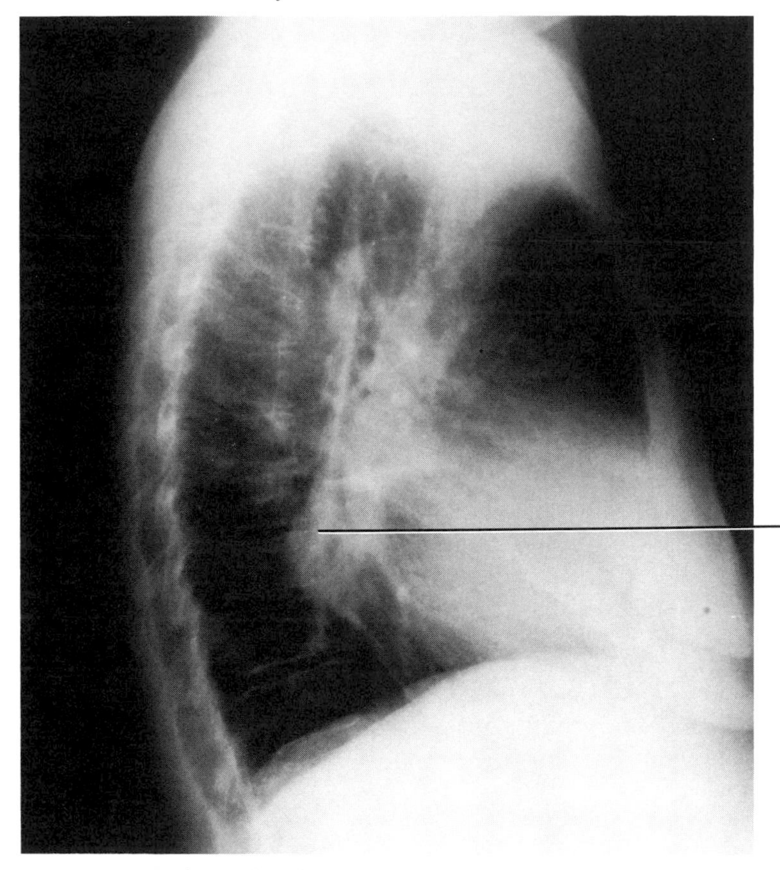

Figure 3.24. Left atrial enlargement.

3.25 ACUTE CHEST TRAUMA

A. Common with automobile accidents, deceleration injury

B. Most common radiographic finding is pulmonary contusion. Represents hemorrhage into the alveoli and interstitium. Is visualized as an area of homogenous opacification dependent on the amount of lung involved. Rib fractures may not be visualized. Initial chest roentgenogram may be clear. Follow-up exam in a few hours demonstrates the contusion. Resolution is usually rapid, within 24 to 48 hours. Patient may have hemoptysis.

C. Rib fractures
   1. The middle ribs (4 to 10) are most commonly fractured.
   2. Fracture of the first three ribs indicates severe trauma because they are well protected by overlying musculature
   3. If at least five ribs are fractured or if at least three ribs are fractured in two different places, a flail chest is present.

D. Hemothorax
   1. Represents hemorrhage into the pleural space
   2. Often associated with rib fractures

E. Pneumothorax (see Sec. 3.05)

F. Aortic rupture
   1. 90% will tear distal to the origin of the left subclavian artery.
   2. Mediastinal widening
      a. Obtain an erect chest roentgenogram if possible.
      b. Supine view of the chest normally looks widened.
   3. Left hemothorax
   4. Left apical cap
      a. Hemorrhage present in the superior aspect of the pleural space
   5. Displacement of mediastinal structures, i.e., esophagus and trachea to the right
   6. Fractures of the first three ribs indicate severe trauma.

G. Diaphragmatic rupture
   1. Almost always the left hemidiaphragm
   2. Herniation of stomach, mesentery, spleen, colon, and small bowel into the left hemithorax
   3. Insertion of nasogastric tube may be diagnostic.

H. Fracture of the sternum
   1. Another indication of severe trauma
   2. Risk of myocardial contusion, arrhythmia, or hemopericardium

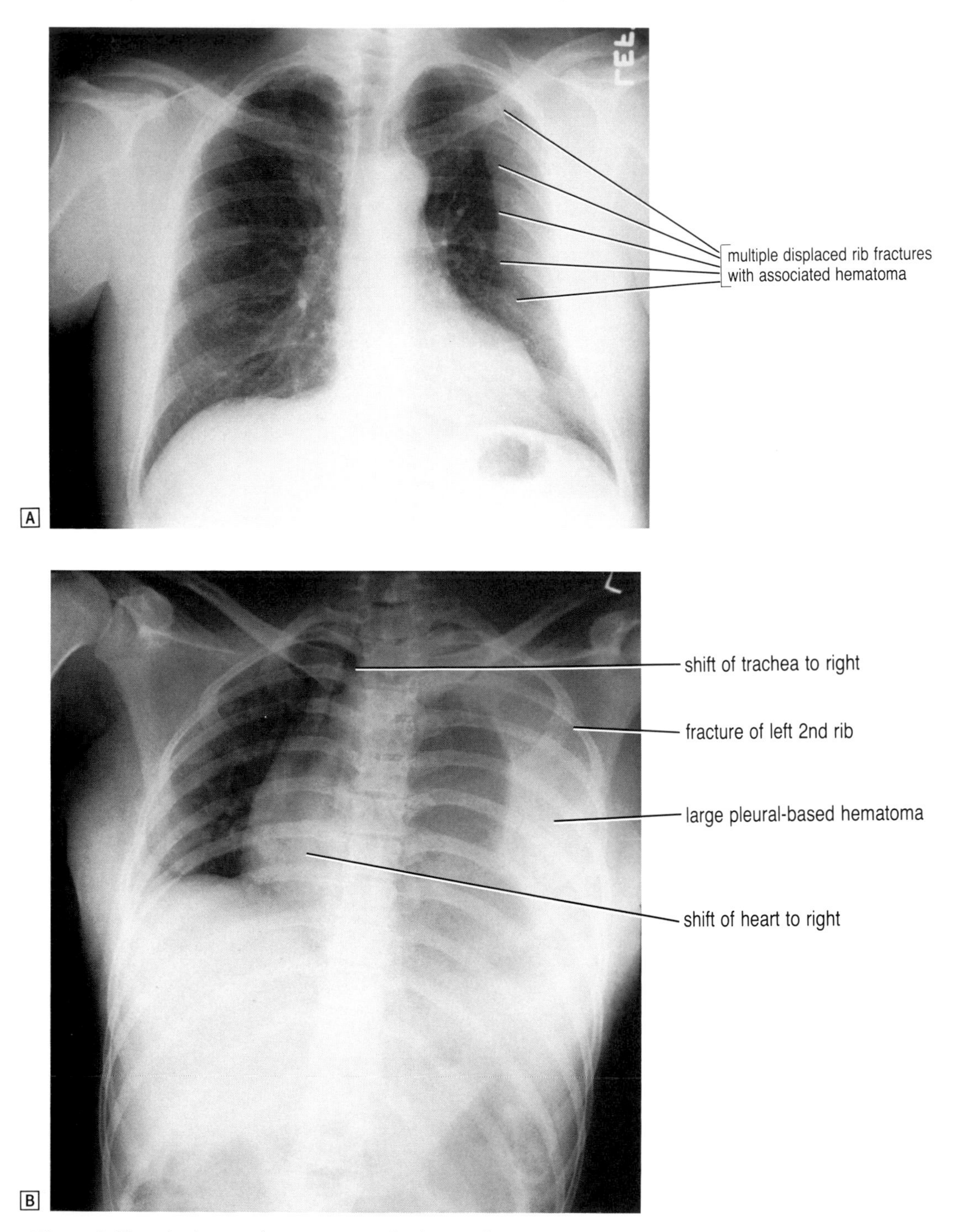

Figure 3.25. *A,* Acute chest trauma. *B,* Acute chest trauma.

3.26 KARTAGENER'S SYNDROME

A. Triad
   1. Situs inversus
   2. Paranasal sinusitus
   3. Bronchiectasis
B. Incidence of 1 in 40,000 with autosomal recessive trait.
C. Dysfunctional cilia predispose to infection of the sinuses and bronchi
D. Affected males are usually sterile because of nonmotile sperm.
E. Abnormal cilia in utero result in situs inversus.
F. An important point needs to be illustrated. If this chest roentgenogram were handed to you, you might put it on the view box the way you perceive a normal chest, thus missing the dextrocardia and situs inversus. The student of radiology must therefore have the power of observation and the knowledge base that such entities do exist. Once again, you must look for something in order to find it.

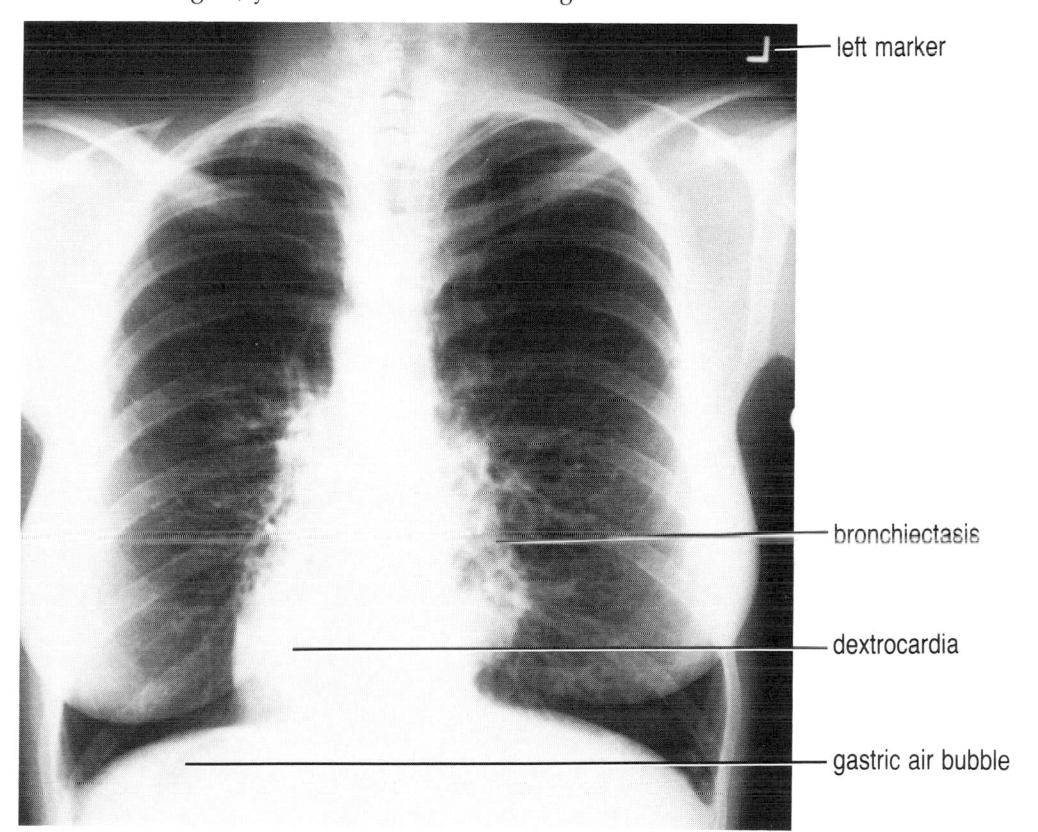

Figure 3.26. Kartagener's syndrome

3.27 AORTIC ANEURYSM

A. An aneurysm represents an abnormal enlargement of a blood vessel.
B. Types of thoracic aneurysms
   1. Arteriosclerotic
   2. Traumatic
   3. Dissecting
   4. Syphilitic
   5. Mycotic
C. A true aneurysm results from a defect in the media layer, and all components of the wall are present in the aneurysm.
D. A false aneurysm results from a rupture of a vessel in which blood is contained within adventitia.
E. Dissecting aneurysms
   1. Type I: involves the entire aorta
   2. Type II: involves the ascending aorta
   3. Type III: involves the descending aorta
F. Marfan's syndrome (cystic medial necrosis) and syphilis usually involve the ascending aorta.
G. Traumatic aneurysms usually occur distal to the origin of the left subclavian artery.
H. Radiographically visualized as enlargement of either the ascending, descending, or entire aorta. Mediastinum may appear widened. A left pleural effusion may be present.
I. Presentation includes chest pain that radiates to the back. May have diminished peripheral pulses or aortic insufficiency.

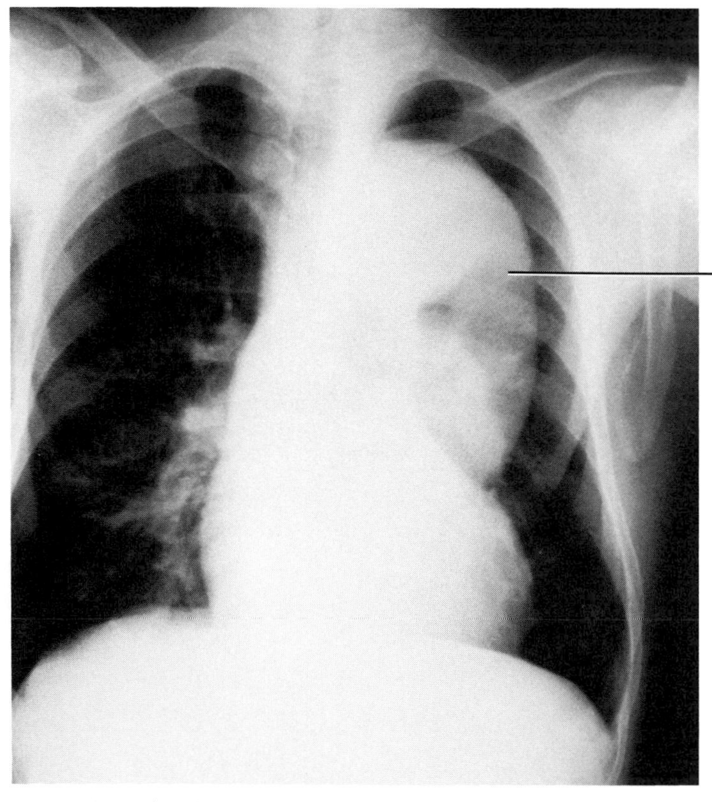

Figure 3.27. Aortic aneurysm.

3.28 LUNG VENTILATION AND PERFUSION SCANS

A. Pulmonary embolus
  1. Presentation
     a. Pleuritic chest pain
     b. Dyspnea
     c. Cough, hemoptysis
     d. Tachycardia
     e. Tachypnea
  2. Differential diagnosis of pulmonary embolus
     a. Pneumonia
     b. Myocardial infarction
     c. Pleurisy
     d. Musculoskeletal pain
     e. Pericarditis
     f. Hyperventilation
  3. Predisposing factors
     a. Deep vein thrombosis
     b. Recent surgery
     c. Bed rest
     d. Severe trauma
     e. Pregnancy
     f. Neoplasm
     g. Previous history
  4. Most pulmonary emboli originate from thrombi of the pelvis and proximal leg.
  5. Majority of pulmonary emboli are multiple and bilateral.
  6. The most common radiographic presentation is a normal chest roentgenogram.
  7. Other radiographic findings
     a. Elevation of left hemidiaphragm
     b. Pleural effusion
     c. Atelectasis
     d. Area of consolidation
     e. Westermark's sign (localized oligemia with associated hyperlucency)
     f. Hampton's hump (wedge-shaped, pleural-based area of increased density)
  8. Evaluation of suspected pulmonary embolus requires correlation of radiographic appearance of the chest, nuclear ventilation, and perfusion studies.
  9. The occurrence of multiple peripheral perfusion defects in the presence of a normal ventilation study and a normal chest is the classic presentation of pulmonary emboli.
  10. Matching ventilation and perfusion defects along with delay washout on the ventilation study are compatible with COPD.
  11. If the clinical findings and radiographic and nuclear medicine studies are equivocal, pulmonary angiography is indicated.

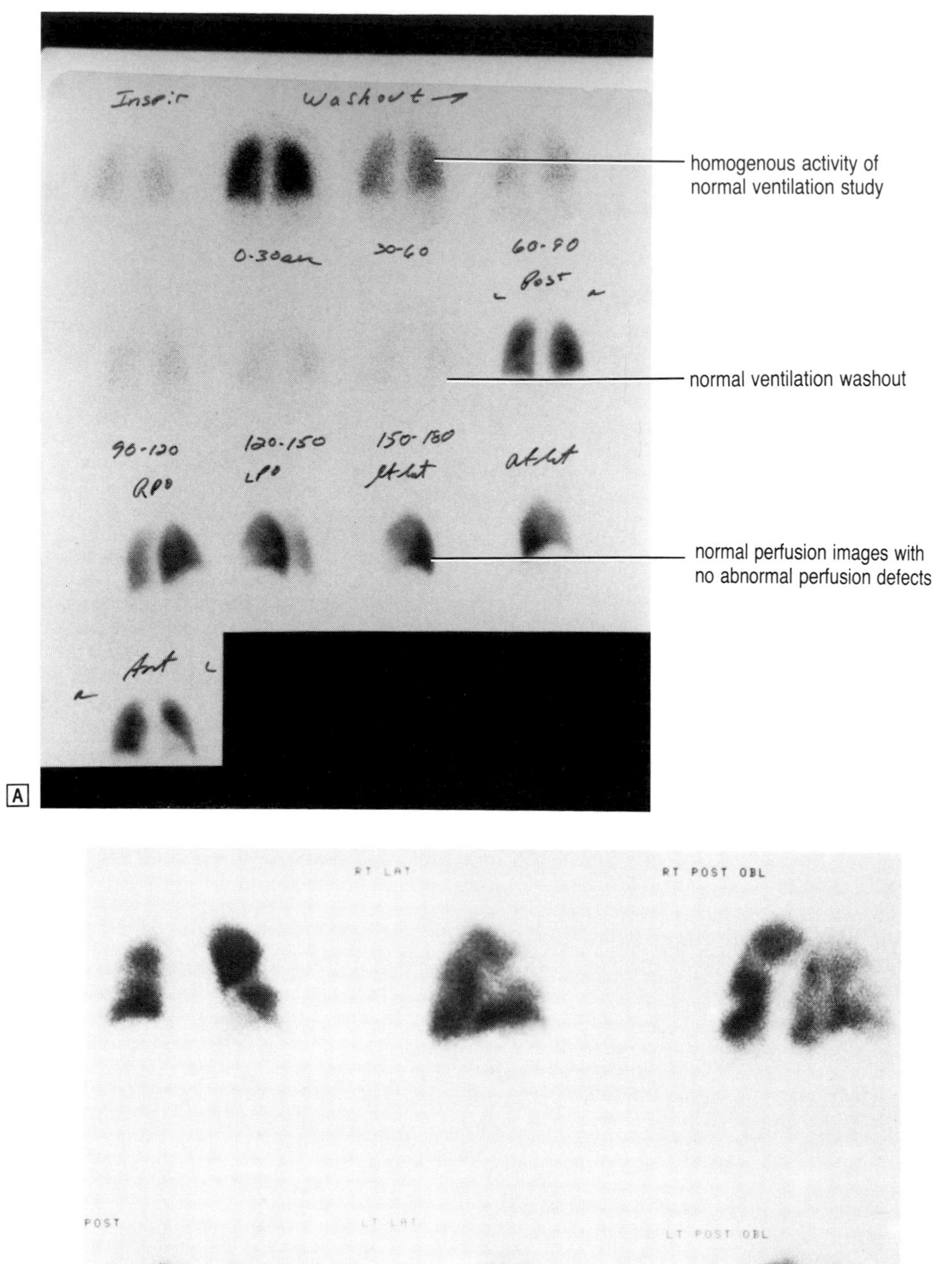

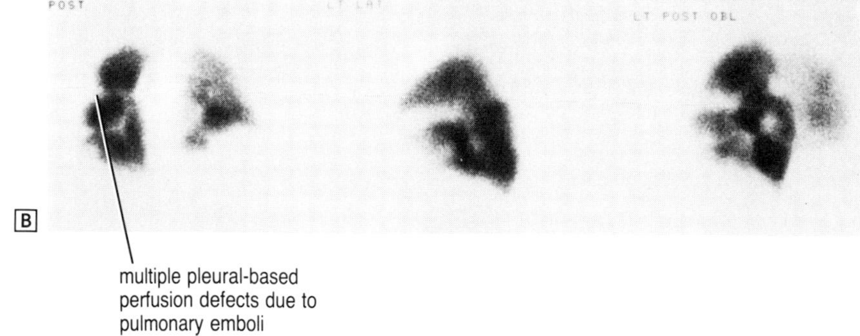

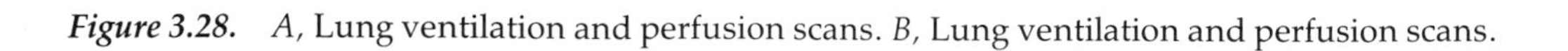
Figure 3.28. *A,* Lung ventilation and perfusion scans. *B,* Lung ventilation and perfusion scans.

3.29 NORMAL CT EXAMINATION OF THE CHEST

A. Demonstration of normal chest anatomy

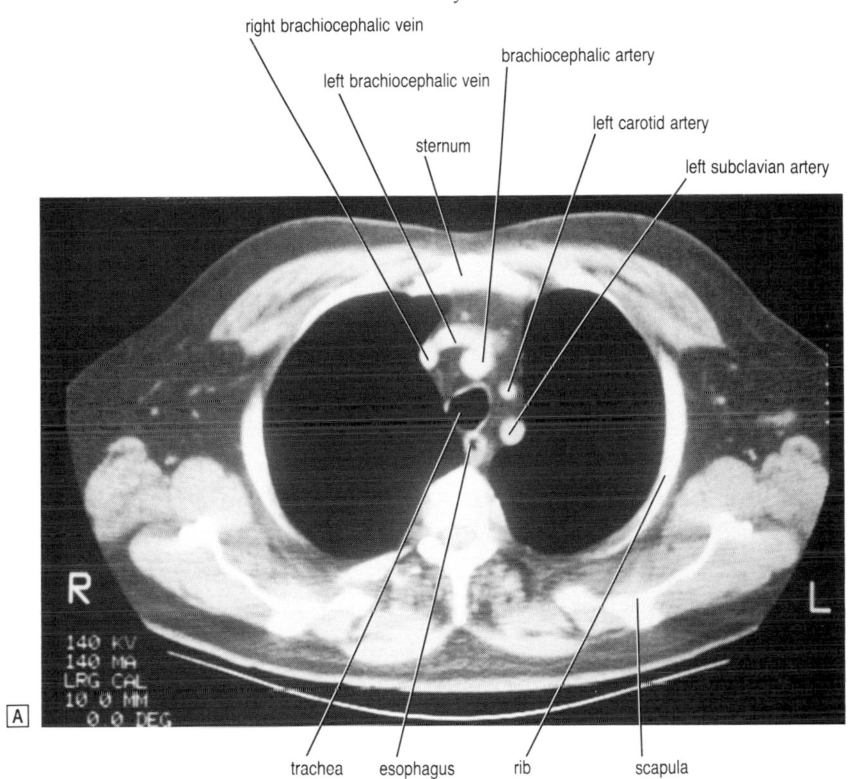

Figure 3.29. *A,* Normal CT of the chest.

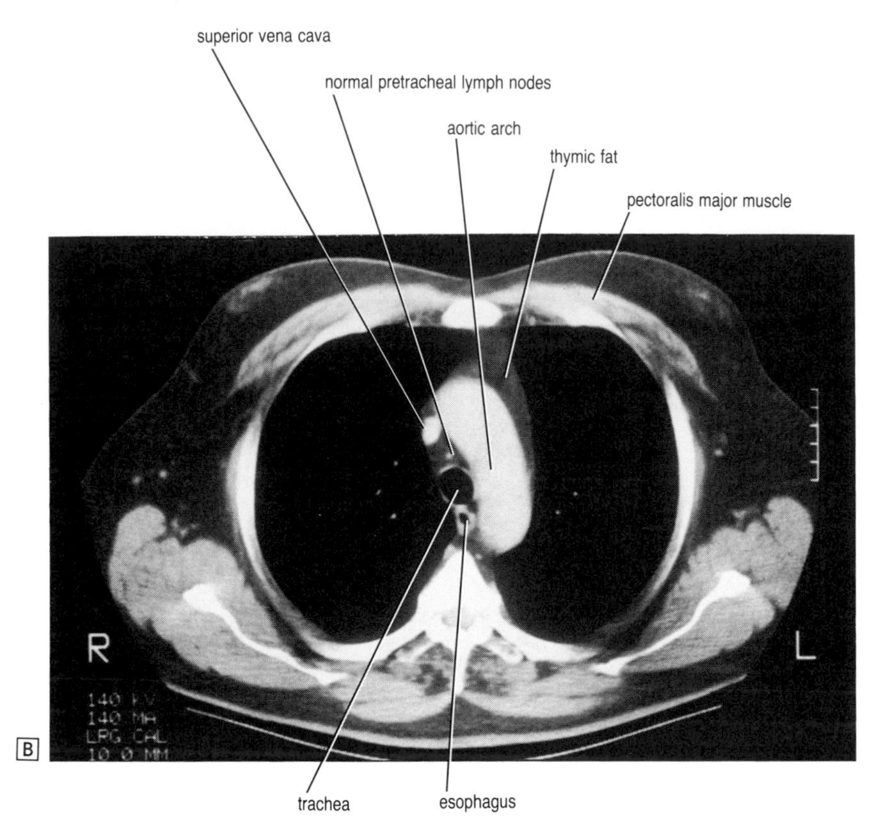

Figure 3.29. *B,* Normal CT of the chest.

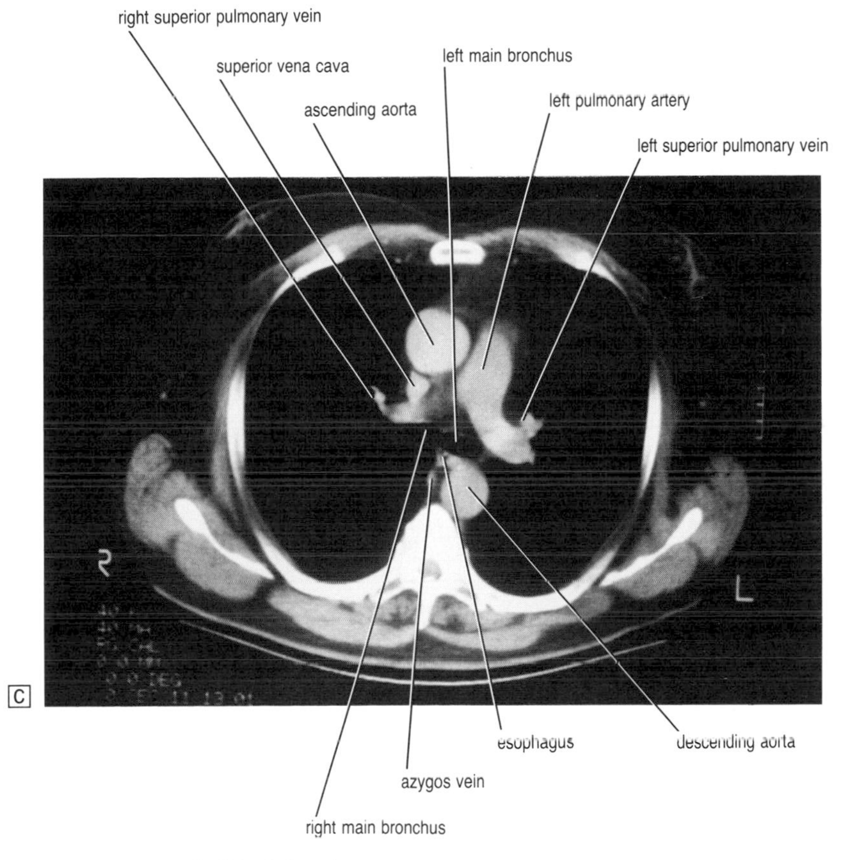

Figure 3.29. C, Normal CT of the chest.

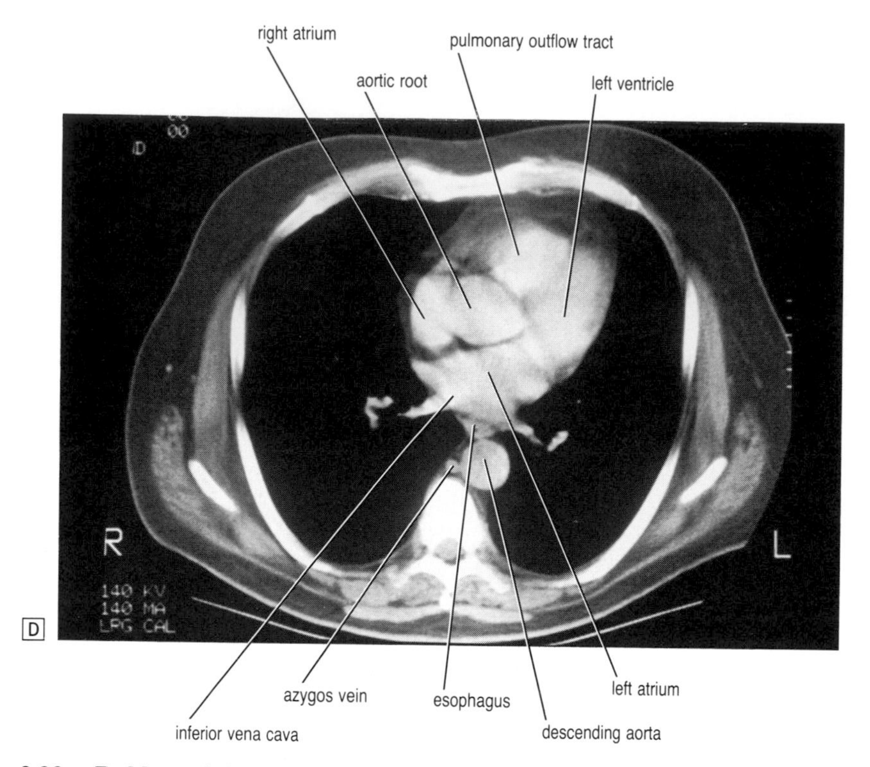

Figure 3.29. *D,* Normal CT of the chest.

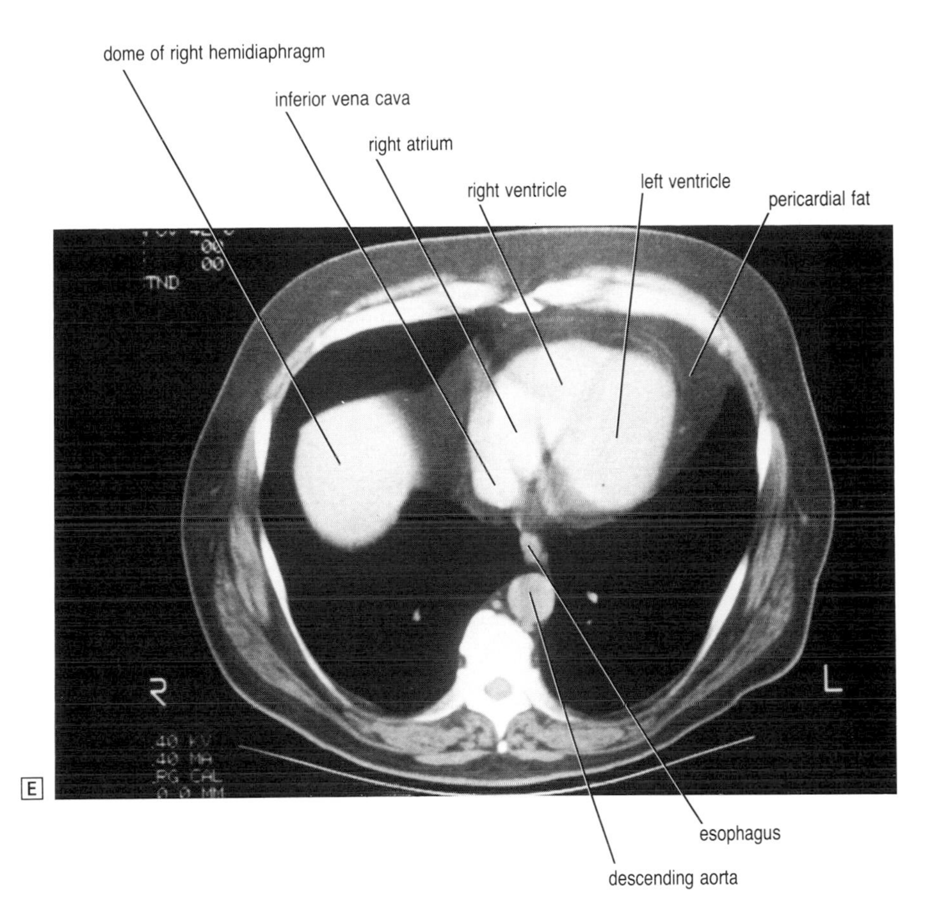

Figure 3.29. *E,* Normal CT of the chest.

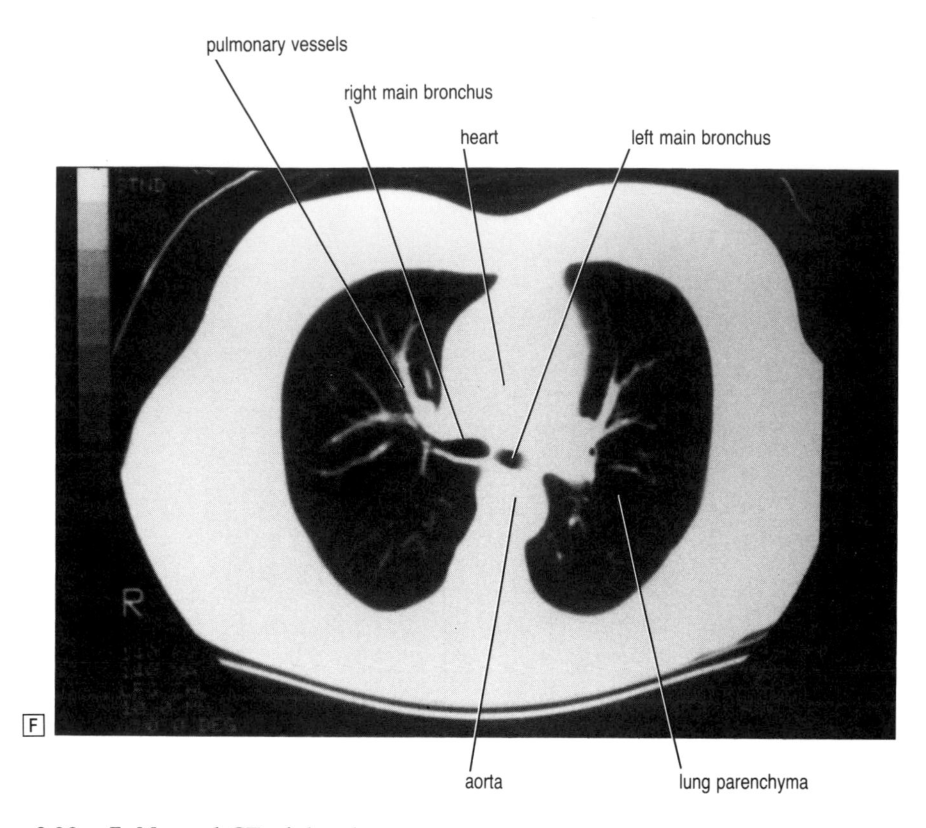

Figure 3.29. *F,* Normal CT of the chest.

References

Eisenberg, R.L.: Diagnostic Imaging in Internal Medicine. New York: McGraw-Hill Book Co., 1985.
Ellis, K.: The adult respiratory distress syndrome. In: Contemporary Diagnostics, Vol. 1. Baltimore: Williams & Wilkins, 1978.
Goodman, L.R., and Putman, C.E.: Intensive Care Radiology: Imaging of the Critically Ill. 2nd Ed. Philadelphia: W.B. Saunders Co., 1983.
Harris, J.H., and Harris, W.H.: The Radiology of Emergency Medicine. 2nd Ed. Baltimore: Williams & Wilkins, 1981.
Juhl, J.H., and Crummy, A.B.: Essentials of Radiologic Imaging. Philadelphia: J.B. Lippincott, 1987.
Pare, J.A.P., and Fraser, R.G.: Synopsis of Diseases of the Chest. Philadelphia: W.B. Saunders Co., 1983.

4

Abdomen and Gastrointestinal Tract

4.01 EVALUATION OF THE ABDOMEN

A. Proper evaluation of the abdomen requires a systematic and repetitive approach.
B. The routine examination of the abdomen is the supine AP view, which should include the domes of the diaphragm and below the symphysis pubis.
C. When complete evaluation of the abdomen is required, additional views include the following.
   1. Erect view to determine the presence of air fluid levels within the bowel
   2. Left-side-down decubitus view to determine the presence of free intraperitoneal air
   3. An erect view of the chest is the most sensitive view for the detection of free intraperitoneal air.
D. Abdomen evaluation
   1. Bowel gas pattern
      a. Distribution of the gas is important. In the normal abdomen, minimal gas is present within the small bowel. Gas can be localized to the small intestine by being centrally located and having parallel indentations completely crossing the bowel loop (valvulae conniventes). Gas can be localized to the large bowel by being peripherally located and having irregular indentations that do not cross the bowel loop (haustral markings).
      b. Small bowel loops greater than 3 cm in width are abnormally distended.
      c. If the transverse colon measures greater than 6 cm, it is abnormally distended.
      d. Above 9 cm in width, the cecum is at risk for perforation.
   2. Organomegaly
      a. The liver, spleen, kidney, and bladder should be evaluated for size, position, and configuration.
   3. Abnormal masses
      a. The abdomen should be evaluated for any abnormal masses that may result in displacement of normal anatomic structures.
   4. Osseous structures
      a. The entire visualized bony skeleton should be evaluated for destructive lesions, fractures, osteoporosis, and degenerative changes.
   5. The presence of free fluid or free intraperitoneal air should be excluded (see Secs. 4.02, 4.03).
   6. Both psoas margins should be visualized and should have a symmetrical appearance.
   7. Abnormal calcifications should also be considered. If calcifications are visualized and their location cannot be determined, additional oblique views will allow accurate localization.
   8. The properitoneal fat line is an important landmark that is visualized as a lucent line on the lateral aspect of the abdomen (see Sec. 4.02).
E. For proper evaluation of the abdomen, remember: bones, stones, masses, and gases.

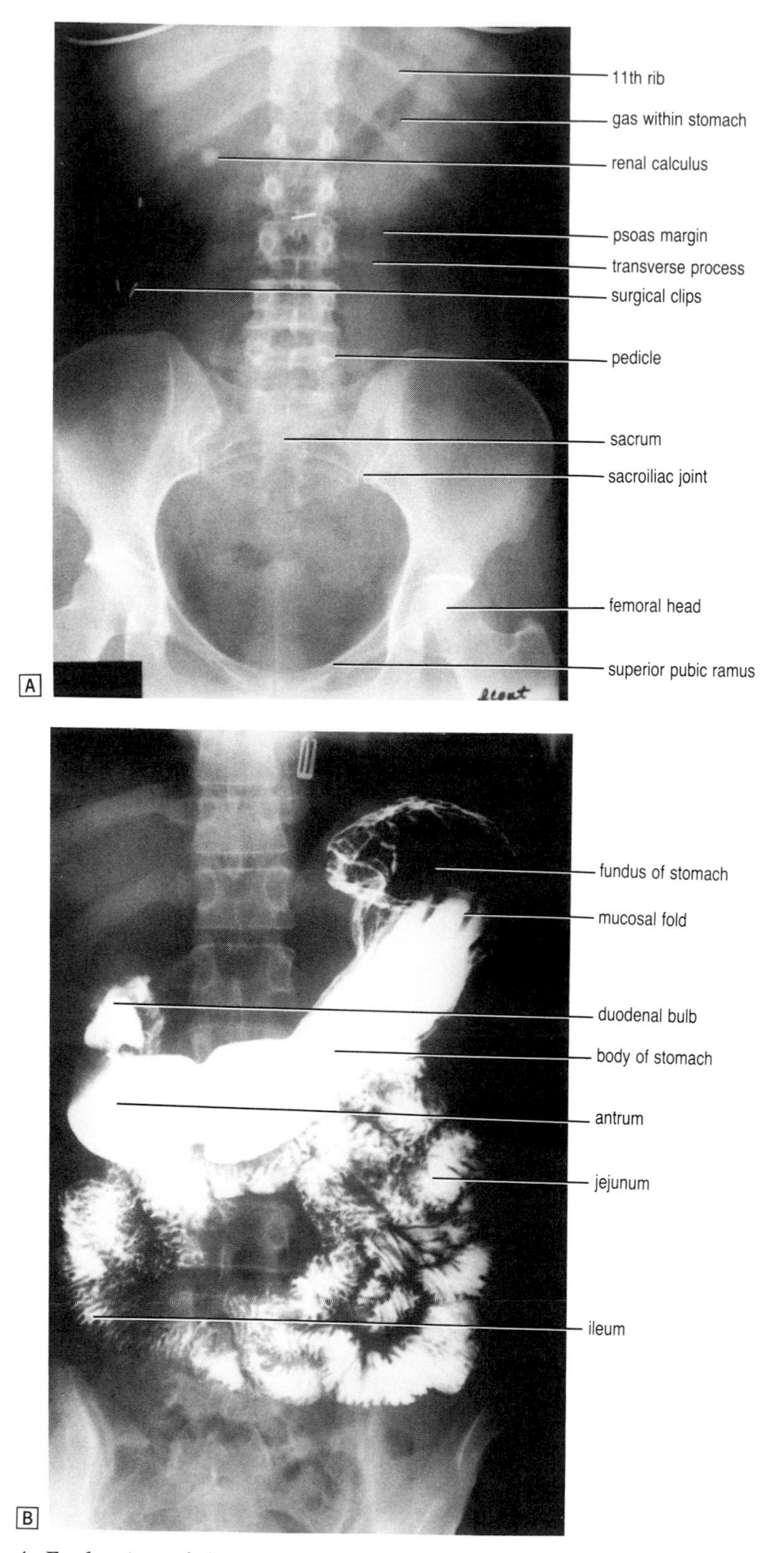

Figure 4.01. *A,* Evaluation of the abdomen. *B,* Evaluation of the abdomen.

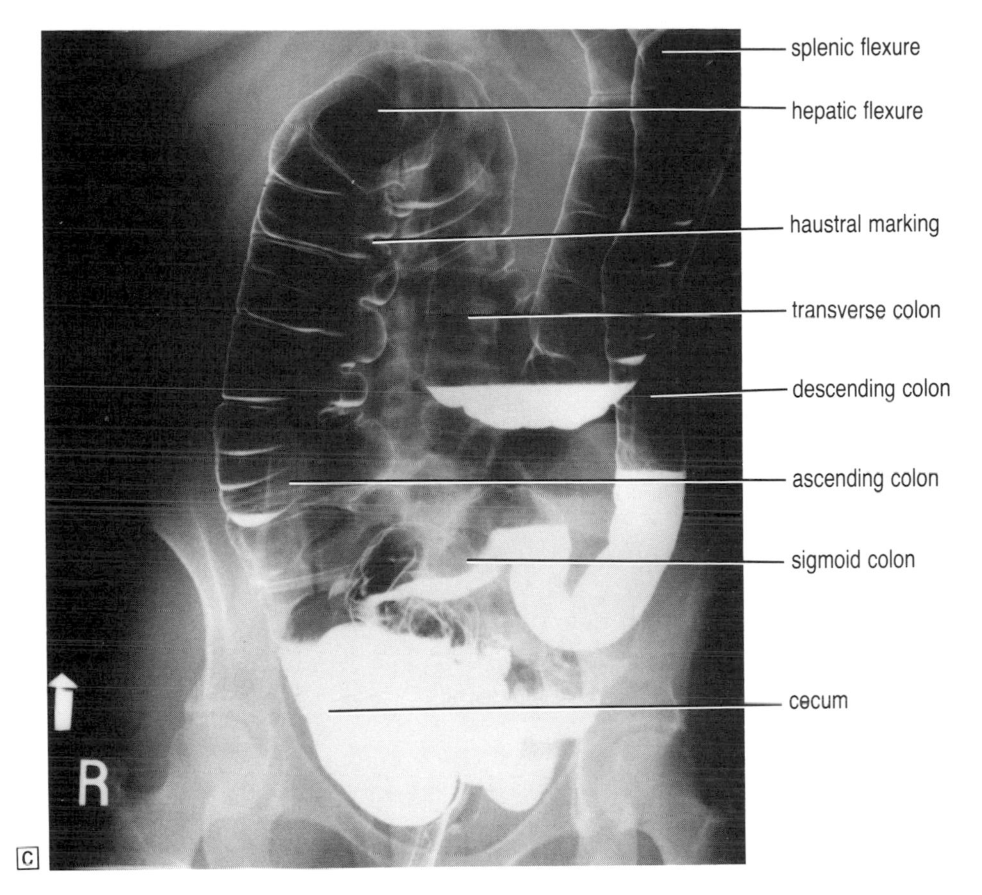

Figure 4.01. C, Evaluation of the abdomen.

4.02 DIFFUSE HAZINESS OF THE ABDOMEN: FREE INTRAPERITONEAL FLUID AND THE GASLESS ABDOMEN

A. Generalized haziness of the abdomen with or without visualized bowel loops is suggestive of free intraperitoneal fluid.

B. Radiographic signs of free fluid
   1. Diffuse haziness results in nonvisualization of normal anatomic landmarks such as obliteration of the psoas margins.
   2. The properitoneal fat line is a lucent line located along the lateral aspect of the abdomen. It lies adjacent to the ascending and descending colon. Free fluid in the paracolic gutters displaces the colon medially. In the presence of a large amount of free fluid, bowel loops appear to be "floating" within the abdomen.
   3. Free fluid within the cul-de-sac appears as soft tissue densities located on the superolateral aspect of the bladder and give the appearance of "Mickey Mouse" or "dog" ears.

C. Remember, improper technique may also result in haziness of the abdomen.

D. Differential diagnosis of free intraperitoneal fluid
   1. Trauma
   2. Neoplasm
   3. Cirrhosis
   4. Peritonitis
   5. Iatrogenic (e.g., peritoneal lavage or peritoneal dialysis)
   6. Lymphatic obstruction

E. Bowel loops may or may not be seen with a large amount of free fluid.

F. Differential diagnosis of a gasless abdomen
   1. Large amount of free intraperitoneal fluid
   2. Large abdominal mass
   3. A high gastrointestinal obstruction
   4. Prolonged emesis
   5. Normal variant
   6. Multiple fluid-filled bowel loops

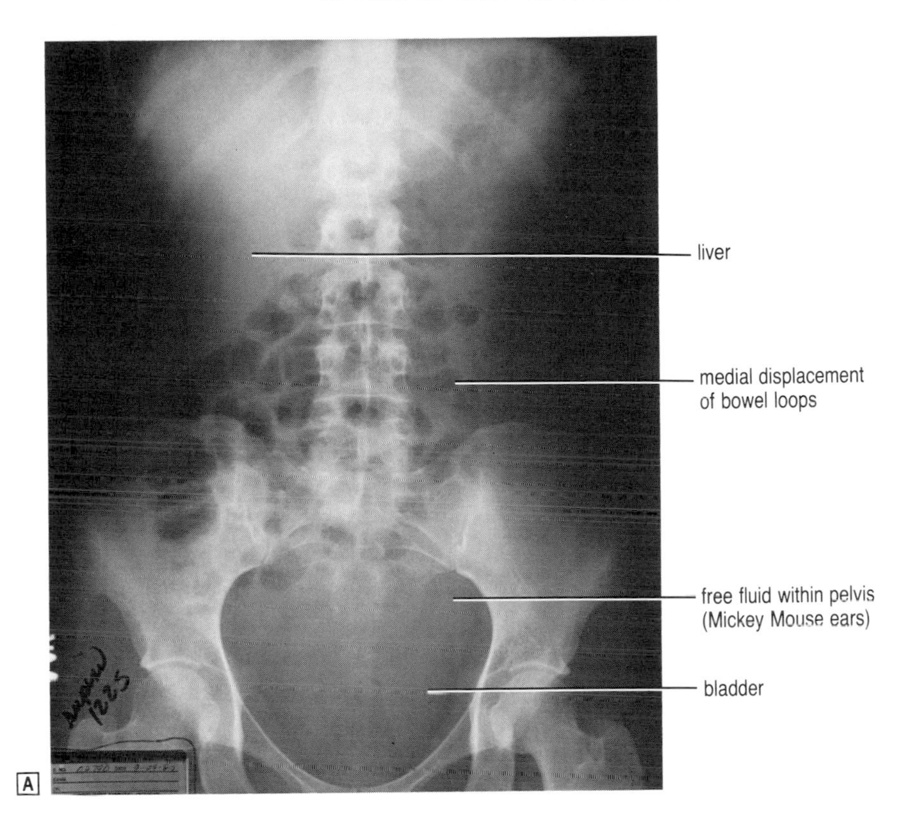

Figure 4.02. *A,* Diffuse haziness of the abdomen: free intraperitoneal fluid and the gasless abdomen.

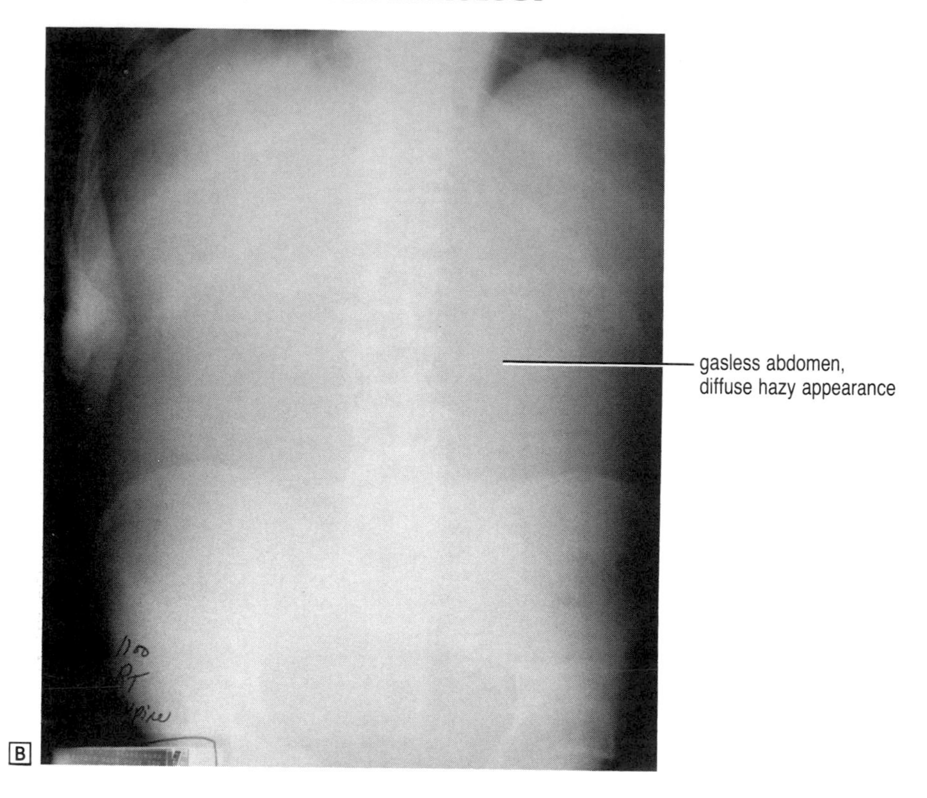

Figure 4.02. *B,* Diffuse haziness of the abdomen: free intraperitoneal fluid and the gasless abdomen.

4.03 PNEUMOPERITONEUM

A. The most sensitive examination for the detection of pneumoperitoneum is the erect chest roentgenogram. Very small amounts of free air can be visualized.
B. If the patient cannot tolerate an erect examination, a right-side-up decubitus view of the abdomen should be obtained.
C. Radiographic signs of pneumoperitoneum
   1. The erect chest roentgenogram demonstrates an abnormal air collection best seen below the right hemidiaphragm.
   2. The right-side-up decubitus view demonstrates layering of air that is not confined within bowel loops.
   3. In the supine view of the abdomen, free air outlines both walls of a bowel loop, resulting in a "double wall" sign as long as the visualized bowel loop is not in contact with another loop. The falciform ligament may become visualized as a curvilinear density in the right upper quadrant. A large amount of free air produces a large central lucency overlying the abdomen known as the "football" sign.
D. Differential diagnosis of pneumoperitoneum
   1. Perforated viscus
      a. Perforated duodenal ulcer. Approximately one third will not demonstrate free air. This is the most common pathologic cause of pneumoperitoneum.
      b. Trauma
      c. Obstruction
      d. Toxic megacolon secondary to ulcerative colitis
      e. Neoplasm
      f. Appendicitis
   2. Iatrogenic
      a. Recent abdominal surgery
      b. Peritoneal dialysis
   3. Entry via vagina, e.g., vaginal douching or oral sex
   4. Pneumomediastinum

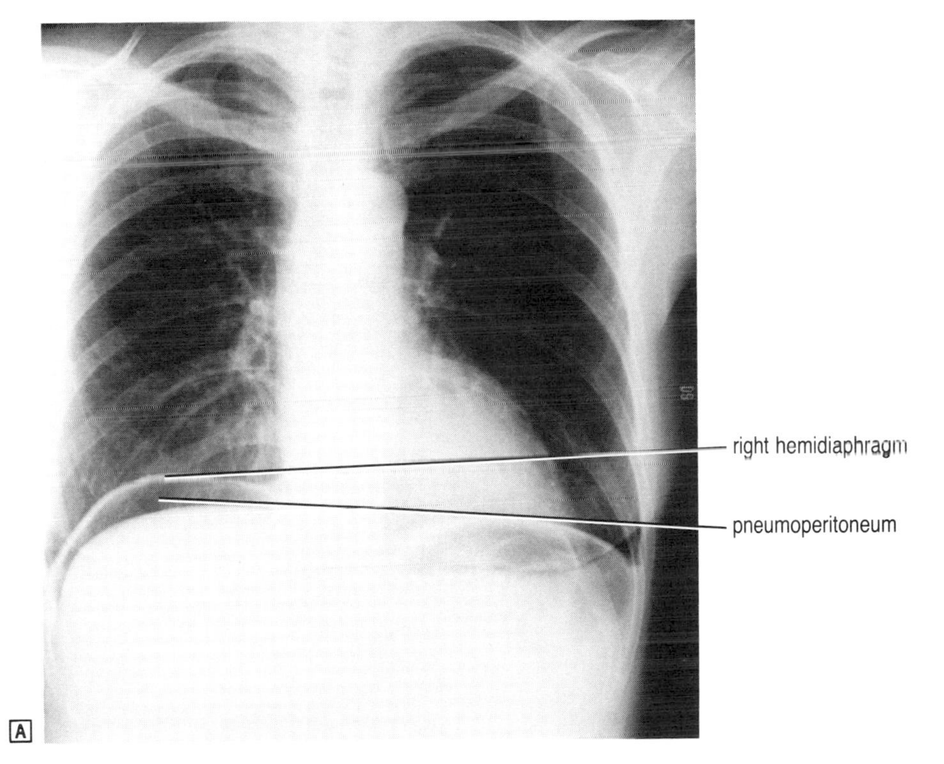

Figure 4.03. *A*, Pneumoperitoneum.

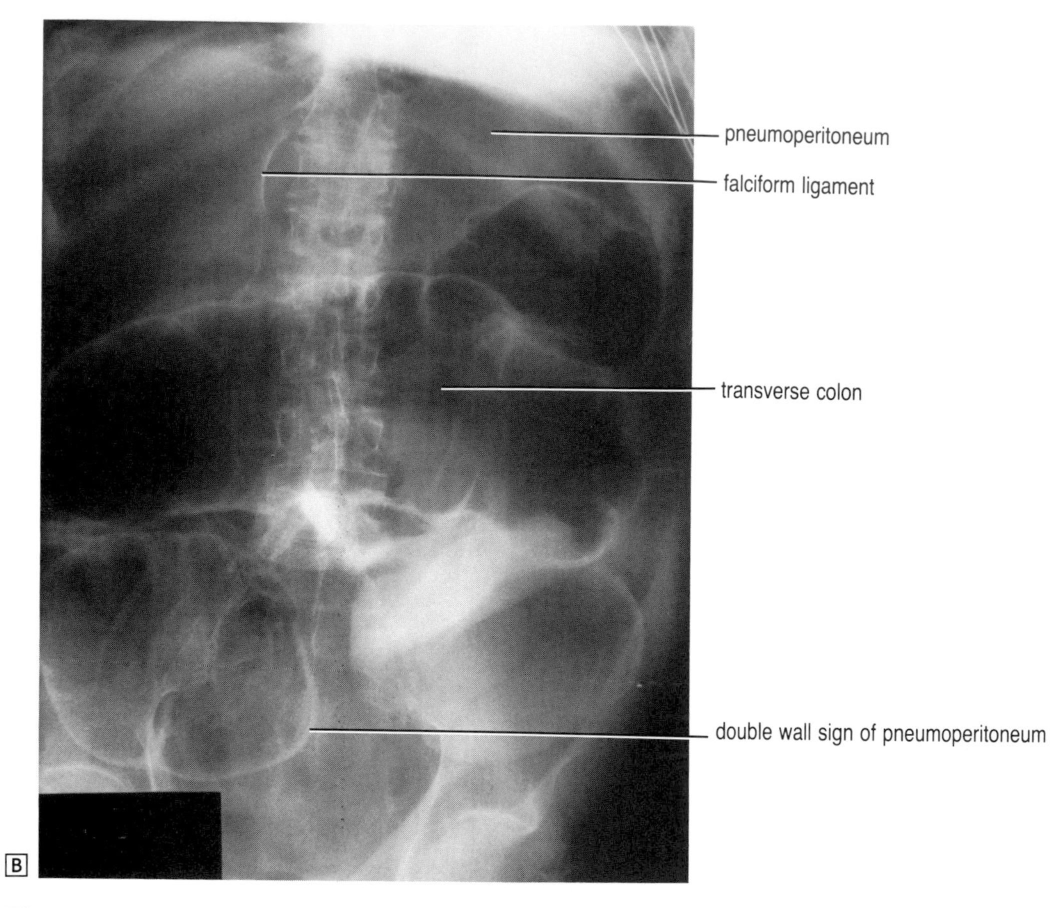

Figure 4.03. *B,* Pneumoperitoneum.

4.04 ABNORMAL ABDOMINAL DENSITIES

A. AP view may often demonstrate abnormal densities in the abdomen. Most represent calcifications, but iatrogenic and self-inflicted conditions may also occur.
   1. Pancreatic calcifications (see Sec. 4.22)
   2. Liver and splenic calcifications
      a. Often visualized as multiple, small, round calcifications in the left and right upper quadrants of the abdomen due to previous granulomatous infection.
   3. Cholelithiasis
      a. Usually visualized as multiple, multifaceted, laminated densities in the right upper quadrant
   4. Mesenteric lymph nodes
      a. When calcified, appear as round or oval densities that move with change in position
   5. Adrenal calcification
      a. Visualized as areas of calcification superior to the kidneys that result from carcinoma, previous infection, previous hemorrhage, Addison's disease, or previous tuberculosis
   6. Appendicolith
      a. Visualized as a laminated calcification in the right lower quadrant in the region of the appendix
   7. Phleboliths
      a. Represent venous calcifications that are usually present in the pelvis and appear smooth and rough. Have a central lucency
   8. Postsurgical changes
   9. Foreign bodies

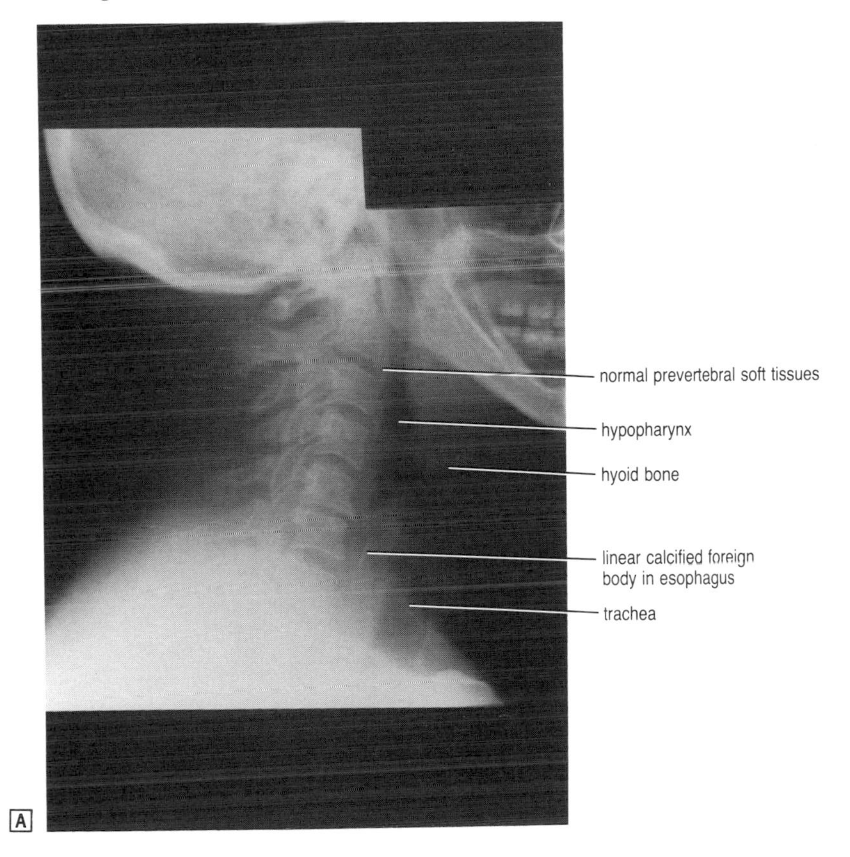

Figure 4.04. *A,* Abnormal abdominal densities.

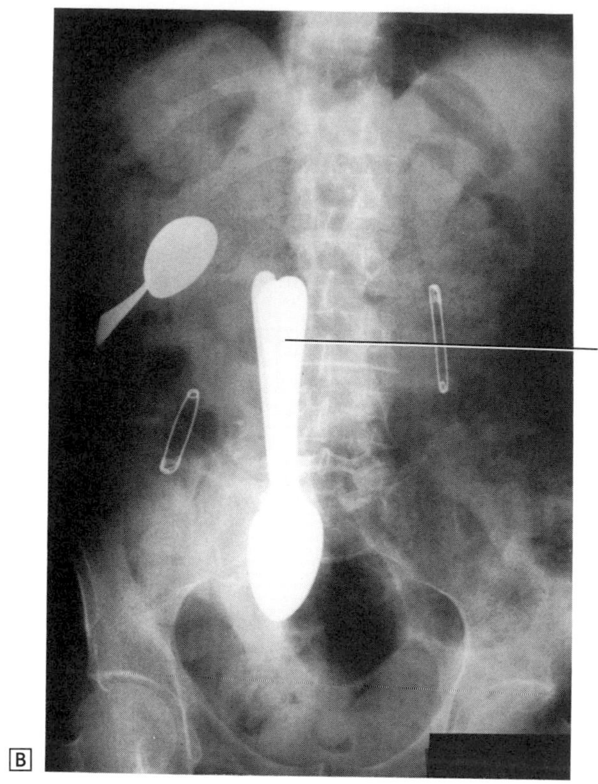

Figure 4.04. *B,* Abnormal abdominal densities.

4.05 ESOPHAGEAL HERNIAS

A. Sliding hiatal hernia
   1. This is the most common condition demonstrated on barium examination of the upper gastrointestinal tract.
   2. Hiatal hernias are variable in size and shape and may be seen on routine chest roentgenogram as round structures commonly with an air fluid level located behind the cardiac silhouette.
   3. This hernia is the result of movement of the gastroesophageal junction into an intrathoracic position as a result of chronic stress and strain.
   4. Schatzki's (B) ring represents the squamocolumnar junction between esophagus and stomach.
   5. Barium examination reveals a Schatzki's ring seen as smooth circular narrowing of the esophagus above the level of the diaphragms. Visualization of folds of the gastric mucosa located in an intrathoracic position above the level of the hemidiaphragm is evidence of a sliding hiatal hernia.

B. Complications of a hiatal hernia are the result of gastroesophageal reflux.
   1. Reflux occurs in approximately 25% of people with hiatal hernia. If reflux occurs, it may lead to esophagitis, esophageal stricture, and Barrett's esophagus, which is associated with adenocarcinoma.
   2. Most people with sliding hiatal hernias are asymptomatic.

C. Paraesophageal hernia (rolling hernia)
   1. In this hernia, the gastroesophageal (GE) junction is undisturbed and remains in normal position.
   2. The fundus of the stomach herniates anteriorly to GE junction through the esophageal hiatus.
   3. Because there is a normal gastroesophageal junction, no reflux occurs.
   4. The major potential complication is volvulus of the herniated fundus.

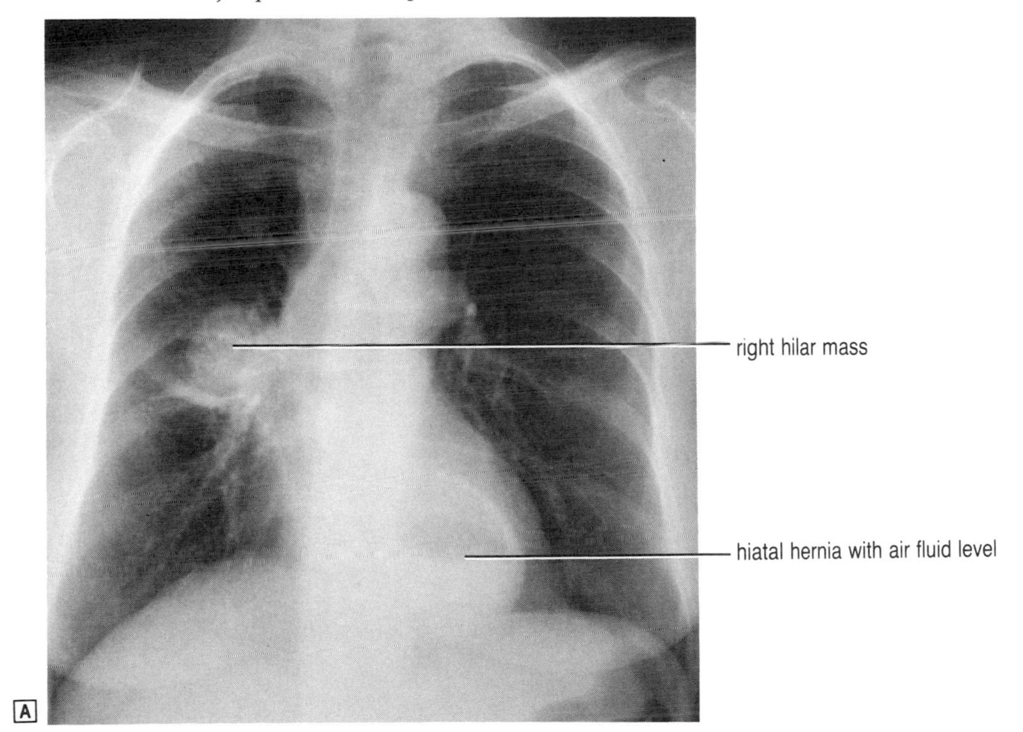

Figure 4.05. *A*, Esophageal hernias.

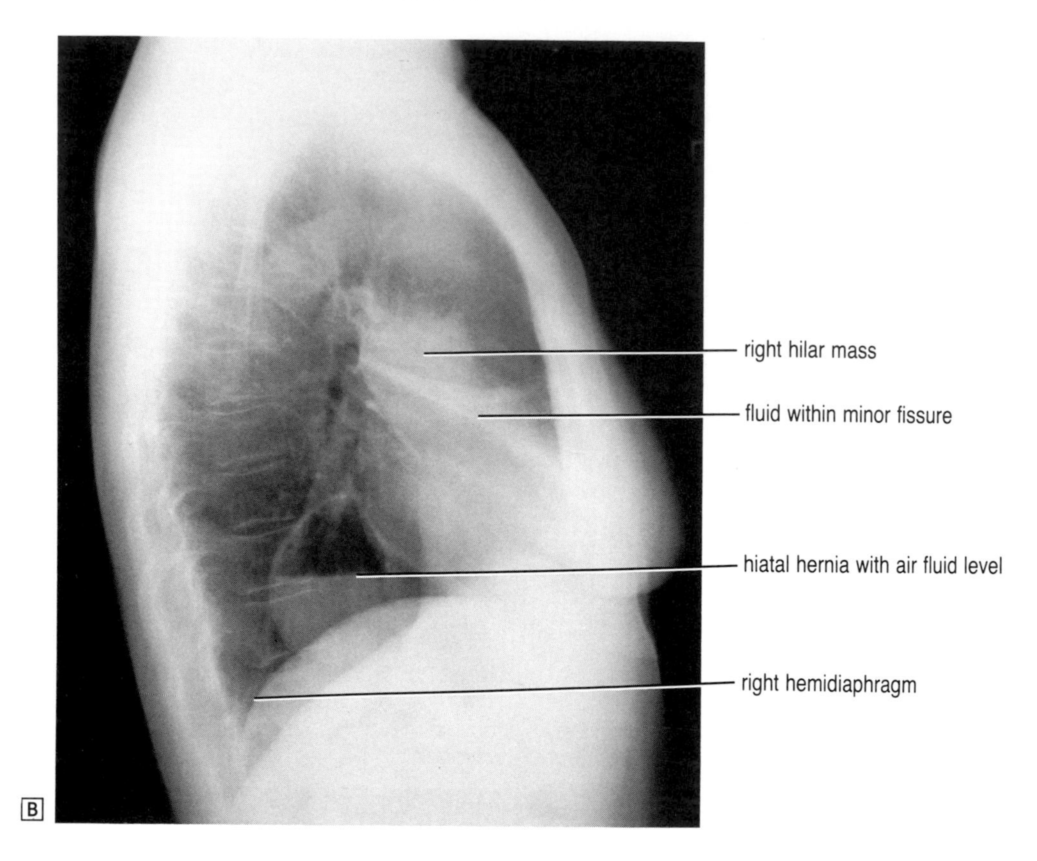

Figure 4.05. *B,* Esophageal hernias.

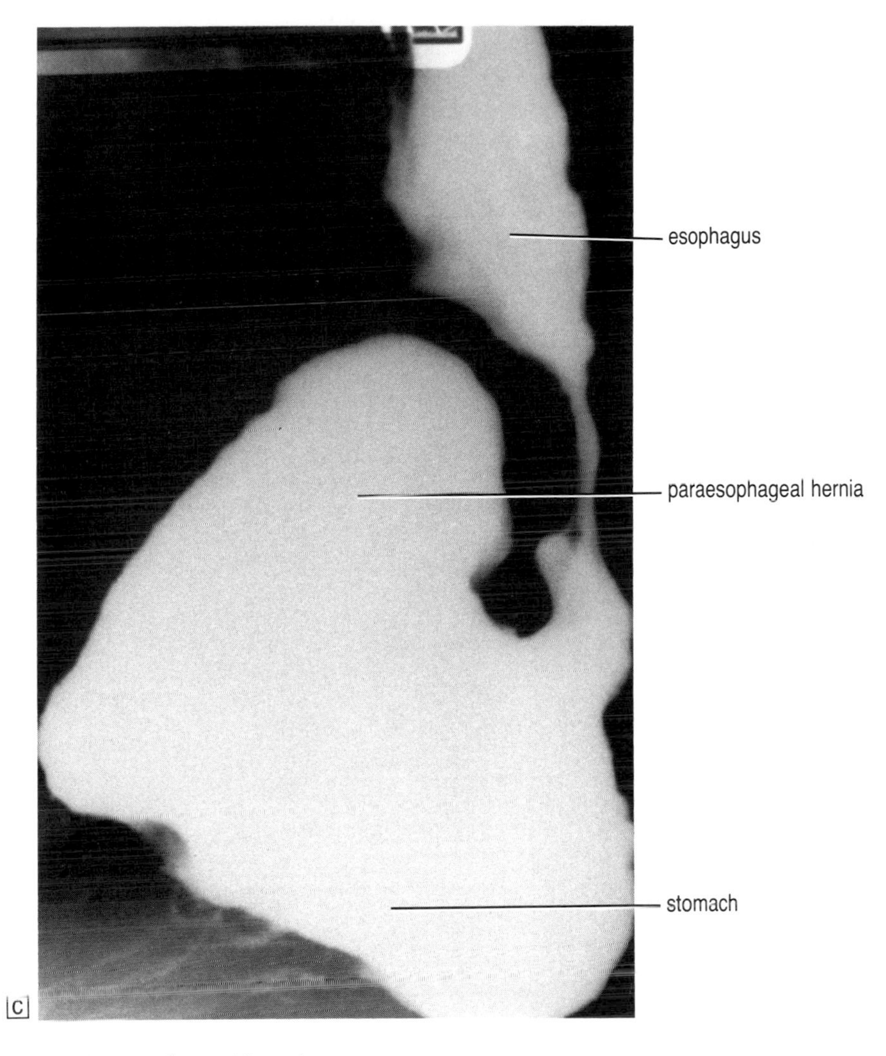

Figure 4.05. C, Esophageal hernias.

4.06 ESOPHAGITIS AND ESOPHAGEAL STRICTURE FORMATION

A. Esophagitis
1. Inflammatory conditions of the esophagus result in ulcer formation, thickening of mucosal folds, and ultimately stricture formation.
2. Ulcers are visualized as linear or small round collections of barium often with surrounding radiating folds. The involved area of the esophagus may appear irregular and indistinct.
3. Eventually there is irregular luminal narrowing due to stricture formation.

B. Differential diagnosis of esophagitis and esophageal stricture
1. Reflux esophagitis
   a. Usually involves the distal esophagus and is associated with a sliding hiatal hernia and reflux
2. Barrett's esophagus
   a. This condition is associated with the presence of a hiatal hernia and reflux. Chronic esophageal irritation results in changing of normal squamous epithelium to columnar epithelium. The area of involvement usually occurs in the mid to distal esophagus with an area of normal esophagus present between this area and the GE junction. Barrett's esophagus is associated with the development of adenocarcinoma in approximately 10% of individuals.
3. Prolonged nasogastric tube placement
4. Inflammatory esophagitis
   a. Candidiasis and herpes result in diffuse multiple ulcerations of the esophagus that usually occur in debilitated patients.
5. Alkali ingestion
   a. Ingestion of corrosives results in ulceration and development of esophageal narrowing.
6. Esophageal carcinoma
   a. Most commonly squamous cell
7. Metastasis
8. Leiomyosarcoma
9. Previous radiation therapy
10. Crohn's disease

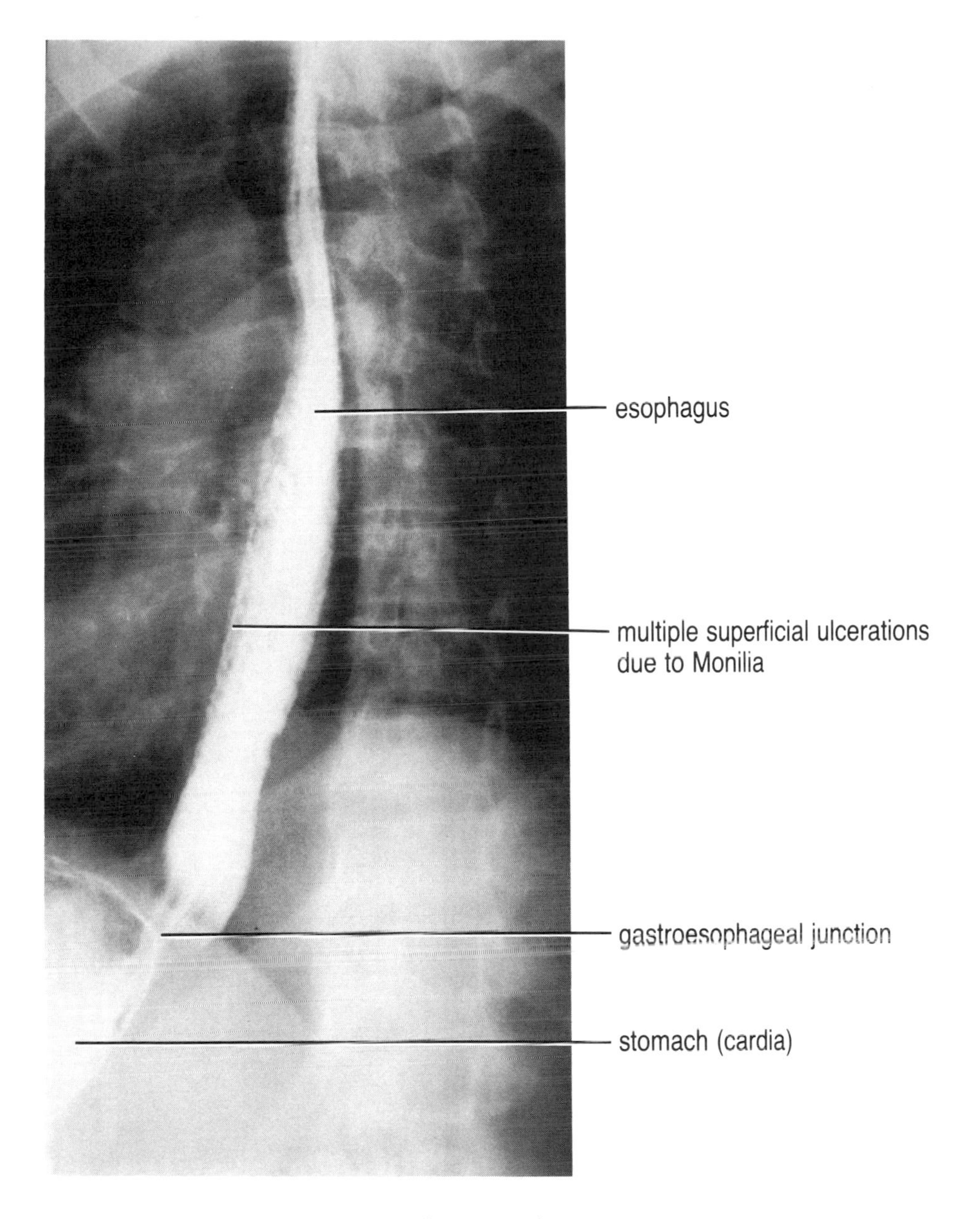

Figure 4.06 Esophagitis and esophageal stricture formation.

4.07 FILLING DEFECT WITHIN THE ESOPHAGUS

A. Differential diagnosis
  1. Foreign body
    a. Diagnosis often made by the history. For example, the patient was eating when a piece of meat became stuck. Anything else the patient ingests regurgitates.
    b. The purpose of the esophagram is to identify the presence of an obstruction, the location and degree of obstruction, and any associated esophageal damage.
    c. Always obtain a soft tissue lateral view of the neck and AP view. This will allow identification of radiopaque foreign bodies, e.g., coins, chicken bones.
    d. Young children often swallow foreign bodies, especially coins. AP and lateral views will determine if the object is located within the esophagus or trachea. On the lateral view, remember the esophagus is located between the vertebral bodies and the air-filled trachea. On the AP view, if a coin is visualized "en face," it is located within the esophagus. If it is seen on edge, it is located in the trachea.
    e. Most foreign bodies become lodged in the upper third of the esophagus.
  2. Neoplasm
    a. The most common benign neoplasm is a leiomyoma, which is visualized as a smooth-filling defect.
    b. Most are intramurally located in the distal third of the esophagus.
    c. The most common malignant neoplasm is squamous cell carcinoma, visualized as an irregular filling defect that may demonstrate ulceration and overhanging margins.
    d. Other benign neoplasms include villous adenoma, polyp, hemangioma, and neurofibroma.
    e. Other malignant neoplasms include adenocarcinoma, which is associated with Barrett's esophagus, metastatic disease, lymphoma, and leiomyosarcoma.
  3. Esophageal varices
    a. Result of portal hypertension
    b. Visualized as dilated, smooth, serpiginous filling defects within the esophagus
  4. Esophagitis
    a. Infection with candidiasis or herpes may result in multiple, nodular filling defects within the esophagus (see Sec. 4.06).

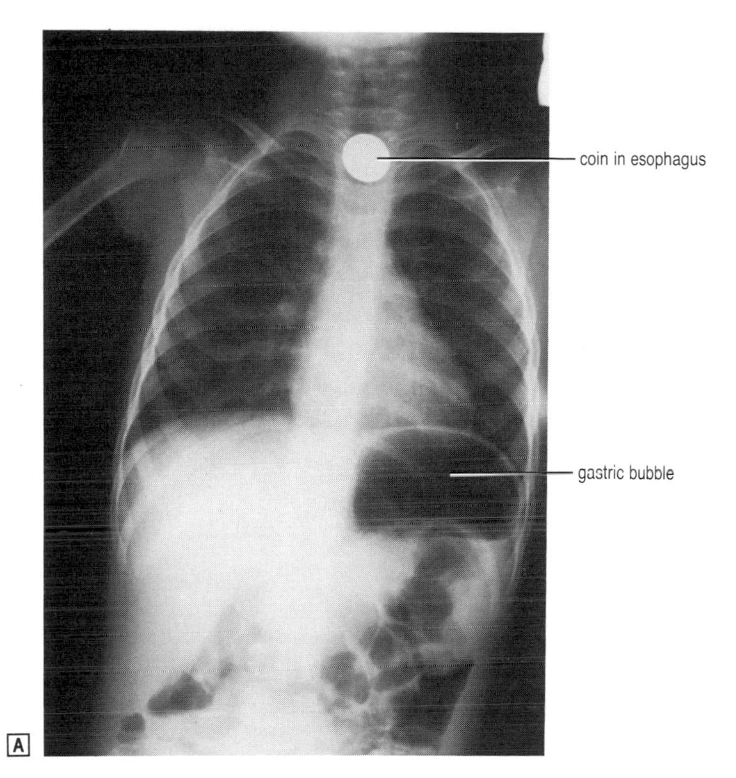

Figure 4.07. *A,* Filling defect within the esophagus.

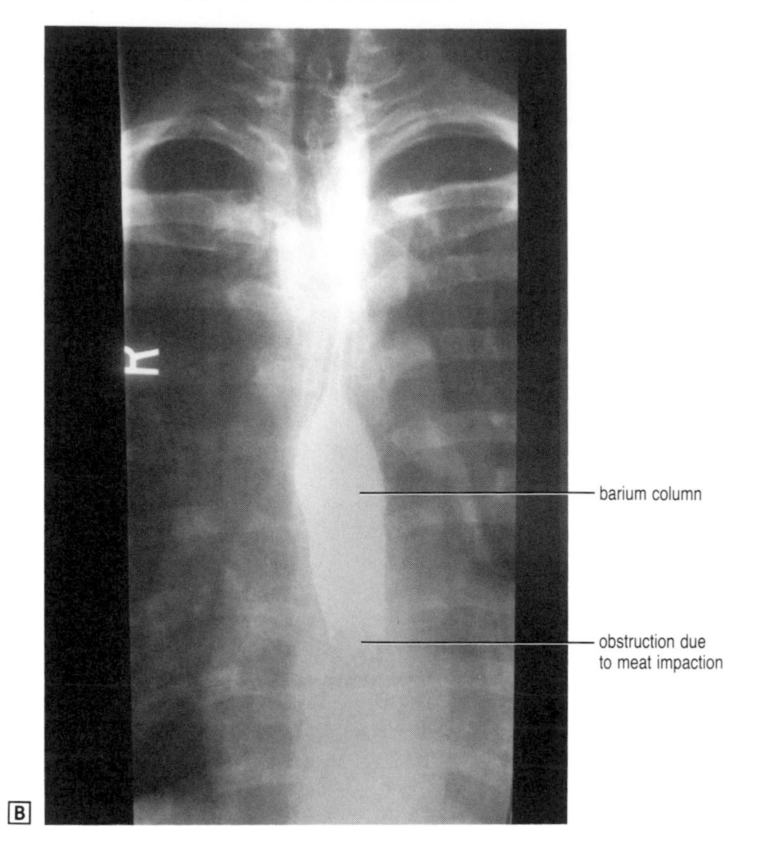

Figure 4.07. *B,* Filling defect within the esophagus.

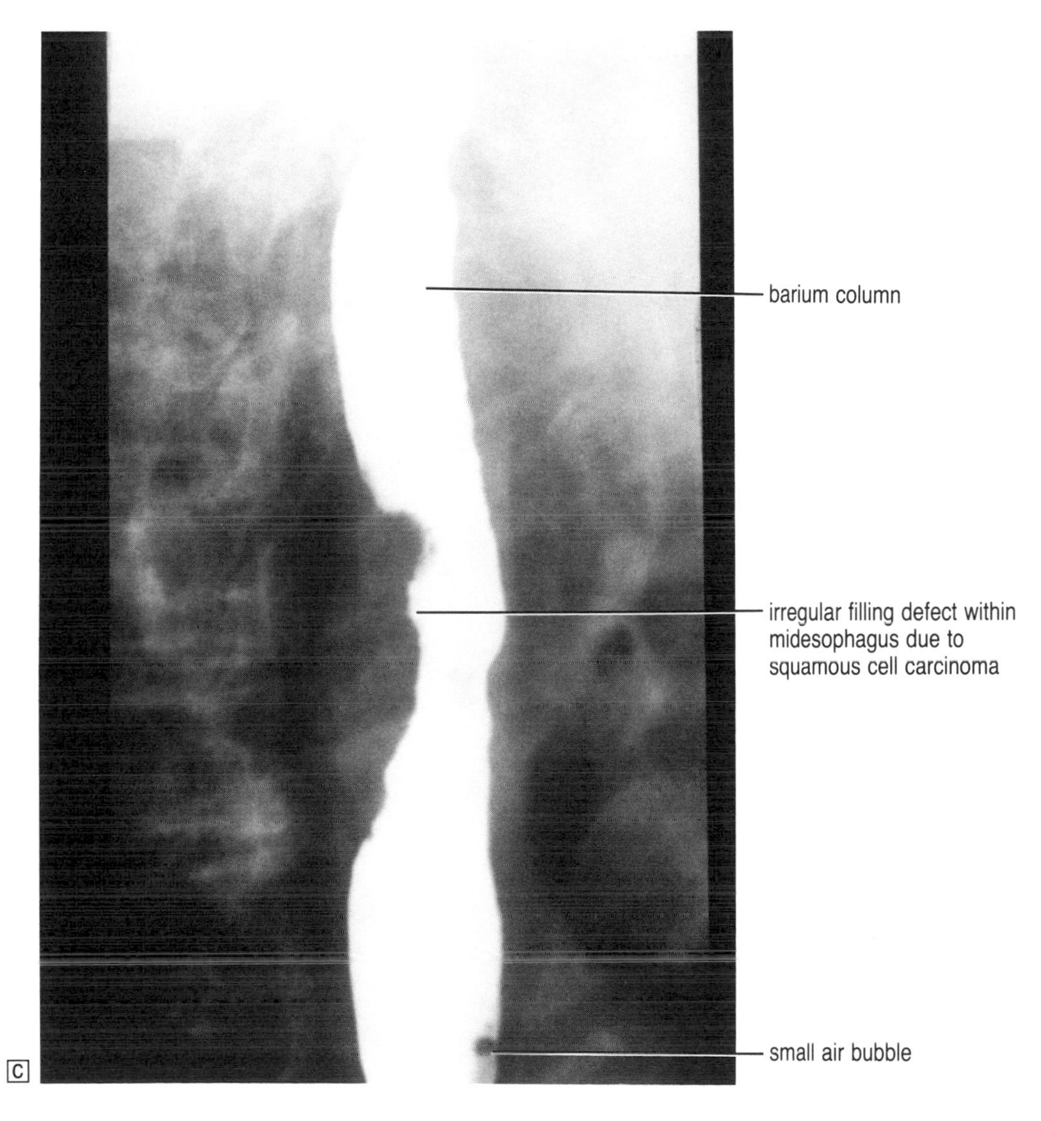

Figure 4.07. C, Filling defect within the esophagus.

4.08 ABNORMAL ESOPHAGEAL MOTILITY

A. Presbyesophagus
   1. This is the most common motility disorder of the esophagus and is related to alteration of swallowing function due to aging.
   2. Radiographically, visualized as impairment of the normal peristaltic wave. Multiple tertiary contractions represent uncoordinated esophageal contractions.

B. Achalasia
   1. This motility disorder results from dysfunction of the lower esophageal sphincter.
   2. This condition results in an enlarged, dilated esophagus that can often be visualized on a chest roentgenogram. A fluid level is often seen.
   3. Radiographically, barium collects within the dilated esophagus. The distal esophagus has a smooth narrowed segment (beak appearance).
   4. Complications of achalasia include aspiration pneumonia and increased risk of esophageal carcinoma.
   5. The differential diagnosis includes causes of esophageal stricture (see Sec 4.06). Always remember the possibility of metastatic disease or primary esophageal carcinoma.

C. Scleroderma (progressive systemic sclerosis)
   1. Smooth muscle is present in the lower two thirds of the esophagus. Scleroderma may impair this smooth muscle activity and may result in atony of the lower two thirds of the esophagus.
   2. Normal swallowing function is present in the upper third of the esophagus owing to the presence of striated muscle.
   3. Impaired peristalsis occurs in the lower esophagus with a wide open (patulous) lower esophageal sphincter. This allows free gastroesophageal reflux, which may lead to esophageal stricture.

D. The CREST syndrome of scleroderma
   1. Calcinosis
   2. Raynaud's phenomenon
   3. Esophageal hypomotility
   4. Sclerodactyly
   5. Telangiectasia

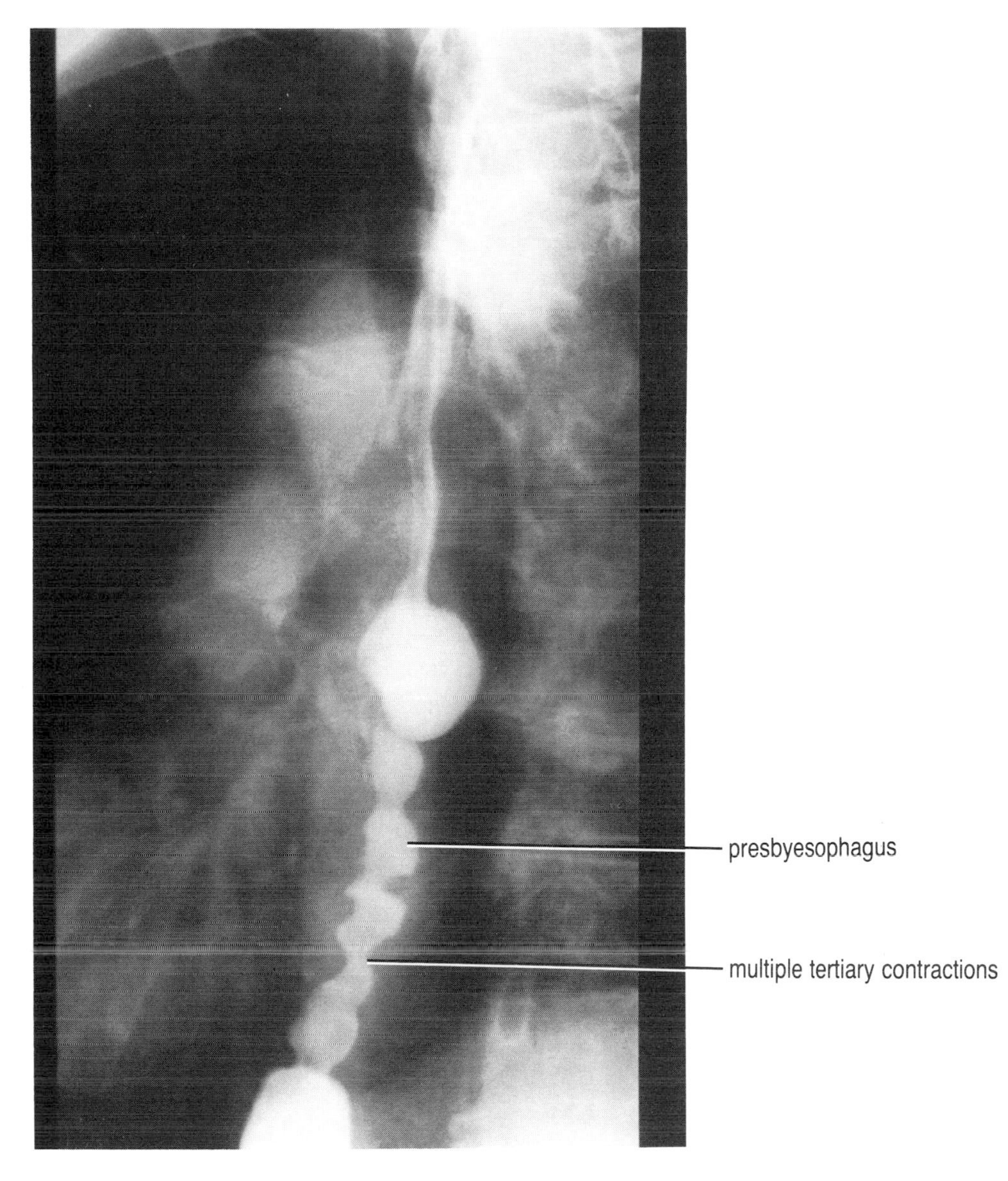

Figure 4.08. Abnormal esophageal motility.

4.09 ENLARGEMENT OF GASTRIC FOLDS

A. The normal rugal folds of the stomach should not exceed 1 cm in width.
B. Differential diagnosis
   1. Acute gastritis may be caused by several conditions
      a. Alcoholic gastritis
      b. Antral gastritis secondary to peptic ulcer disease
      c. Gastritis secondary to ingestion of corrosive agents
      d. Inflammatory gastritis secondary to bacterial infection
   2. Lymphoma
   3. Menetrier's disease
      a. This is a protein-losing enteropathy that results in large mucosal folds predominantly in the body and fundus of the stomach.
   4. Adenocarcinoma
   5. Gastric varices
      a. Visualized as multiple, serpiginous filling defects present in the fundus. Usually are associated with esophageal varices. As an isolated finding may suggest splenic vein thrombosis.
   6. Lymphoid hyperplasia (pseudolymphoma)
   7. Eosinophilic gastroenteritis
   8. Crohn's disease

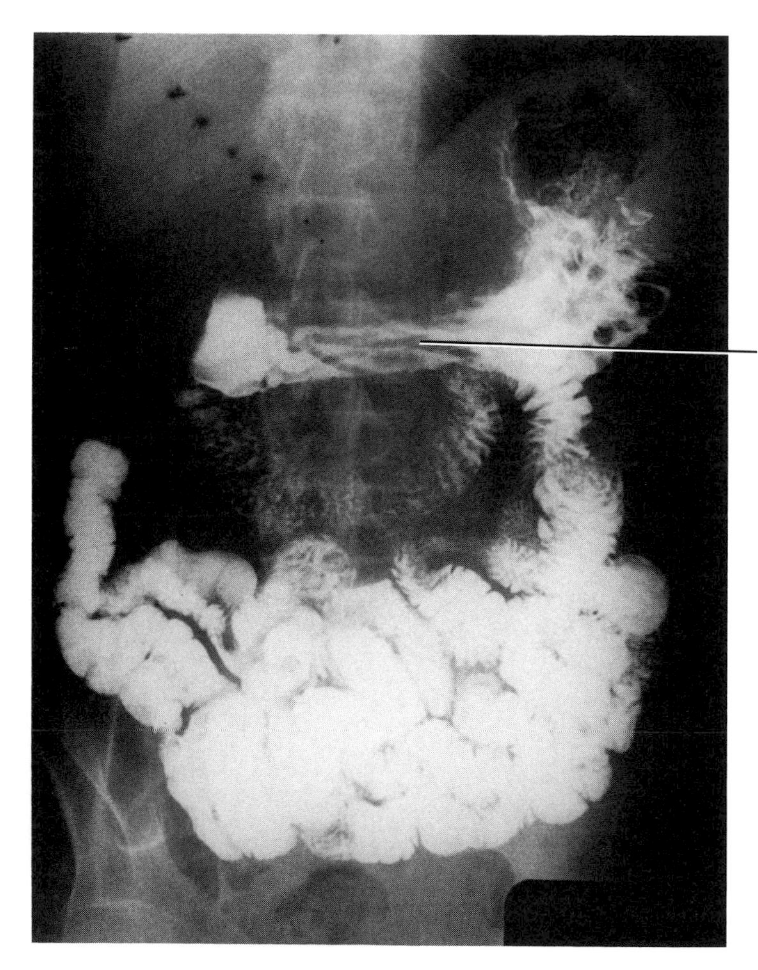

Figure 4.09. Enlargement of gastric folds.

4.10 FILLING DEFECTS WITHIN THE STOMACH

A. Differential diagnosis
   1. Neoplasm
      a. Benign
         (1) Most common is a hyperplastic polyp—a well-defined lesion, often multiple, that results from chronic gastritis.
         (2) Hamartoma results in multiple defects. Hamartomas are associated with Peutz-Jeghers syndrome.
         (3) Adenomatous polyp may undergo malignant transformation and is usually greater than 2 cm. Adenomatous polyps are associated with familial polyposis syndrome and with pernicious anemia.
         (4) Other benign lesions include leiomyoma, lipoma, and neurofibroma.
      b. Malignant
         (1) Metastatic lesions are often multiple and tend to ulcerate centrally, resulting in a "target" appearance. They are most often due to melanoma, lung carcinoma, breast carcinoma, and Kaposi's sarcoma.
         (2) Adenocarcinoma has a variable appearance, but the presence of irregularity and possible ulceration are suggestive of a malignant nature.
         (3) Lymphoma often appears similar to adenocarcinoma.
         (4) Leiomyosarcoma is usually a large neoplasm that affects the body of the stomach.
   2. Foreign body
   3. Ectopic pancreas presents as a "target" lesion (central collection of barium) usually within the gastric antrum along the greater curvature.
   4. Bezoars are large masses secondary to hairballs (trichobezoar) or vegetable matter (phytobezoar).
   5. Previous surgery, e.g., Nissen fundoplication for hiatal hernia repair

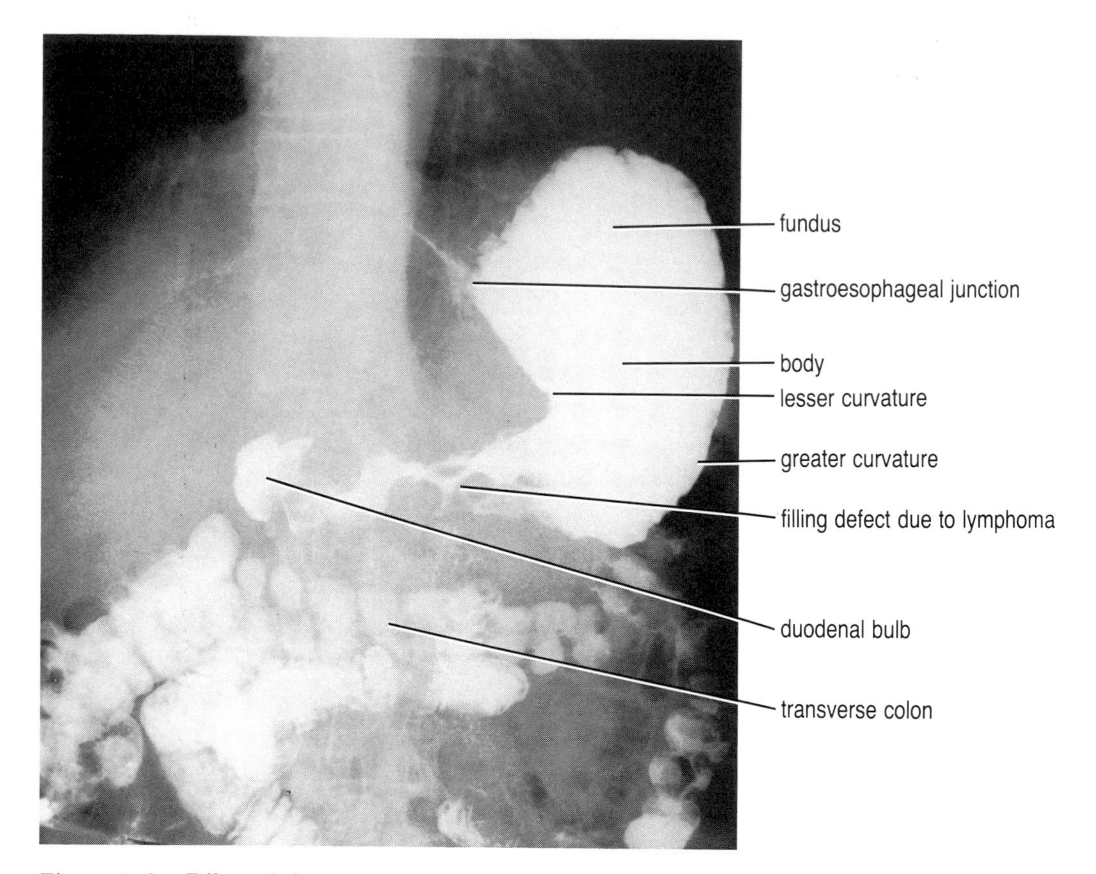

Figure 4.10. Filling defects within the stomach.

4.11 GASTRIC OUTLET OBSTRUCTION AND DILATATION

A. Dilatation of the stomach results in gaseous distention and often a mottled appearance owing to retained food particles and secretions.
B. Differential diagnosis
   1. Peptic ulcer disease
      a. This is the most common cause of gastric outlet obstruction in the adult population. Obstruction results from edema and spasm of the duodenal bulb.
   2. Malignant neoplasm
   3. Diabetes mellitus
      a. Chronic gastric dilatation, known as gastric paresis, may result from neuropathy.
   4. Metastasis
   5. Gastric volvulus
      a. May occur in the presence of a paraesophageal hernia
   6. Hypertrophic pyloric stenosis
   7. Neuromuscular dysfunction
   8. Status postvagotomy
   9. Postoperative ileus
   10. Abdominal trauma
   11. Annular pancreas

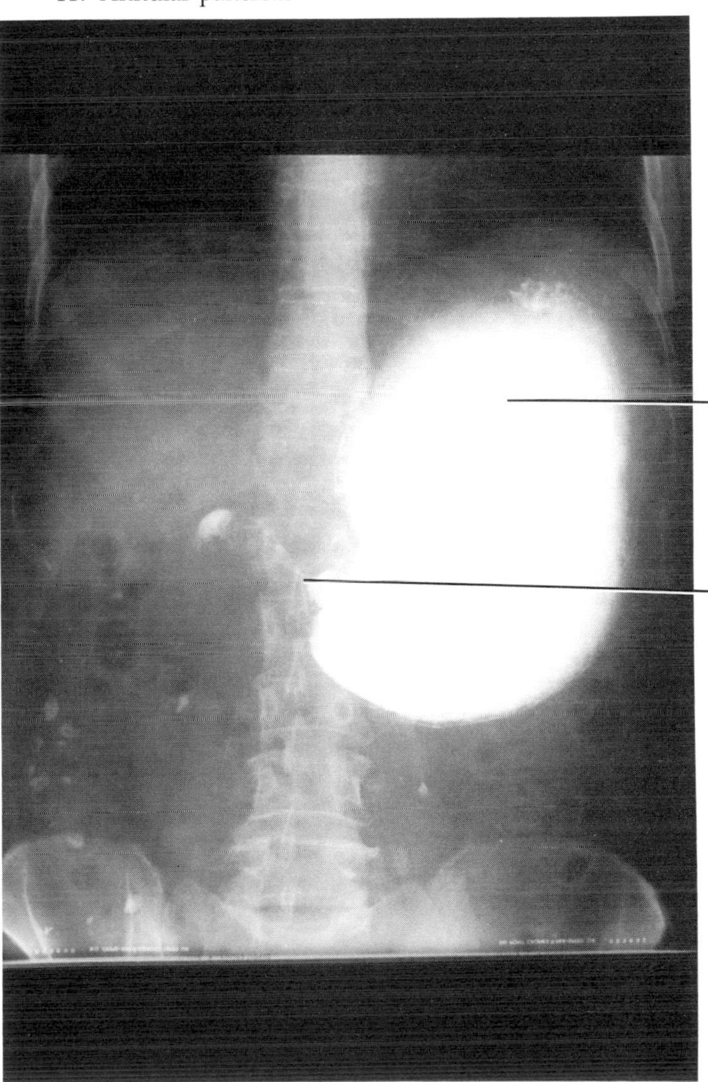

Figure 4.11. Gastric outlet obstruction and dilatation.

4.12 GASTRIC AND DUODENAL ULCERS

A. Peptic ulcer disease is a common condition that most often affects men. It is composed of duodenal ulcers, gastric ulcers, and Zollinger-Ellison syndrome.
B. Duodenal ulcers
   1. These account for most peptic ulcers.
   2. Most duodenal ulcers occur within the duodenal bulb.
C. Approximately 5% of the ulcers are postbulbar.
D. Radiographic signs of duodenal ulcers on UGI examination
   1. Deformity of the duodenal bulb due to spasm and edema
   2. The presence of an ulcer crater. Visualized in profile as a collection of barium that extends beyond the lumen. Visualized en face as a central collection of barium with a surrounding radiolucent rim of edema. Linear streaks of barium are seen radiating to the ulcer.
   3. Thickened duodenal folds greater than 4 mm are suggestive of duodenitis.
E. Clinical signs include epigastric pain that occurs several hours after a meal. The pain is often relieved by eating.
F. Gastric ulcers
   1. Most gastric ulcers are benign, but the presence of malignancy must be excluded.
   2. Most gastric ulcers occur along the lesser curvature of the stomach in the region of the antrum.
   3. Benign gastric ulcers appear similar to duodenal ulcers on UGI exam.
   4. If the ulcer crater does not extend beyond the lumen and if there is irregularity or nodularity of the folds and they do not radiate to the ulcer, a malignant ulcer should be considered.
   5. Clinical signs also include epigastric pain, but there may be no relief with eating and possibly exacerbation of the pain.
G. Zollinger-Ellison syndrome
   1. This is a non-beta islet cell tumor that secretes excessive gastrin resulting in multiple ulcers in atypical locations.
   2. Mucosal folds of both the stomach and duodenum may be thickened.
H. Complications of peptic ulcer disease
   1. Perforation: most perforations occur through the anterior portion of the duodenal bulb.
   2. Hemorrhage
   3. Gastric outlet obstruction
   4. Pancreatitis

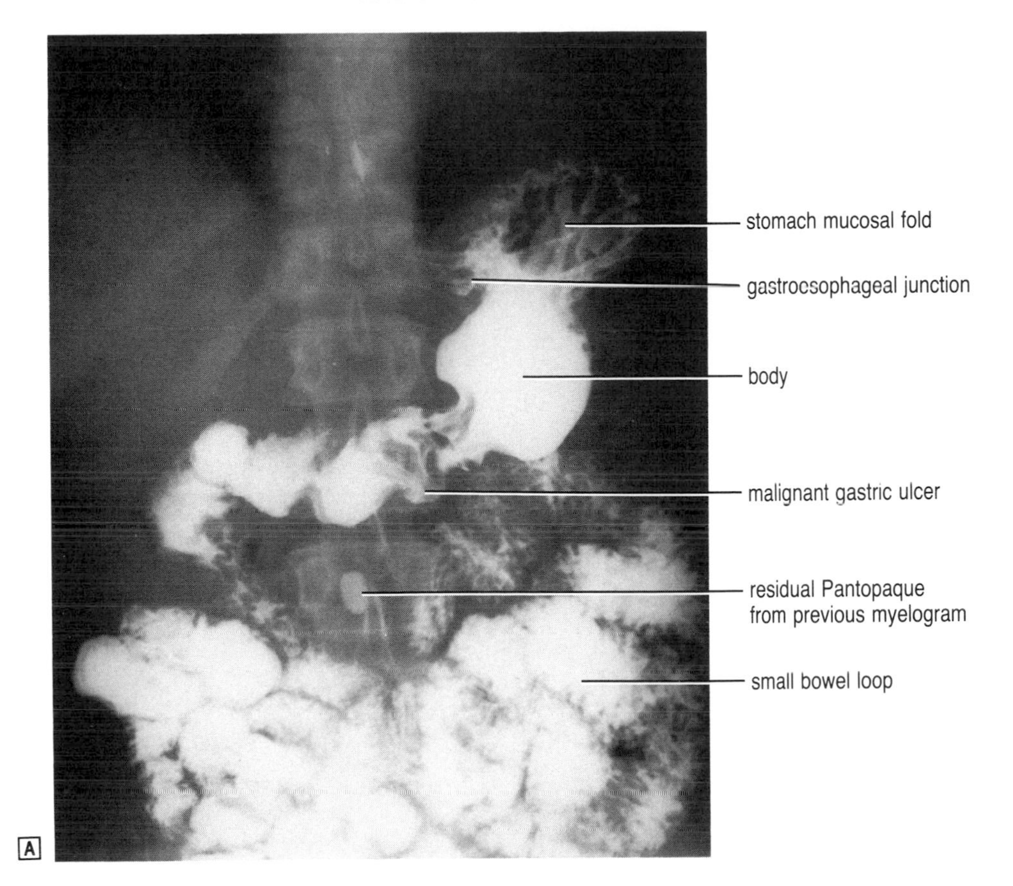

Figure 4.12. *A,* Gastric and duodenal ulcers.

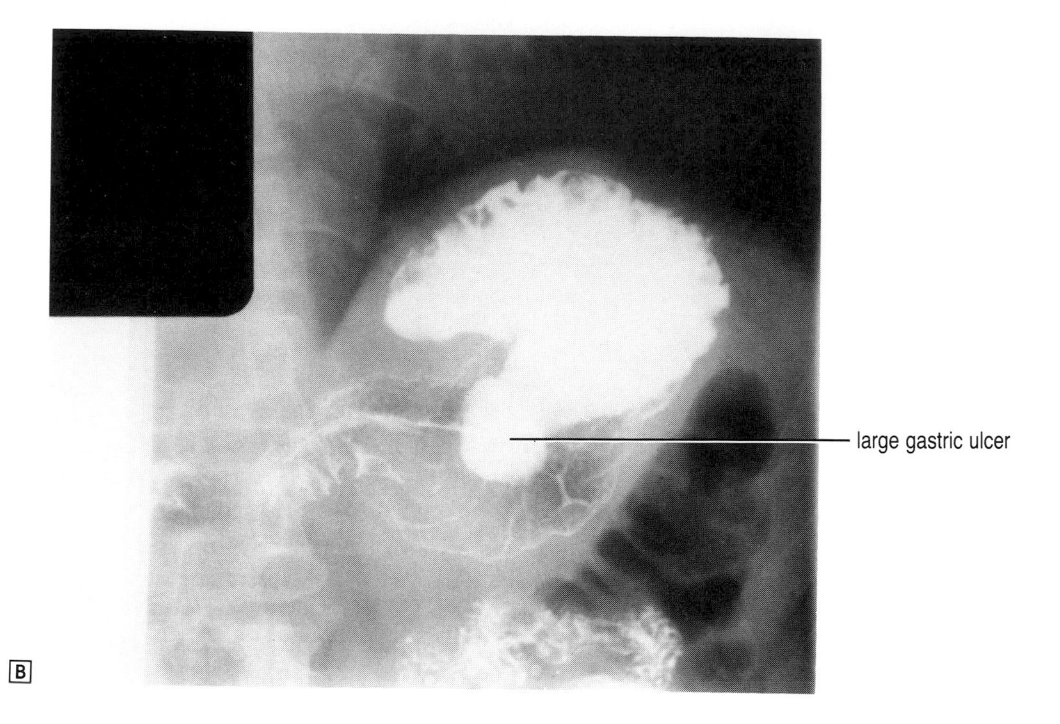

Figure 4.12. *B,* Gastric and duodenal ulcers.

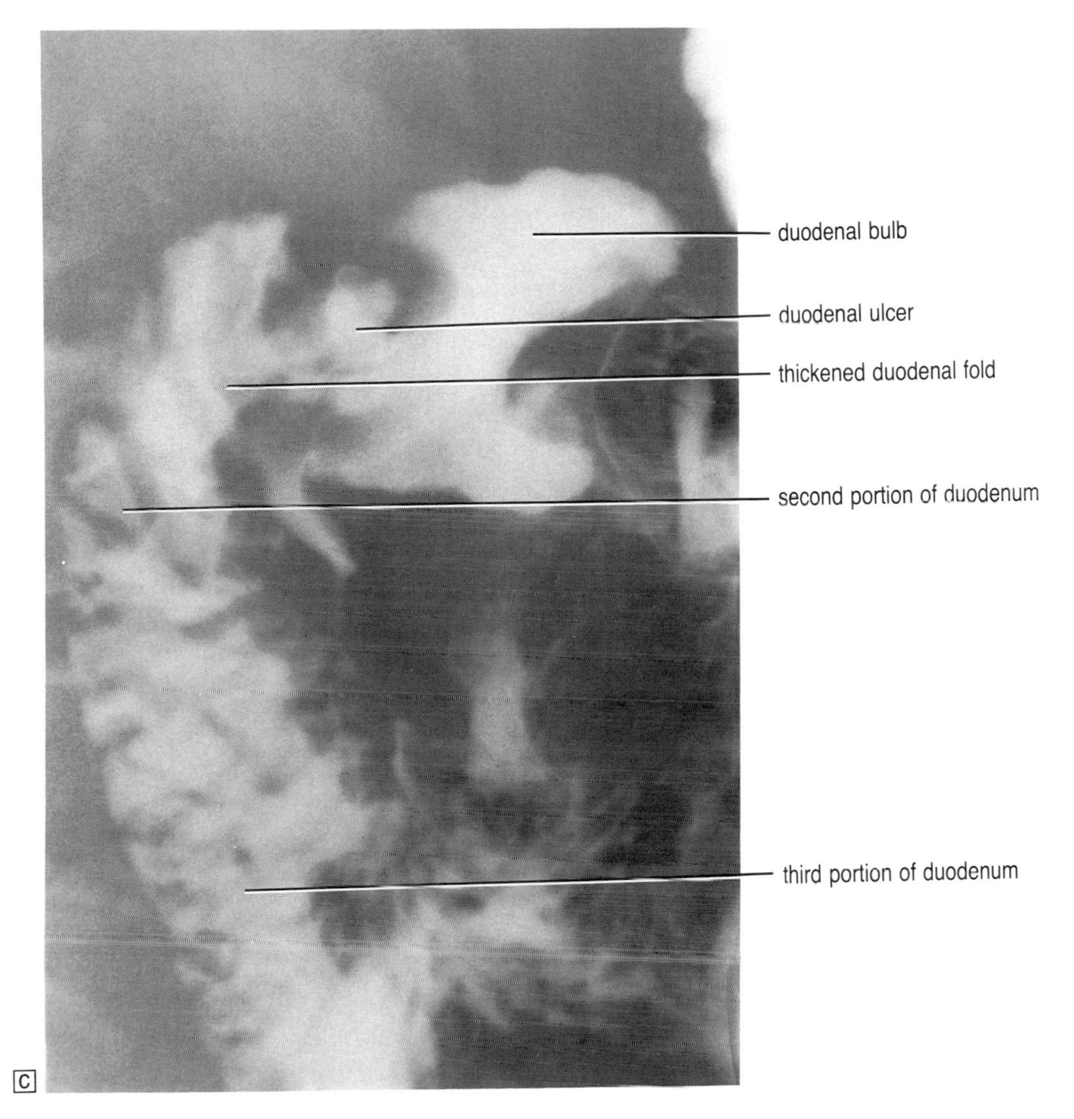

Figure 4.12. C, Gastric and duodenal ulcers.

4.13 GALLBLADDER DISEASE

A. Most gallstones are radiolucent because they are composed of cholesterol. Approximately 20% are radiopaque because they contain calcium bilirubinate. Plain films of the abdomen demonstrate the gallstones in the right upper quadrant of the abdomen. Additional oblique views may help localize the calcifications and exclude renal stones.

B. Gallstone ileus is the result of erosion of a gallstone through the wall of the gallbladder and formation of a fistula with the small bowel. If the stone is large enough, it may result in mechanical obstruction of the small bowel (see Sec. 4.15). Multiple loops of dilated small bowel are present with air in the biliary tree.

C. A porcelain gallbladder is visualized as widespread calcification of the gallbladder wall due to chronic inflammation. This condition is most common in women and is associated with a significant risk of gallbladder carcinoma.

D. Emphysematous cholecystitis, most often seen in diabetics, is visualized as air within the gallbladder wall due to infection. There is an increased risk of perforation of the gallbladder.

E. Acute cholecystitis
   1. The clinical setting of acute cholecystitis consists of acute onset of right upper quadrant pain, fever, and elevated white count. The patient may experience nausea, vomiting, and anorexia.
   2. Acute cholecystitis results from cystic duct obstruction by a calculus. Approximately 10% of the cases are due to acalculous cholecystitis.
   3. The radiologic diagnosis of acute cholecystitis can be made when ultrasound examination of the gallbladder reveals the presence of calculi in combination with the appropriate clinical presentation.
   4. Hepatobiliary imaging is an excellent modality for detection of acute cholecystitis. This is a nuclear medicine test in which technetium 99m is labeled to iminodiacetic acid. In the normal patient, the radionuclide is rapidly excreted by the liver and activity is normally present in the gallbladder by 30 minutes. Activity is also identified within the biliary tree. It is present within the common bile duct and is seen entering the duodenum.
   5. In the presence of acute cholecystitis, the radionuclide is not able to enter the gallbladder because of obstruction of the cystic duct and inflammation. The hepatobiliary scan reveals nonvisualization of the gallbladder.
   6. Delayed visualization of the gallbladder is compatible with chronic cholecystitis.

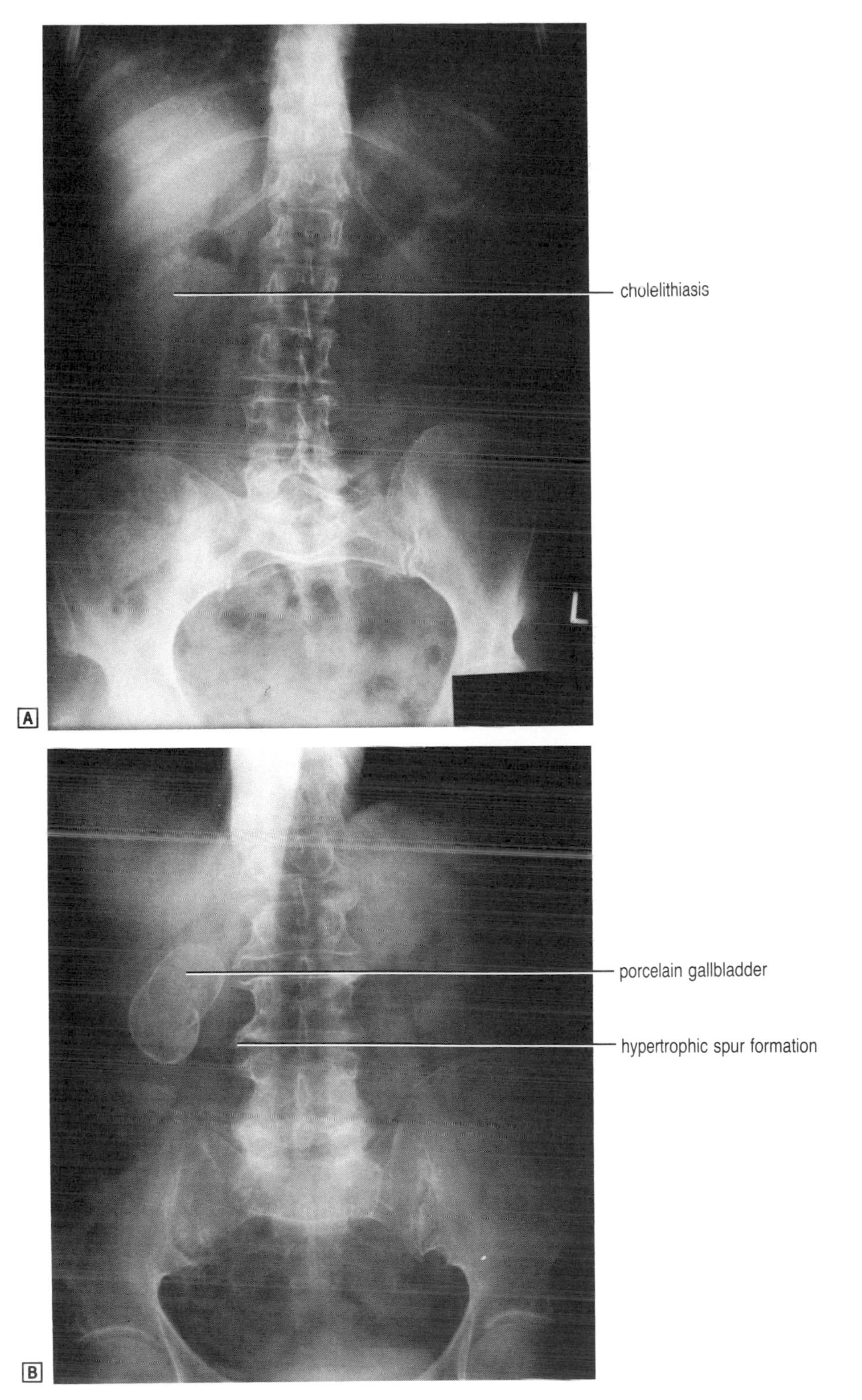

Figure 4.13. *A*, Gallbladder disease. *B*, Gallbladder disease.

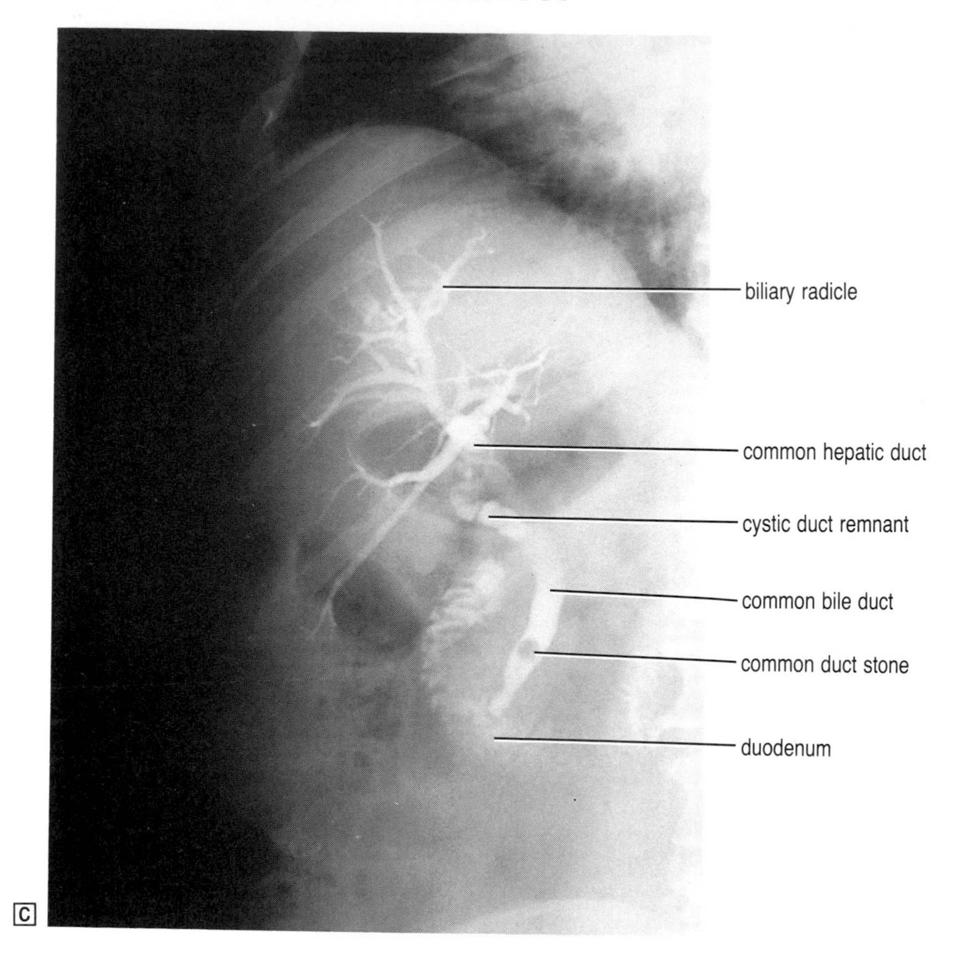

Figure 4.13. C, Gallbladder disease.

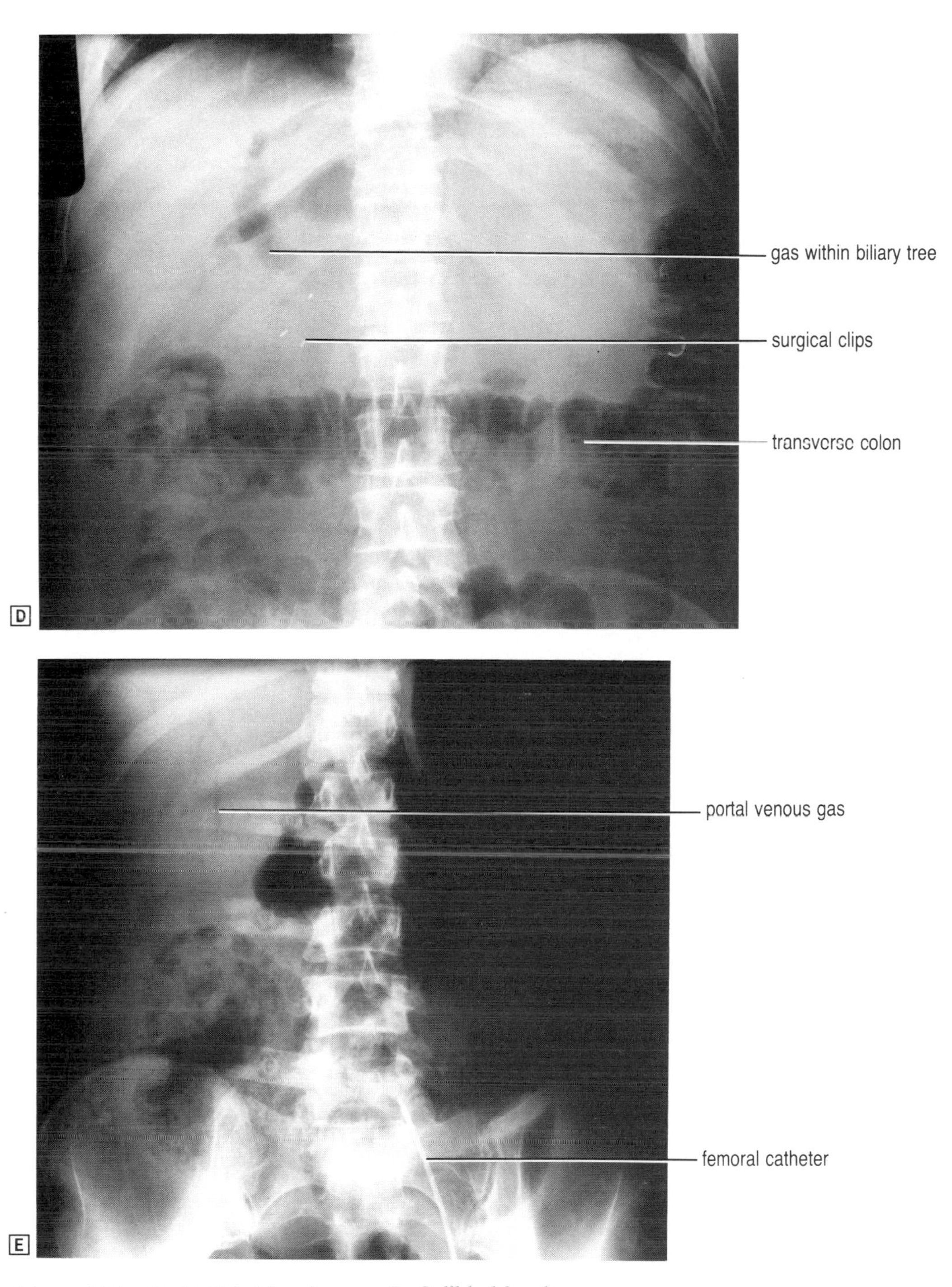

Figure 4.13. *D,* Gallbladder disease. *E,* Gallbladder disease.

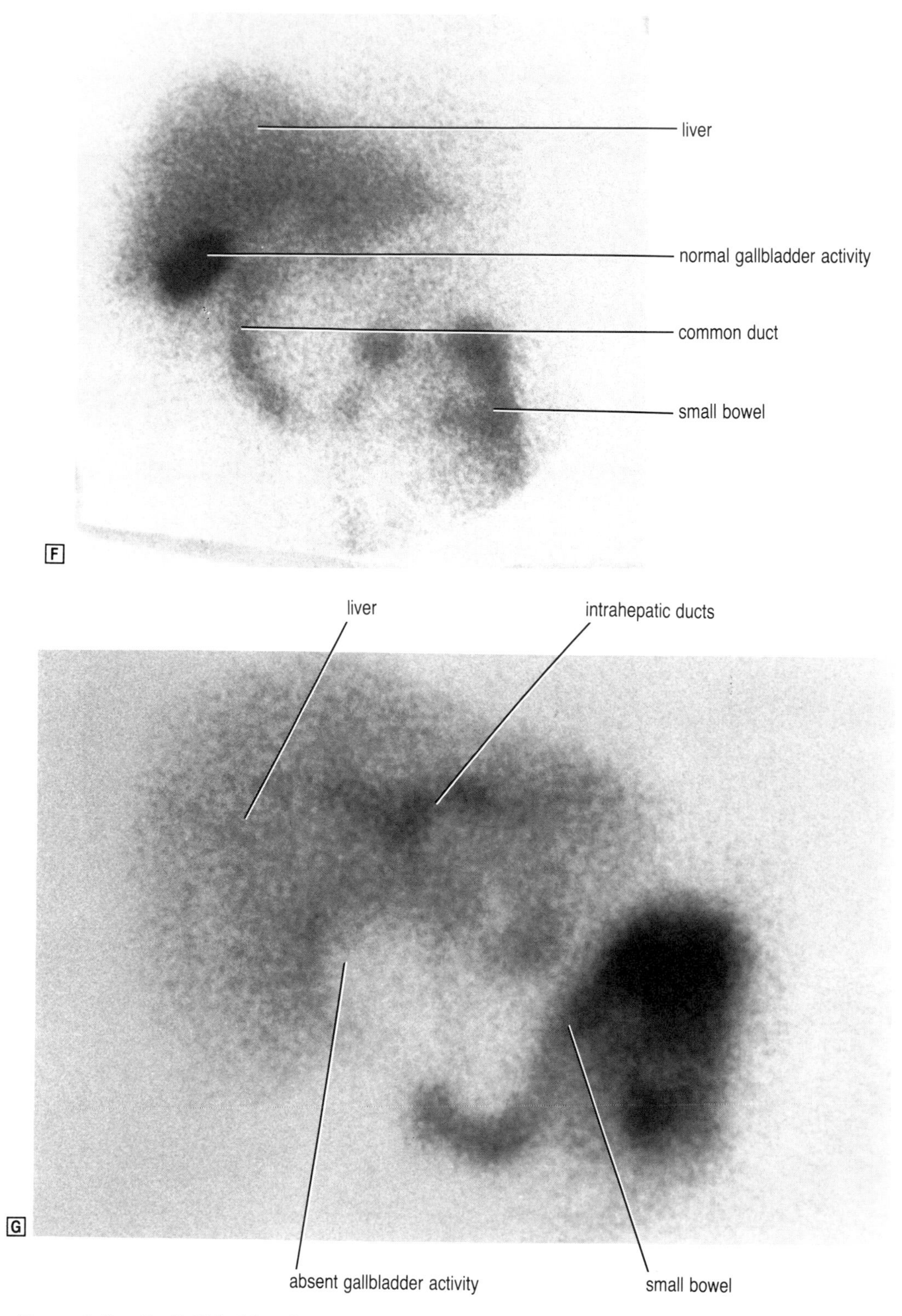

Figure 4.13. *F*, Gallbladder disease. *G*, Gallbladder disease.

4.14 CROHN'S DISEASE (REGIONAL ENTERITIS)

A. Is an inflammatory bowel disease that usually affects individuals between 20 and 30 years of age
   1. Most often involves the terminal ileum and other areas of the small bowel
   2. May also involve colon, esophagus, and stomach

B. Radiographically visualized as mucosal thickening with narrowing of the bowel lumen due to spasm and later development of fibrosis, known as the "string sign"

C. Ulcers occur that are transmural lesions.

D. Involvement produces a "cobblestone" appearance.

E. Areas of involvement are interrupted by normal-appearing bowel, resulting in "skip" lesions.

F. The rectum is uninvolved in most cases.

G. Complications
   1. Fistula formation
   2. Abscess formation
   3. Bowel obstruction
   4. Cholelithiasis
   5. Renal lithiasis
   6. Hydronephrosis
   7. Ankylosing spondylitis
   8. Cholangitis

H. Presentation
   1. Abdominal pain
   2. Episodic diarrhea
   3. Occult blood in stool
   4. Weight loss
   5. Fever

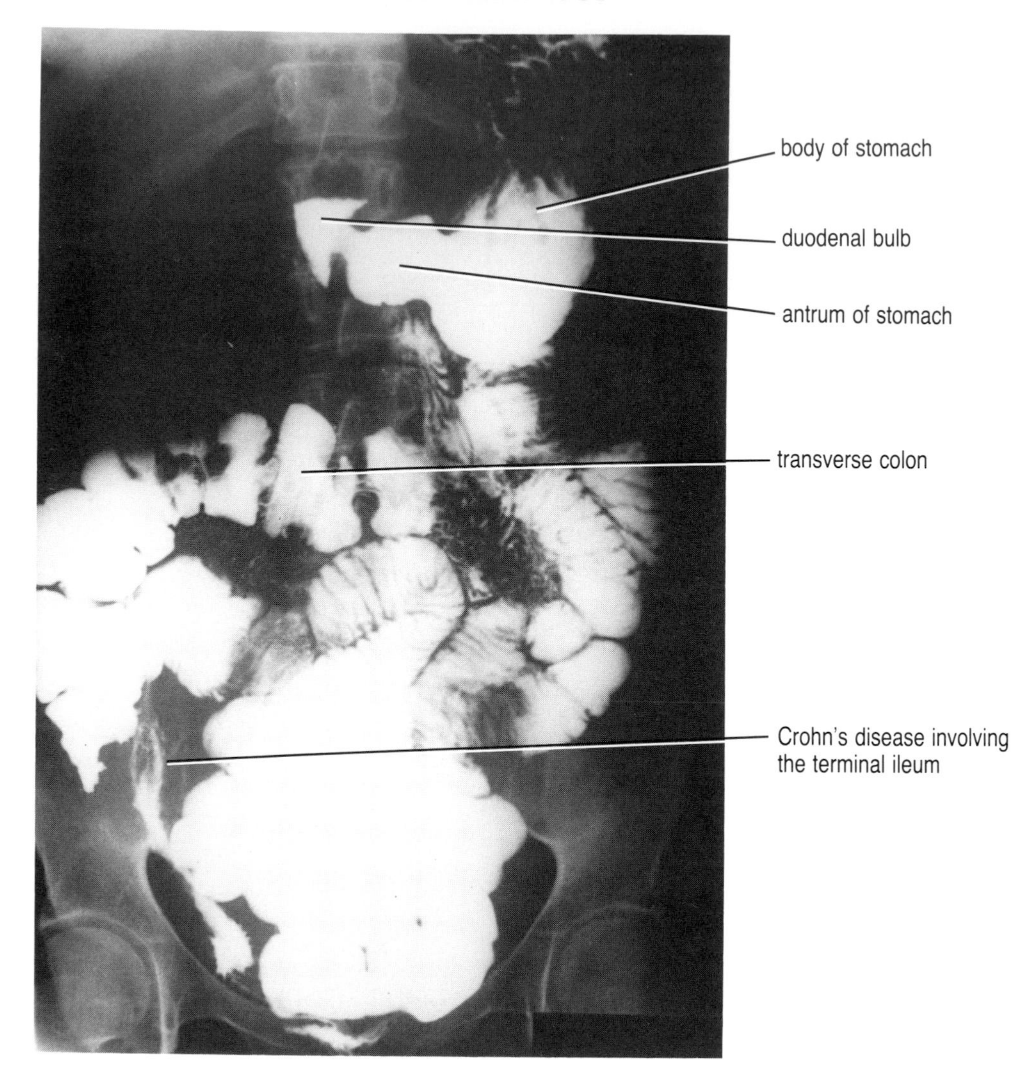

Figure 4.14. Crohn's disease (regional enteritis).

4.15 BOWEL OBSTRUCTION AND ILEUS

A. Small bowel obstruction
   1. Mechanical obstruction of the small bowel results in gaseous distention of the small bowel proximal to the obstruction.
   2. If a complete obstruction is present, gas is only visualized distal to the obstruction early in the course.
   3. Distended small bowel loops are greater than 3 cm in width, are centrally located within the abdomen, have parallel indentations known as valvulae conniventes, and form a stepladder configuration when obstructed.
   4. An erect view of the abdomen demonstrates the presence of air fluid levels that are located at different levels.
   5. A paralytic (adynamic) ileus can be excluded because of the lack of large bowel gas.

B. Differential diagnosis
   1. Adhesions from previous abdominal surgery are the most common cause.
   2. Hernias (inguinal, umbilical, femoral, and incisional) are the next most common cause.
   3. Neoplasm
   4. Gallstone ileus
   5. Stricture (Crohn's disease, ichemia, tuberculosis)
   6. Intussusception

C. Large bowel obstruction
   1. The most common cause of large bowel obstruction is colon carcinoma.
   2. Mechanical obstruction of the large bowel results in gaseous distention of the large bowel proximal to the obstruction.
   3. The transverse colon is abnormally distended if its width is greater than 6 cm.
   4. The cecum is at risk for perforation in the acute setting if it measures greater than 9 cm.
   5. Colonic gas is identified by its peripheral location and the presence of irregularly spaced indentations known as haustral markings.
   6. If the ileocecal valve is competent, the entire colon proximal to the obstruction dilates and the cecum is at risk for perforation. An incompetent valve results in dilatation of small bowel loops as well.
   7. Cecal volvulus
      a. The cecum may twist on its mesentery and result in obstruction. Most often visualized as an air-distended bean-shaped mass in the left upper quadrant of the abdomen.
   8. Sigmoid volvulus
      a. A redundant loop of sigmoid colon may twist on its mesentery and also result in obstruction. Is usually visualized as an air-distended inverted "U"-shaped mass that extends out of the pelvis.
      b. If bowel obstruction is suspected, a barium enema allows diagnosis and localization of the obstruction, and possible therapeutic reduction.

D. Ileus
      a. A paralytic ileus (adynamic) results in diffuse gaseous distention of the small and large bowel.
      b. Air fluid levels may be present on an erect view, but the fluid levels are located on the same plane.
      c. Differential diagnosis
         (1) Postoperative ileus
         (2) Trauma
         (3) Secondary to medication
         (4) Peritonitis
         (5) Electrolyte imbalance
      d. A localized ileus (sentinel loop) may result in response to an inflammatory process such as appendicitis, pancreatitis, or cholecystitis.

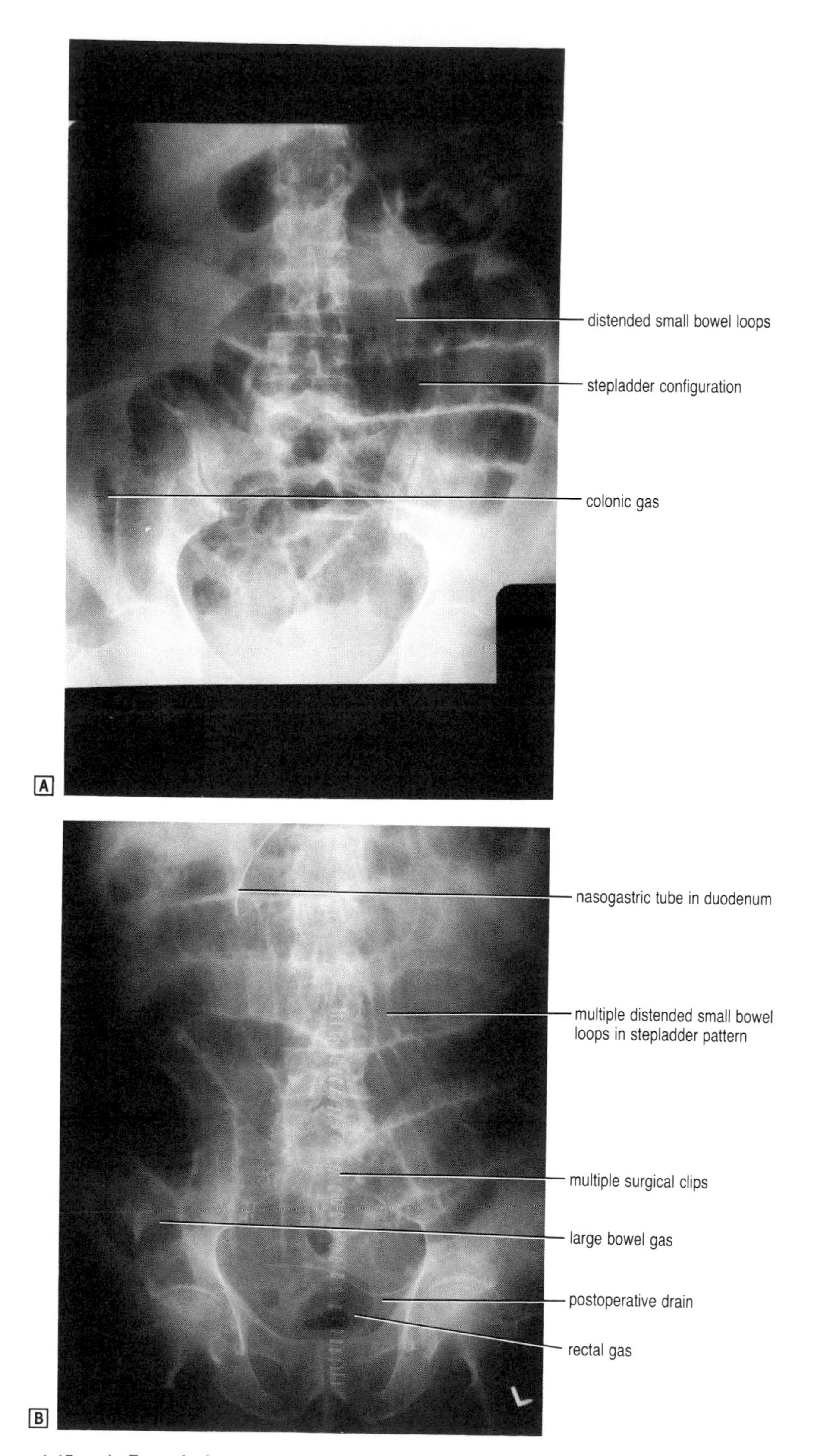

Figure 4.15. *A,* Bowel obstruction and ileus. *B,* Bowel obstruction and ileus.

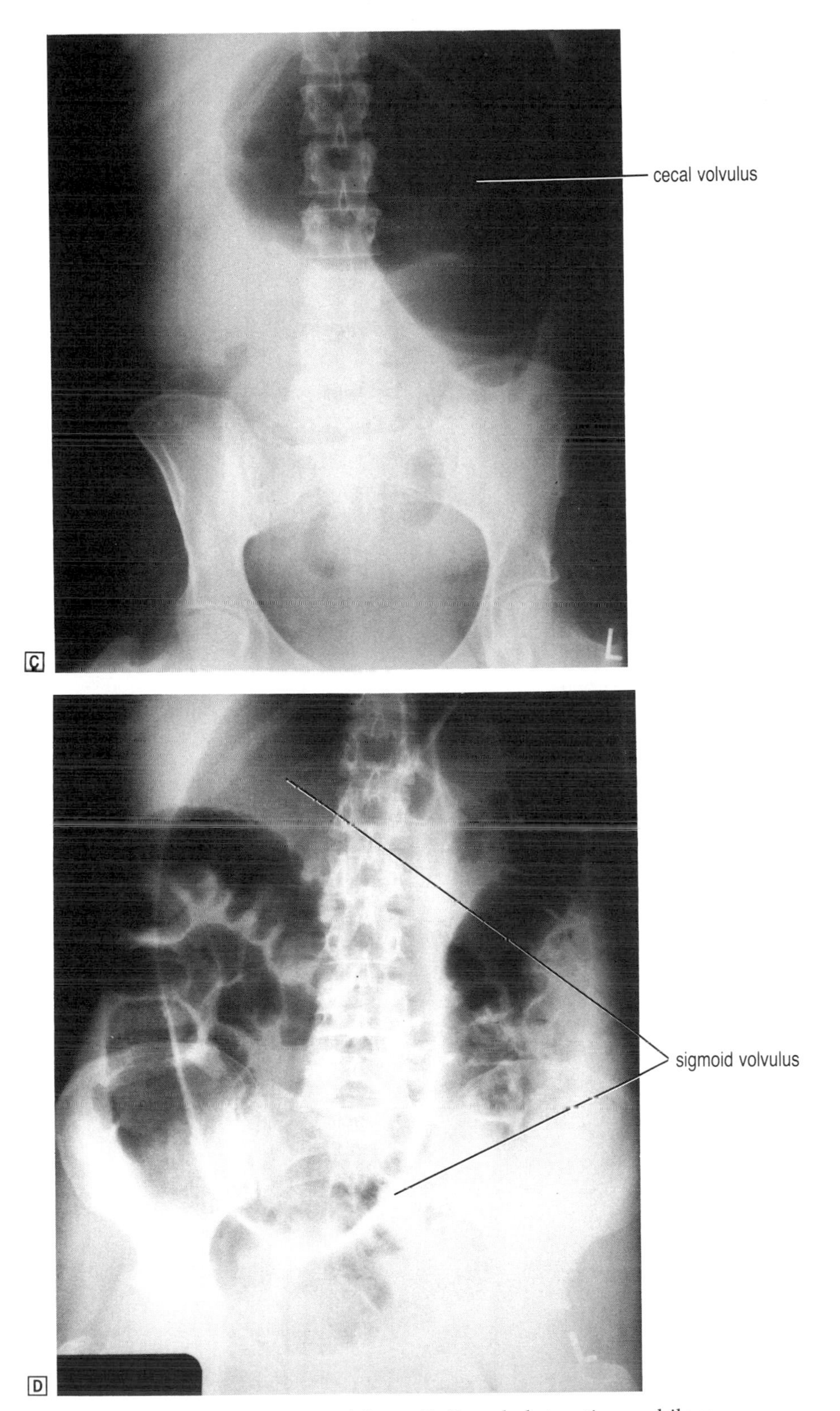

Figure 4.15. *C*, Bowel obstruction and ileus. *D*, Bowel obstruction and ileus.

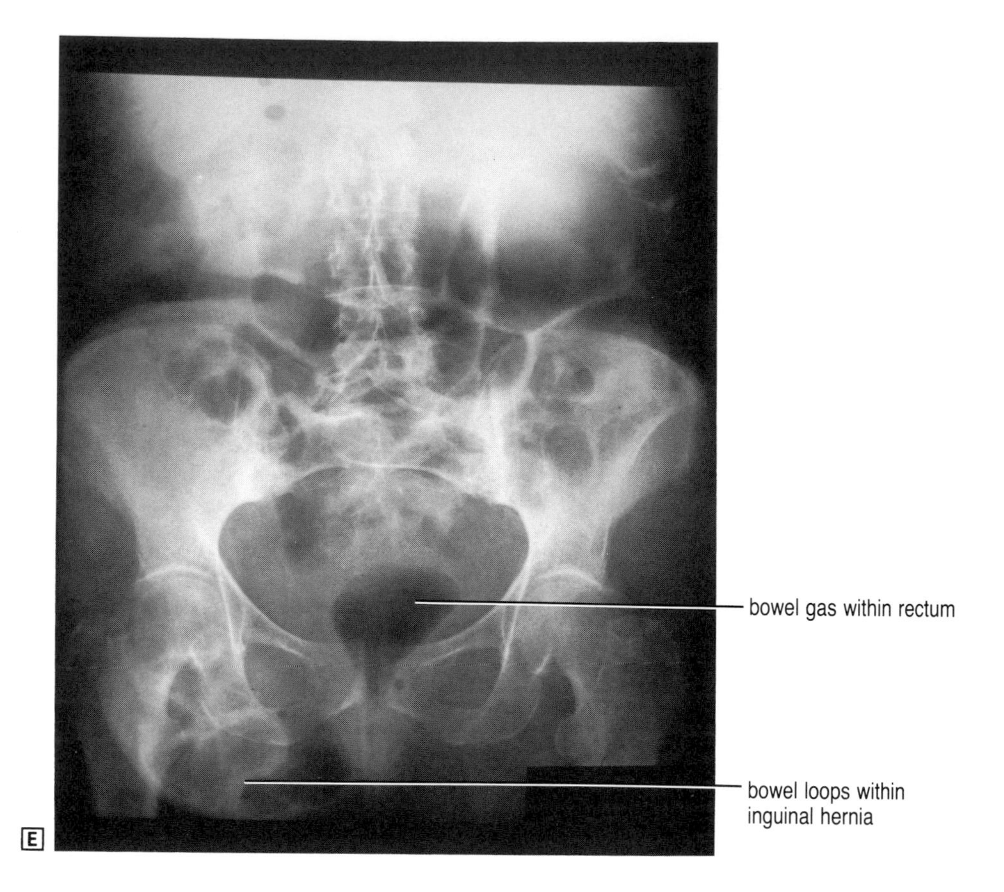

Figure 4.15. *E*, Bowel obstruction and ileus.

4.16 ULCERATIVE COLITIS

A. Is an inflammatory bowel disease that usually affects individuals between 20 and 40 years of age.
B. Most often originates in the rectum
C. The disease process affects the colon in a continuous fashion and may involve the terminal ileum ("backwash ileitis").
D. Roentgenograms may demonstrate a normal gas pattern or may reveal gaseous distention of the colon with mucosal edema manifested by "thumbprinting" (see Sec. 4.19). Pneumoperitoneum (see Sec. 4.03) or pneumatosis (see Sec. 4.21) may also be visualized.
E. Barium enema reveals multiple superficial ulcerations seen as multiple small pinpoint collections of barium. The ulcerations are superficial, involving the mucosa.
F. Pseudopolyps representing hypertrophy of normal mucosa as superficial ulcerations heal may be visualized.
G. Complications
   1. Increased risk of colon cancer
   2. Toxic megacolon
   3. Stricture formation
   4. Fistula formation
   5. Ankylosing spondylitis
   6. Arthritis
   7. Cholangitis
H. Presentation
   1. Episodic attacks
   2. Abdominal pain
   3. Bloody diarrhea
   4. Weight loss
   5. Fever
I. Toxic megacolon is a life-threatening complication of ulcerative colitis. The colon appears distended (width is greater than 6 cm). Mucosal edema visualized as "thumbprinting" may be seen. Pneumatosis coli may also be visualized indicating impending perforation. The colon is at great risk for perforation owing to its fragile state. Barium enema is contraindicated in the acute phase. Toxic megacolon is associated with systemic toxicity.

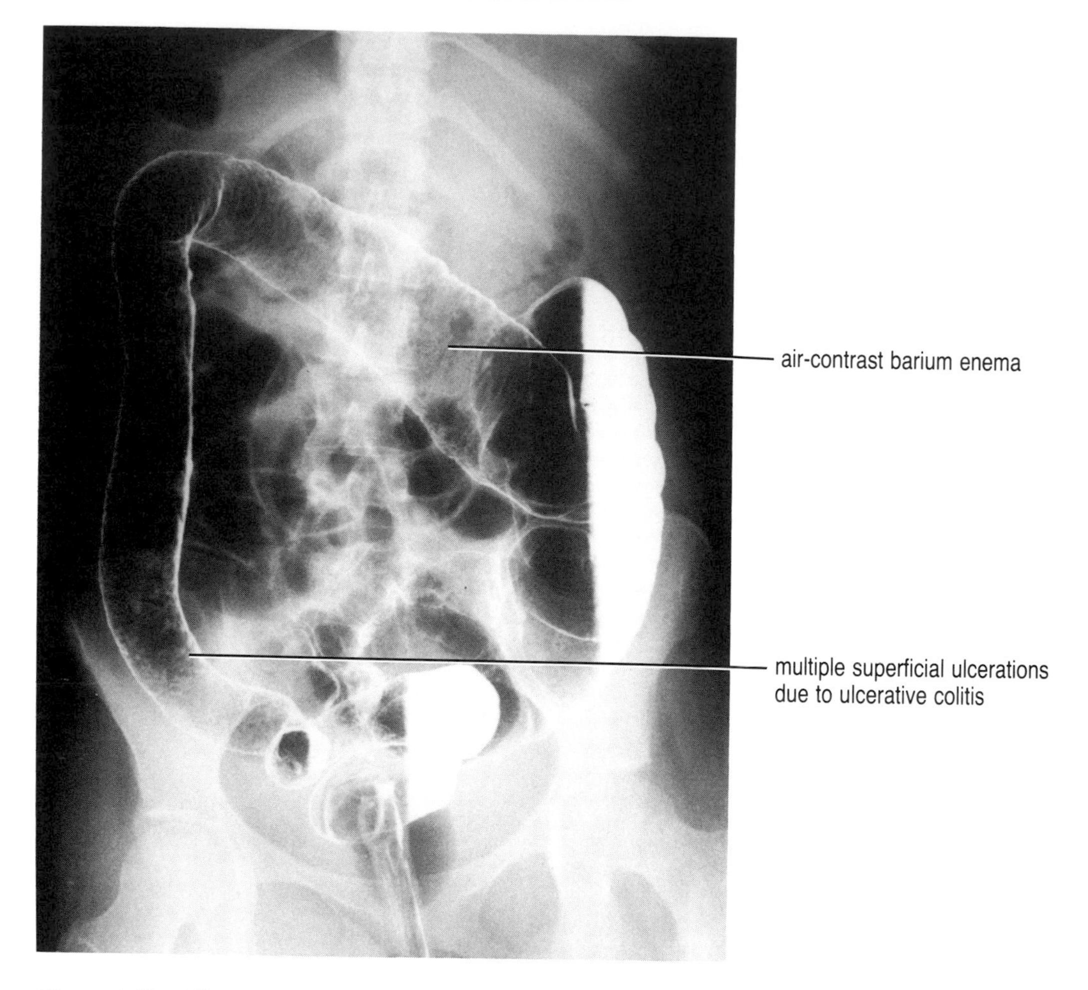

Figure 4.16. Ulcerative colitis.

4.17 COLONIC POLYPS

A. Colonic polyps are a common finding on barium examination of the colon. The colon must be thoroughly cleansed prior to examination because retained fecal debris may mask the presence of polypoid lesions.
B. Polyps are visualized on a single contrast barium enema as filling defects. A double contrast exam reveals a barium-coated filling defect.
C. Diverticula seen en face may mimic a polyp.
D. Polyps may have a stalk (pedunculated) or may be sessile.
E. Types of polyps
   1. Most common polyp is the hyperplastic polyp, which is less than 5 mm in size and represents a benign lesion.
   2. Adenomatous polyp is usually larger in size and is a premalignant lesion.
   3. Villous adenomas are usually larger than 2 cm and appear irregular and bulky. These are premalignant lesions most often found in the rectosigmoid region.
   4. Other benign lesions include hamartoma, inflammatory polyps, and lipomas.
F. The larger the polyp, the greater the chance of malignancy.
G. Most individuals with polyps are asymptomatic, but they may present with rectal bleeding or occult blood in the stool.
H. Polyposis syndromes
   1. A polyposis syndrome should be considered if a polyp is identified in a young individual, if multiple polyps are present, or if colon cancer occurs before the age of 40.
      a. Gardner's syndrome
         (1) Multiple adenomatous polyps most often present in the rectum.
         (2) Autosomal dominant
         (3) A premalignant condition
         (4) Associated with lipomas, leiomyomas, osteomas of the paranasal sinuses
      b. Familial polyposis syndrome
         (1) Multiple adenomatous polyps most often present in the rectosigmoid colon.
         (2) Autosomal dominant
         (3) Affects young adults
         (4) A premalignant condition
      c. Peutz-Jegher's syndrome
         (1) Multiple hamartomatous polyps most often in small bowel, less likely in stomach and colon
         (2) Autosomal dominant
         (3) Affects young children
         (4) Associated mucocutaneous pigmentation due to melanin deposition
      d. Juvenile polyposis
         (1) Multiple hamartomatous polyps are present within the large and small bowel.
         (2) Affects children
      e. Cronkhite-Canada syndrome
         (1) Multiple inflammatory polyps present within the stomach and colon
         (2) Affects middle-age adults
         (3) Associated with hair loss, hyperpigmentation, and atrophy of the fingernails and toenails
         (4) The polyps are benign, but the disease is ultimately fatal.

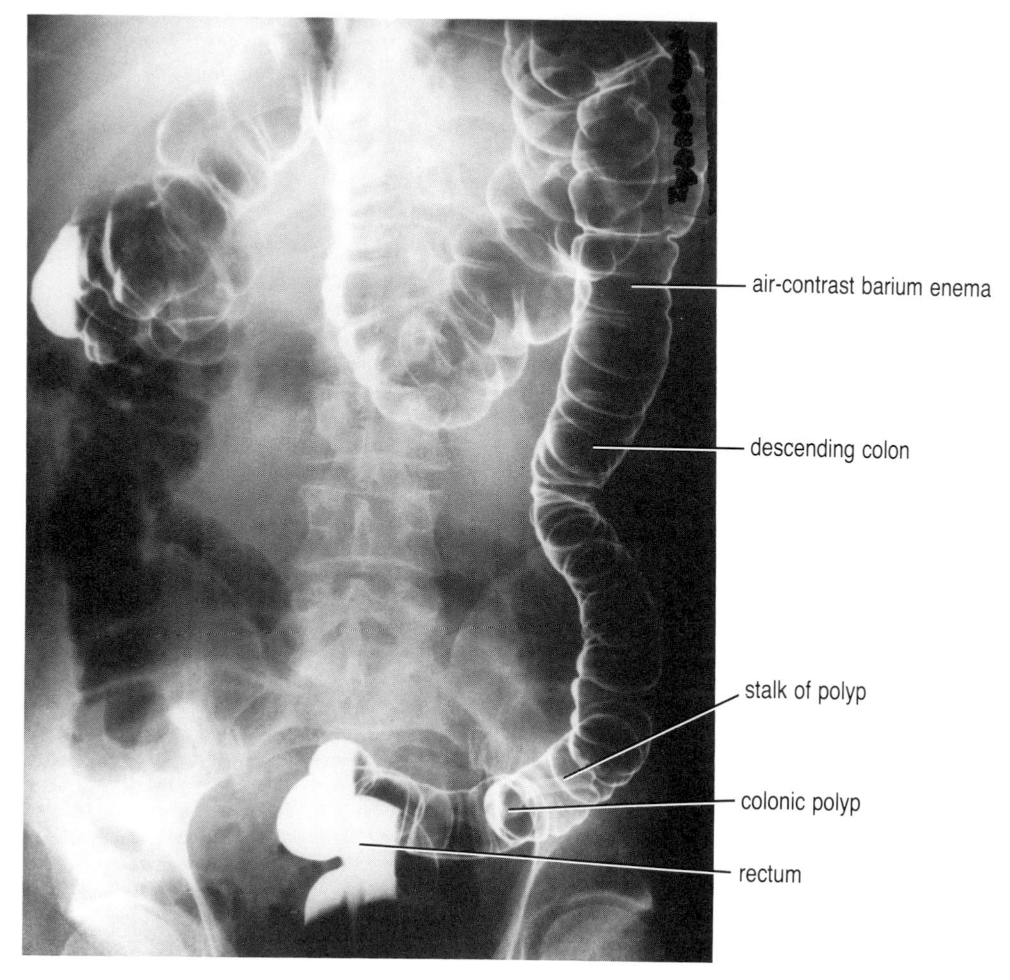

Figure 4.17. Colonic polyps.

4.18 COLONIC DIVERTICULOSIS/DIVERTICULITIS

A. Diverticulosis is one of the most common types of colonic disease demonstrated.
B. A diverticulum is an outpouching of mucosa and submucosa that herniates through the muscle wall at weak points where blood vessels penetrate the muscle layer.
C. A plain abdominal film may reveal residual contrast from a previous barium examination located within the diverticula.
D. Barium enema reveals multiple round collections of barium located outside the lumen.
E. Most often found in the sigmoid colon
F. Diverticula may simulate a polyp when visualized en face.
G. Most are asymptomatic, but patient may complain of intermittent abdominal pain
H. Complications
   1. Bleeding
      a. Diverticula of the ascending colon tend to bleed more than those of the descending colon.
   2. Diverticulitis
      a. Perforation of a diverticulum results in a localized inflammatory response
      b. Approximatley 20% of the individuals with diverticulosis will develop diverticulitis at some time.
      c. The involved segment of colon is narrowed due to inflammation and spasm. Area of involvement may resemble carcinoma.
      d. May result in abscess formation or a fistulous tract with the bladder, ureter, or vagina
      e. Ileus or colonic obstruction may also develop.
      f. Signs include fever, low abdominal pain, elevated white blood count, and possible palpable mass.

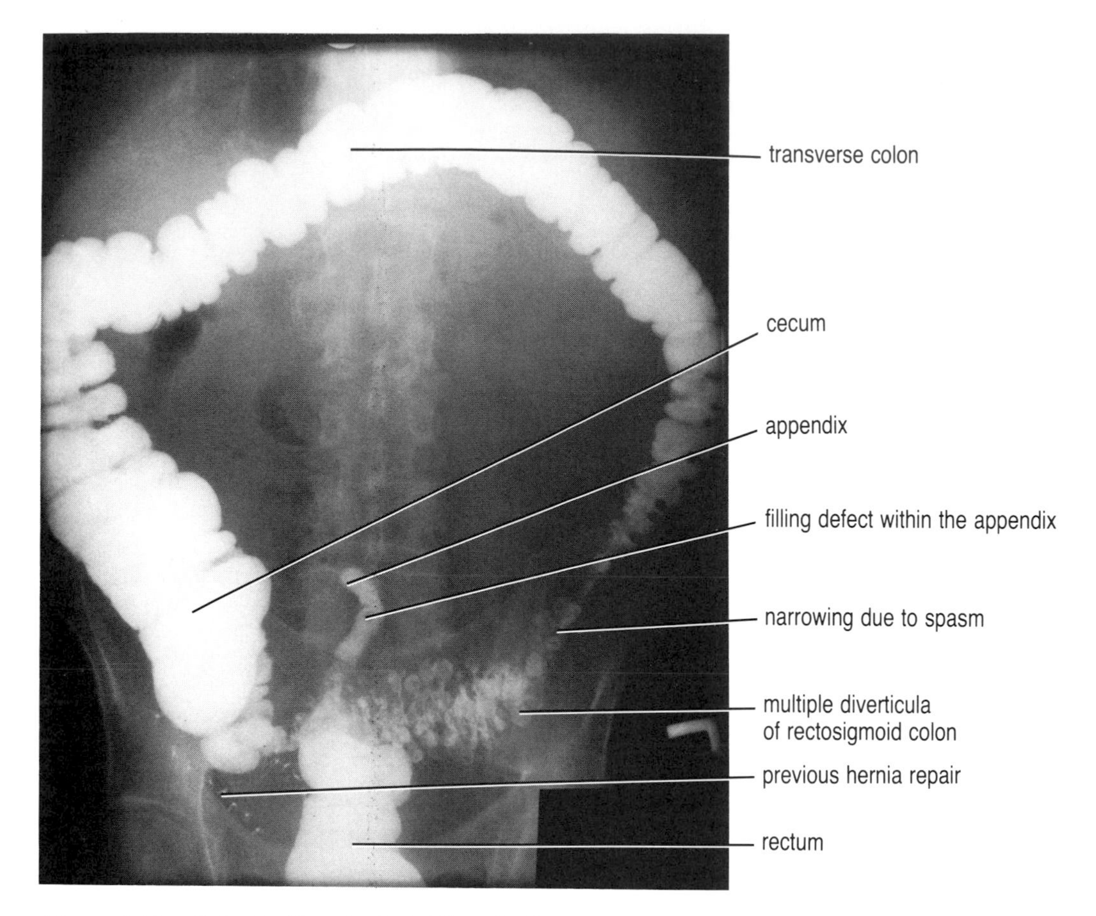

Figure 4.18. Colonic diverticulosis/diverticulitis.

4.19 COLON CANCER

A. Carcinoma of the colon is a common malignancy and is the third most frequent in occurrence behind carcinoma of the lung and breast.
B. Adenocarcinoma is the most common type of colon cancer.
C. Most individuals are over age 50.
D. Rectosigmoid colon is the most common site. The descending colon is the second most common followed by the cecum and ascending colon.
E. Lesions within the ascending colon tend to bleed and may produce an iron-deficiency anemia.
F. Lesions of the descending and rectosigmoid colon are more prone to cause obstruction and bloody stools.
G. The barium enema examination is an excellent cost-effective method of evaluation of the colon.
H. Thorough cleansing of the colon must be achieved before examination. Retained fecal debris impairs the ability to detect small polypoid lesions.
I. The colon may be examined with a single-contrast (solid column) or double-contrast (air contrast) method. The single-contrast exam is utilized in older less cooperative patients and in emergency situations in an unprepared colon, to exclude obstruction. The double-contrast exam provides excellent mucosal detail and can be utilized in most individuals following thorough cleansing of the colon.
J. Radiographically, carcinoma may be detected as small polypoid lesions, irregularity of the lumen, or the classic annular carcinoma that produces the "apple core" or "napkin ring" lesion.
K. Signs of colon cancer and predisposing factors
   1. Bloody stools
   2. Anemia
   3. Significant weight loss
   4. Abdominal pain
   5. New-onset constipation or diarrhea
   6. History of previous colon cancer, ulcerative colitis, or polyps
   7. Positive family history
L. Dukes' classification
   A. Involves the mucosa and submucosa but does not extend into the muscle layer
   B. Extends into the muscle layer
   C. Involves the serosa and lymph nodes
   D. Distant metastases

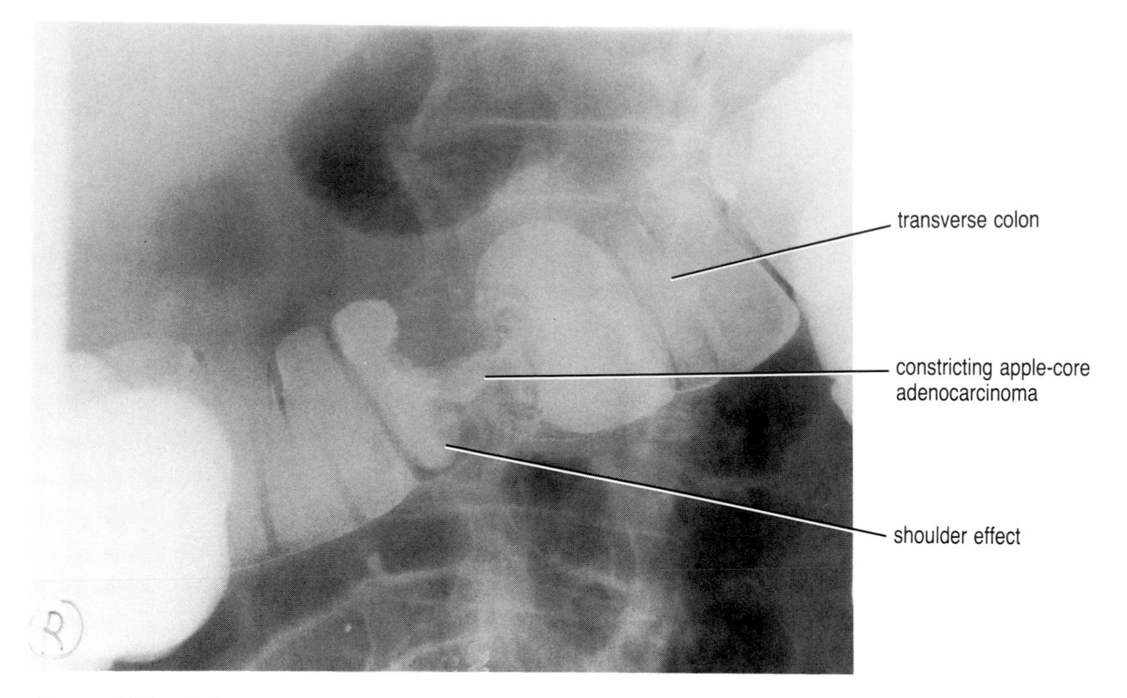

Figure 4.19. Colon cancer.

4.20 PNEUMATOSIS INTESTINALIS AND THUMBPRINTING OF THE COLON

I.

A. Pneumatosis is visualized as abnormal air collections that are located within the bowel wall and follow the contour of the involved loop.
B. May be visualized as linear lucencies in the bowel wall that parallel the bowel loop. Pneumatosis may also be seen as multiple, round, cystic air collections within the bowel wall.
C. Differential diagnosis
   1. Bowel infarction secondary to vascular occlusion
   2. Toxic megacolon secondary to ulcerative colitis (see Sec. 4.16)
   3. Necrotizing enterocolitis, seen in debilitated neonates
   4. Idiopathic—benign condition
   5. Secondary to COPD. Rupture of bleb with dissection of air along interstitium into the mediastinum and finally through diaphragmatic openings.

II.

A. Thumbprinting of the colon is visualized as multiple round indentations resembling thumbprints that follow the contour of the bowel loop.
B. Thumbprinting results from mucosal edema and submucosal hemorrhage.
C. Differential diagnosis
   1. Ischemic colitis or mesenteric infarction
   2. Submucosal hemorrhage secondary to abdominal trauma or iatrogenic anticoagulation
   3. Metastatic disease
   4. Lymphoma
   5. Inflammatory bowel disease
D. Ischemic colitis
   1. Vascular occlusion of the superior mesenteric or inferior mesenteric artery may result in bowel ischemia or infarction.
   2. Condition is most often due to occlusion of the inferior mesenteric artery that supplies the splenic flexure and descending colon.
   3. Radiographically visualized as thumbprinting as described previously. The involved segment of bowel may demonstrate gaseous distention or thickening of the bowel wall. Pneumatosis coli may be visualized.
   4. The development of portal venous gas is an ominous sign.
   5. Signs of ischemic colitis
      a. Abdominal pain
      b. Bloody diarrhea
      c. Emesis
      d. Abdominal distention

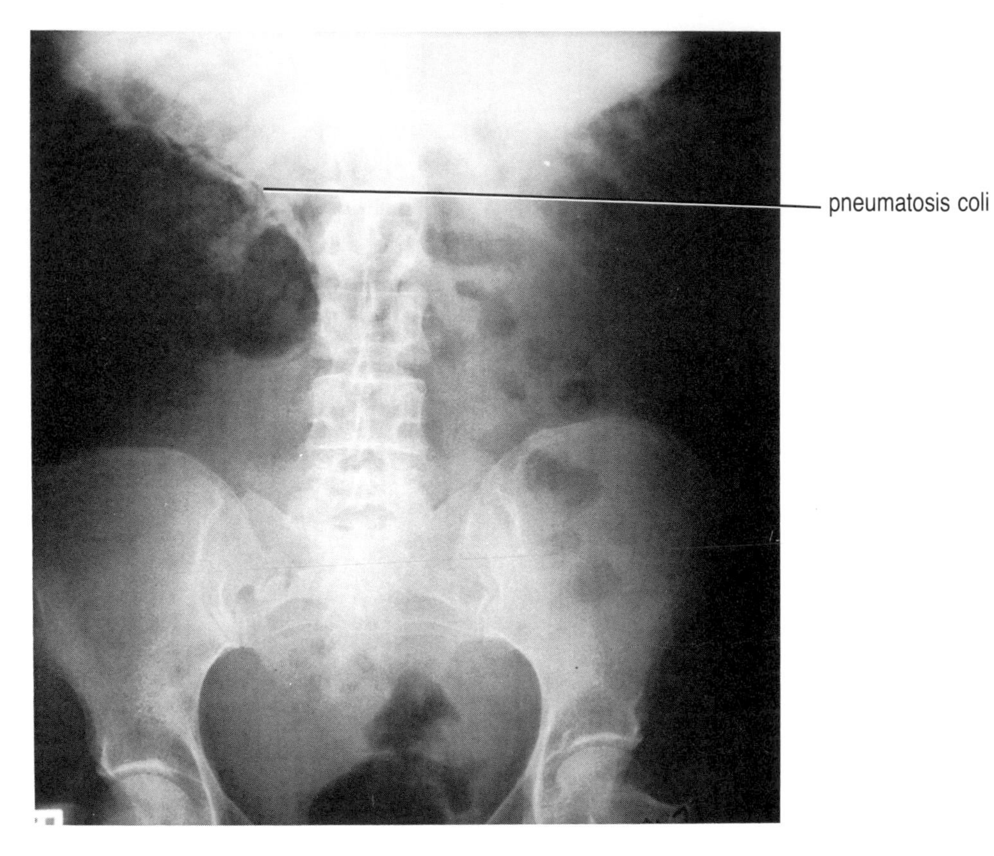

Figure 4.20. Pneumatosis intestinalis and thumbprinting of the colon.

4.21 PANCREATIC CALCIFICATIONS

A. The pancreas overlies the upper abdomen in the region of L1 and L2. The head of the pancreas lies to the right of L1 and L2.
B. Differential diagnosis
   1. Chronic alcoholic pancreatitis
      a. Most common cause of pancreatic calcifications
      b. Visualized as multiple irregular calcifications distributed through the gland
   2. Hyperparathyroidism
      a. Approximately 15% of these individuals develop chronic pancreatitis. Radiographic appearance of calcifications is similar to that of chronic alcoholic pancreatitis.
   3. Cystic fibrosis
      a. Visualized as a diffuse fine granular pattern
   4. Carcinoma
      a. Association between adenocarcinoma and chronic pancreatitis. The visualized calcifications are due to chronic pancreatitis.
   5. Pancreatic pseudocyst
      a. May demonstrate curvilinear calcification of the wall
   6. Hereditary pancreatitis
      a. Autosomal dominant transmission
      b. Visualized as coarse irregular calcifications throughout the pancreas
   7. Kwashiorkor
   8. Idiopathic disease

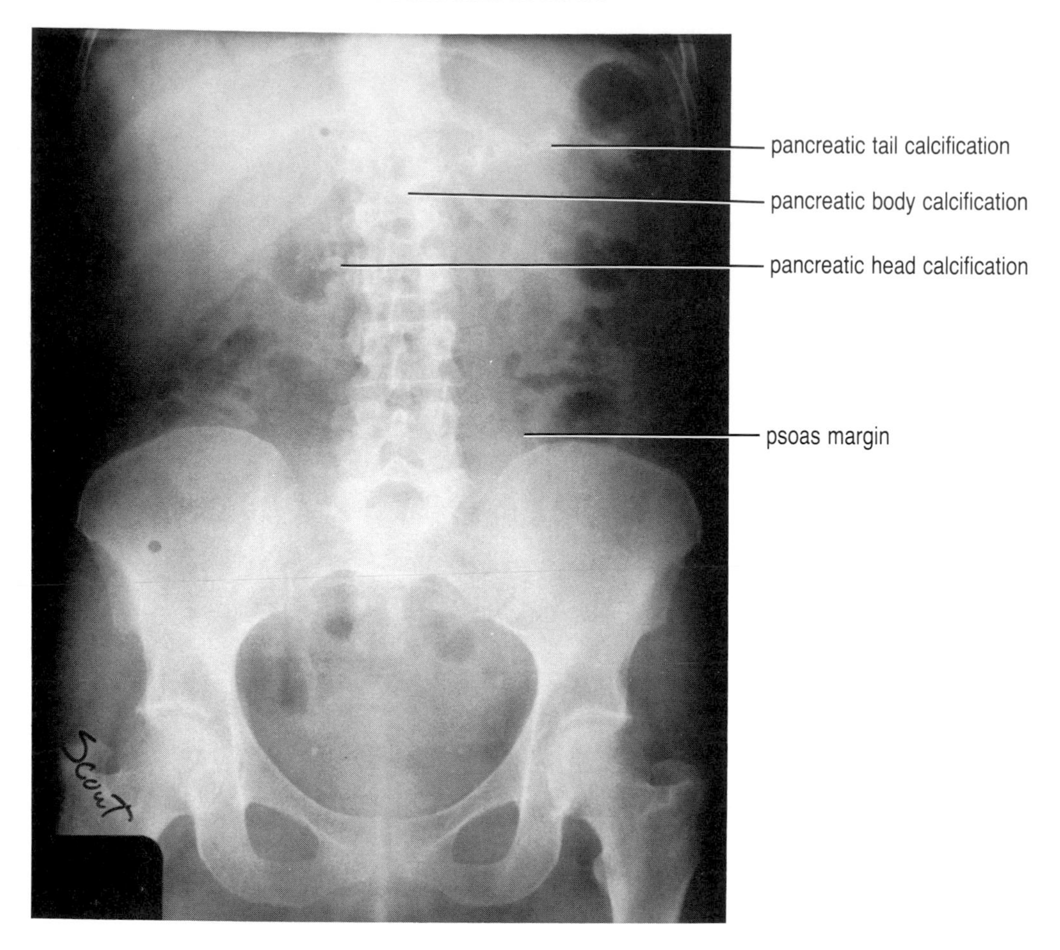

Figure 4.21. Pancreatic calcifications.

4.22 NORMAL CT EXAMINATION OF THE ABDOMEN

A. CT examination of the abdomen is best accomplished by utilizing intravenous and oral-contrast media. Tomographic scans should be obtained from the level of the diaphragms to the pubic symphysis. CT is an excellent method of evaluating the abdominal contents.

B. Normal CT anatomy of the abdomen

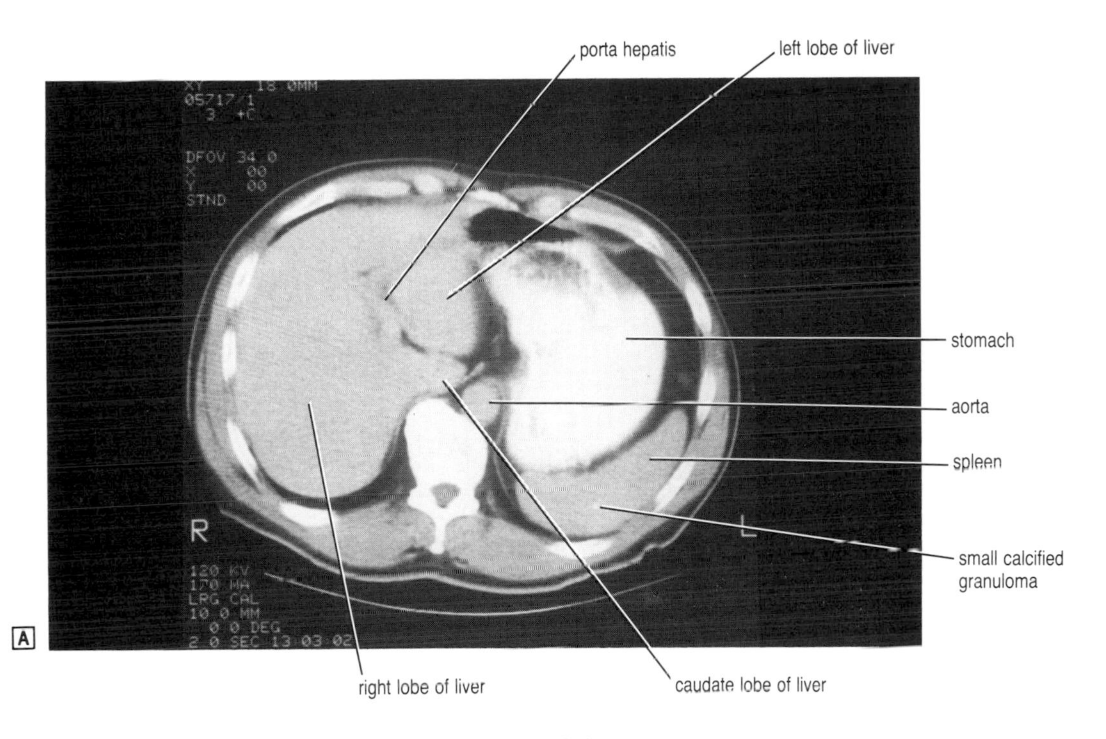

Figure 4.22. *A*, Normal CT examination of the abdomen.

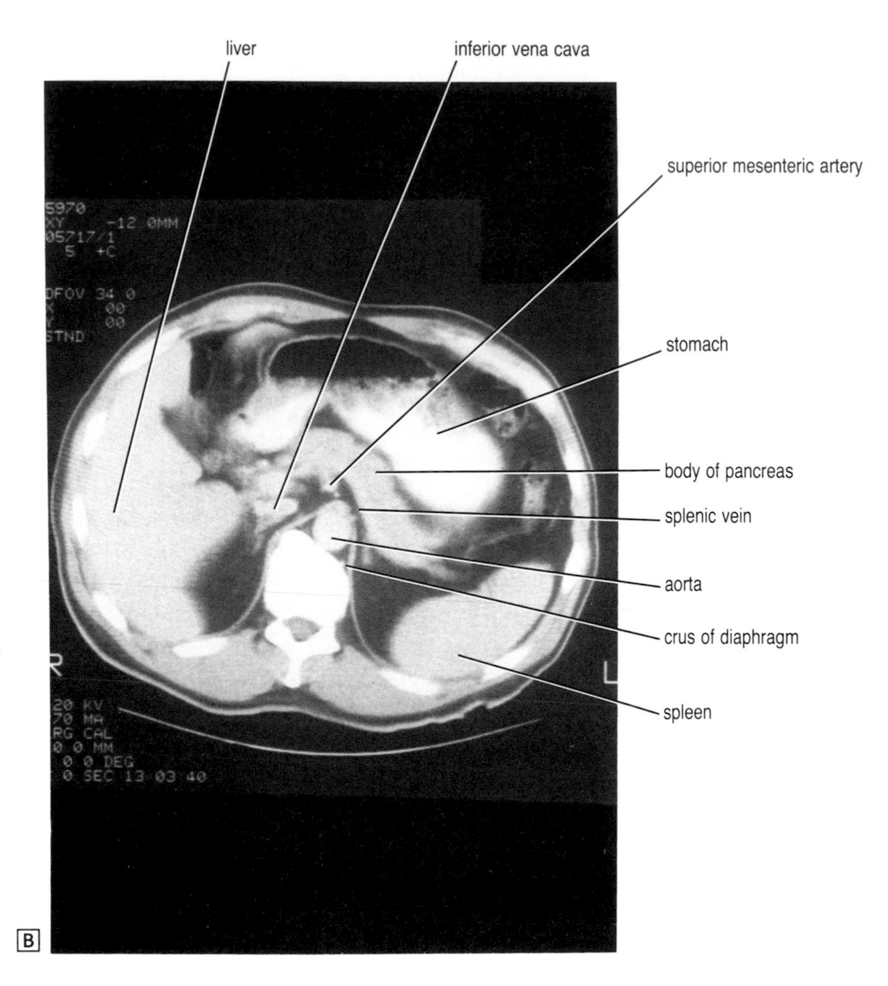

Figure 4.22. *B,* Normal CT examination of the abdomen.

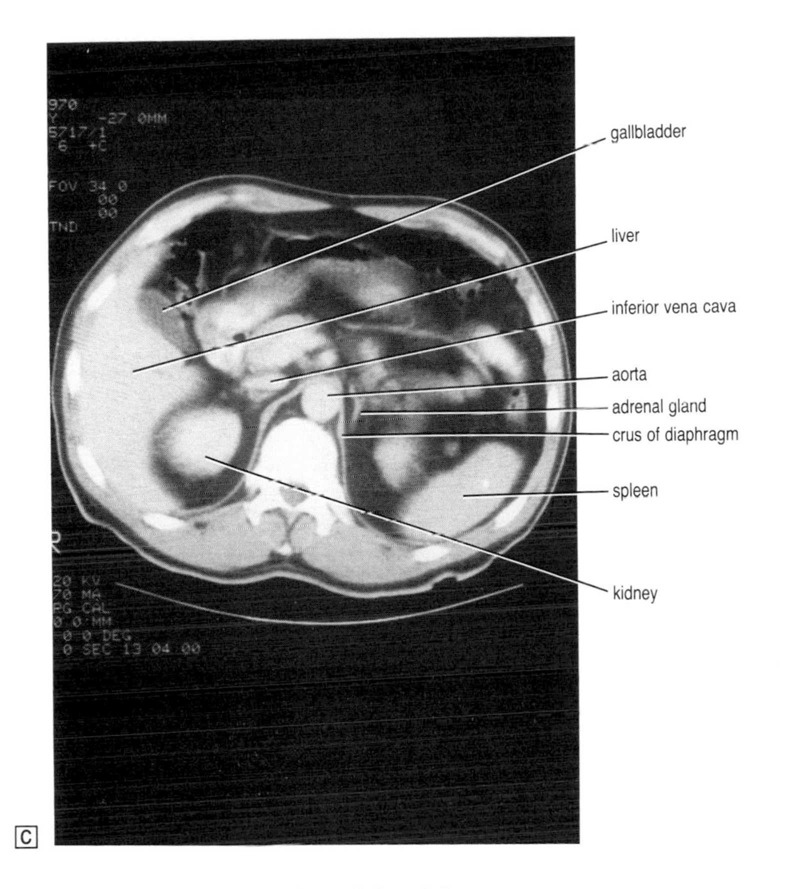

Figure 4.22. C, Normal CT examination of the abdomen.

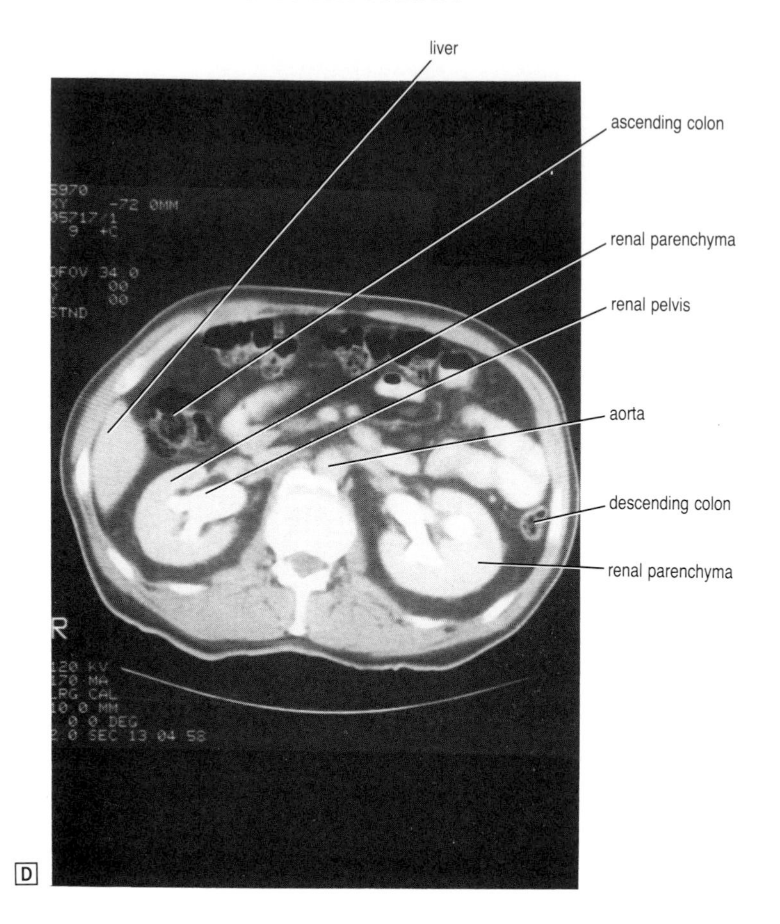

Figure 4.22. *D,* Normal CT examination of the abdomen.

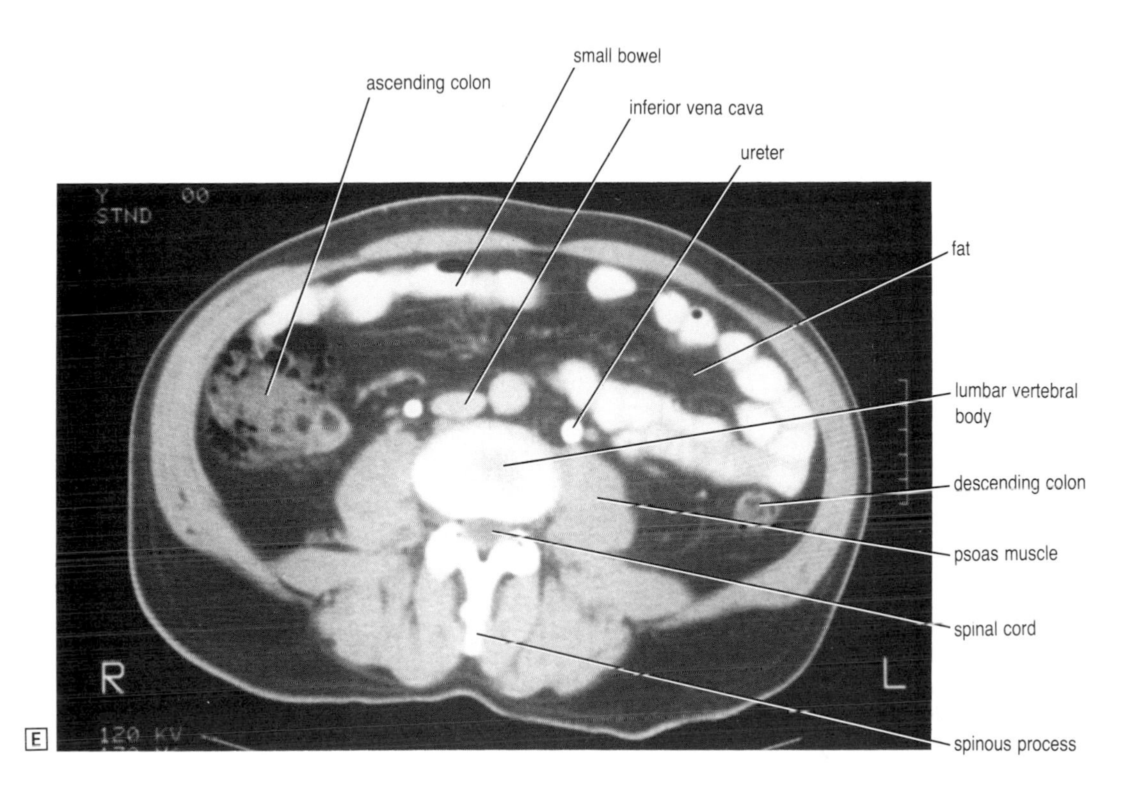

Figure 4.22. *E,* Normal CT examination of the abdomen.

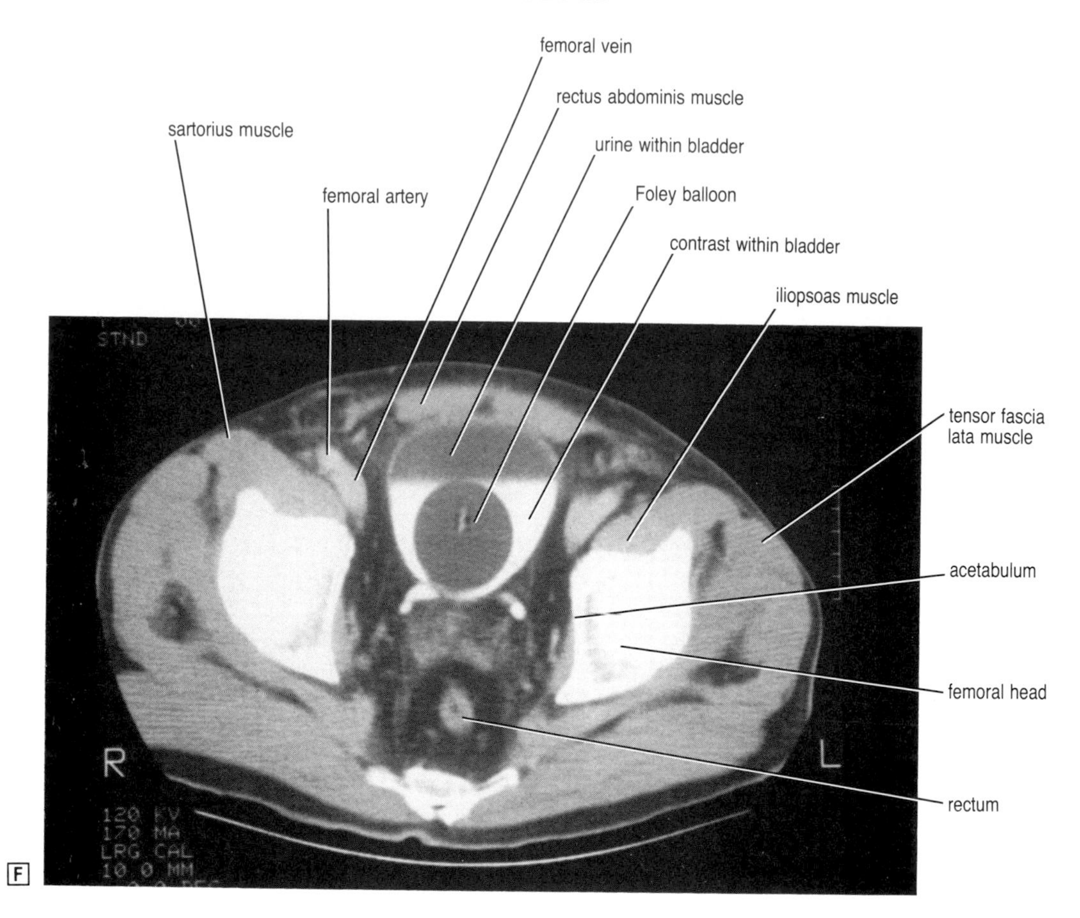

Figure 4.22. *F,* Normal CT examination of the abdomen.

4.23 CT OF ABDOMINAL TRAUMA

A. In the presence of abdominal trauma, CT is an excellent modality for evaluation of the abdomen. Intravenous contrast is helpful in the setting of trauma. Contrast shows assessment of renal function and delineation of areas of contusion and laceration.
B. Free intraperitoneal fluid from acute hemorrhage or even peritoneal lavage appears as an area of low attenuation (density). Free fluid may produce a rim of low attenuation around the liver, layered within the paracolic gutters or low within the pelvis.
C. The liver, spleen, and kidneys have a homogenous density. Acute hemorrhage appears as an area of low attenuation that may be focal and intraparenchymal, representing a contusion. Larger areas of low density suggest the presence of laceration.
D. Cysts and areas of infarct are also low-attenuation areas that may mimic acute hemorrhage.
E. Subcapsular hematomas appear as areas of low attenuation at the periphery of an organ. These areas result in displacement of the normal parenchyma and appear lenticular in configuration.
F. Injuries to the bowel and mesentery may not be visualized on CT.

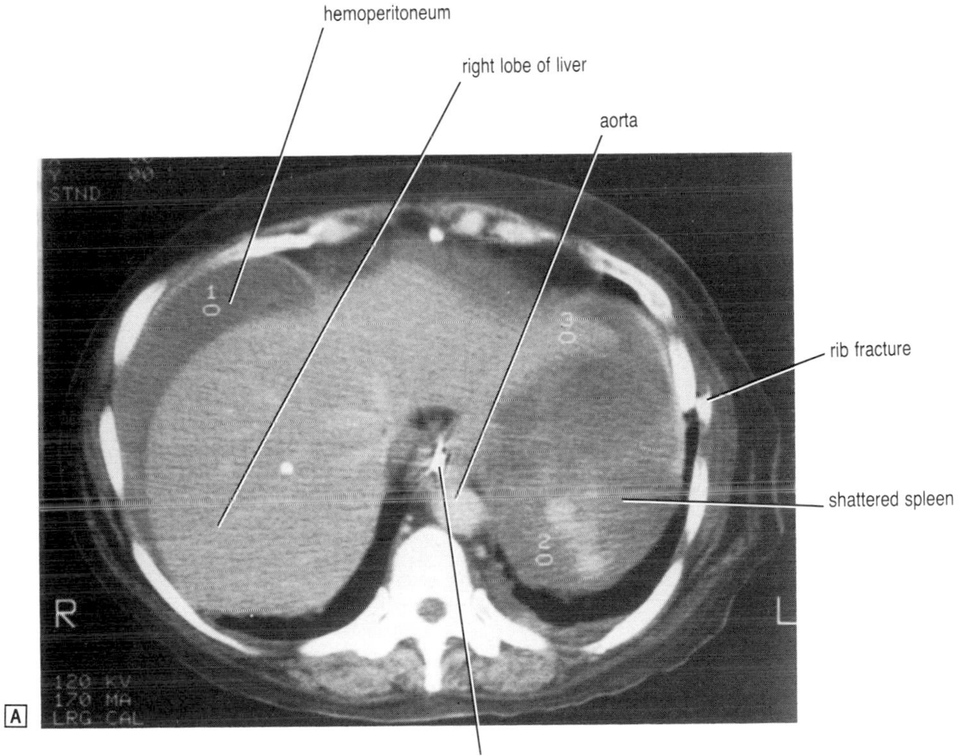

Figure 4.23. *A,* CT of abdominal trauma.

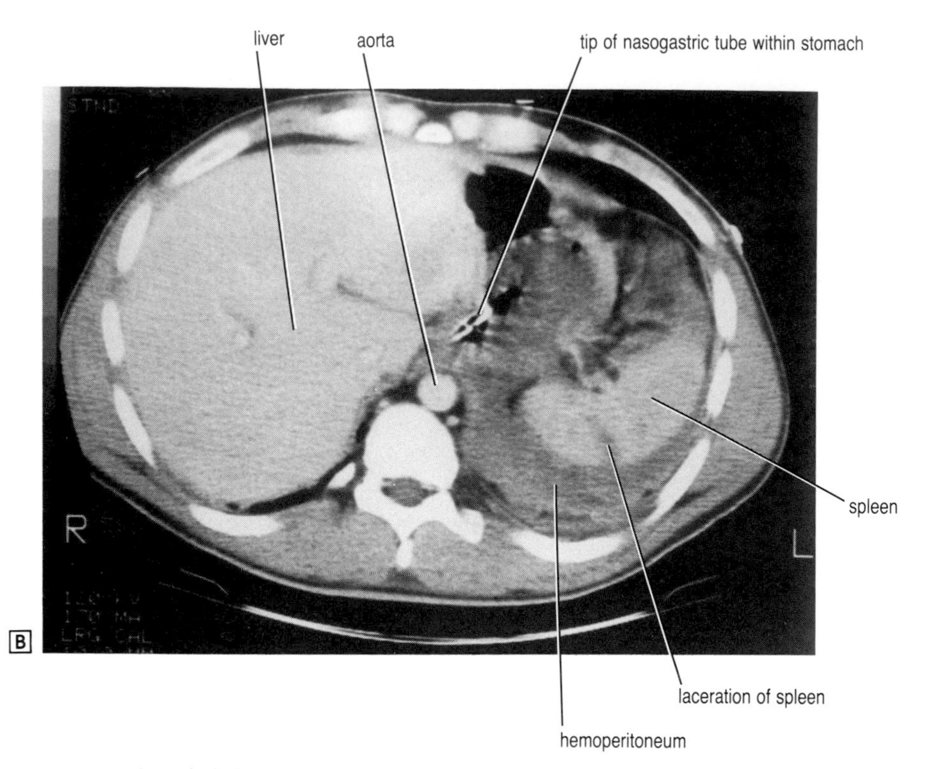

Figure 4.23. *B,* CT of abdominal trauma.

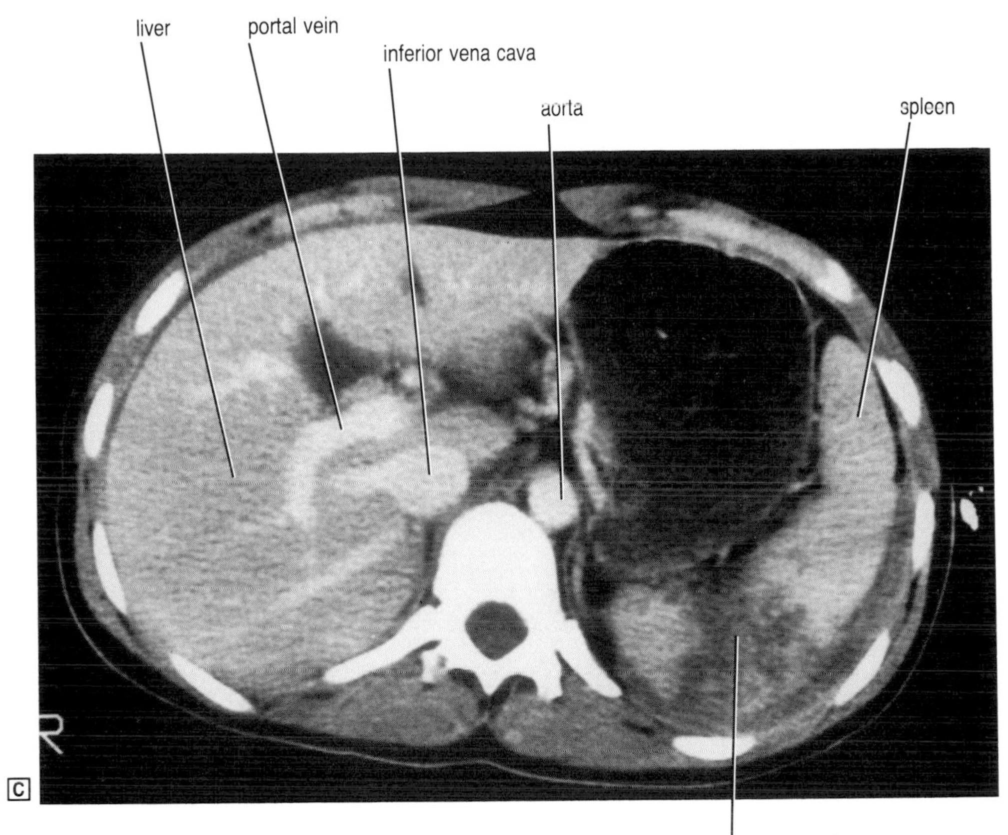

Figure 4.23. C, CT of abdominal trauma.

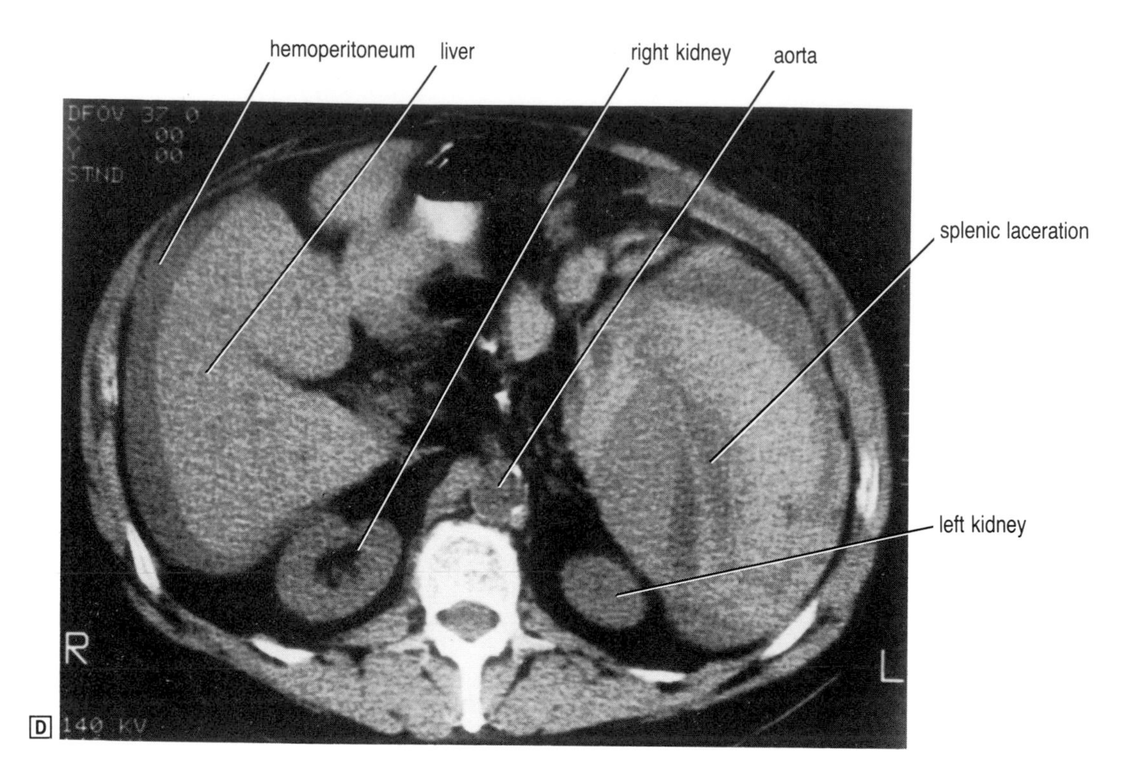

Figure 4.23. *D,* CT of abdominal trauma.

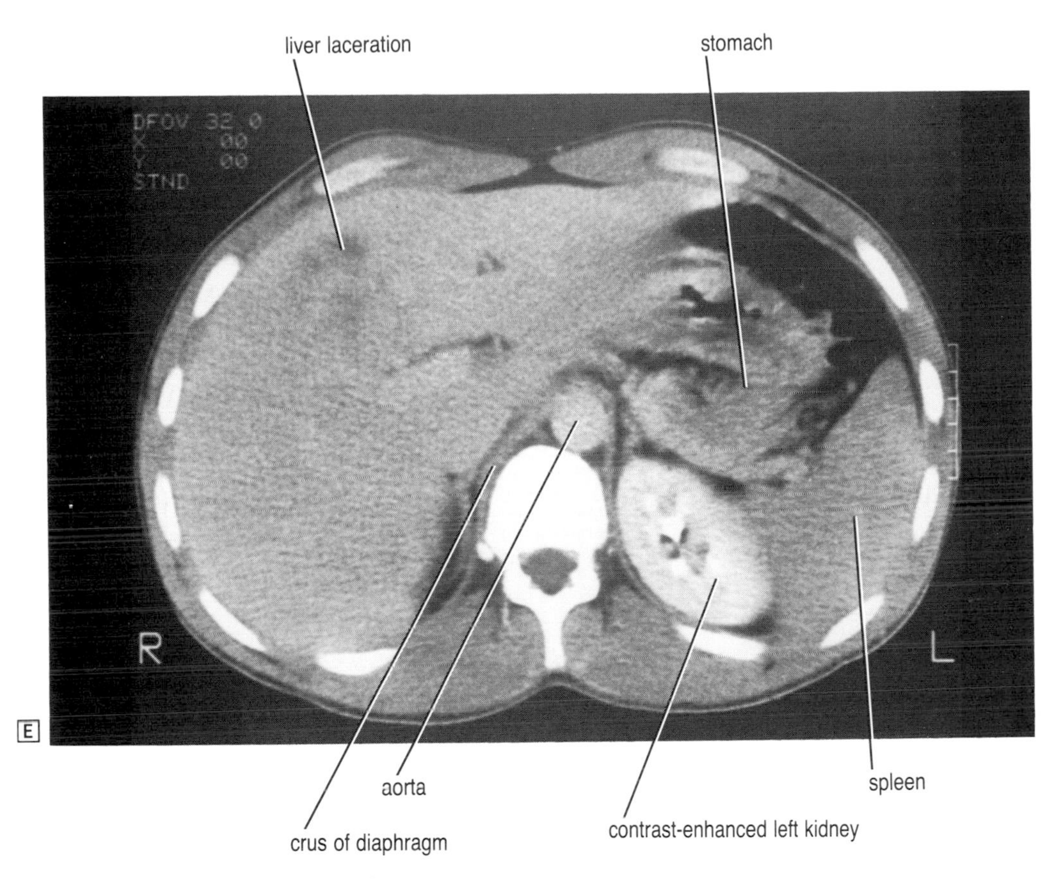

Figure 4.23. *E,* CT of abdominal trauma.

References

Eisenberg, R.L.: Diagnostic Imaging in Internal Medicine. New York: McGraw-Hill Book Co., 1985.

Harris, J.H., and Harris, W.H.: The Radiology of Emergency Medicine. 2nd Ed. Baltimore: Williams & Wilkins, 1981.

Jones, B., and Braver, J.M.: Essentials of Gastrointestinal Radiology. Philadelphia: W.B. Saunders Co., 1982.

Juhl, J.H., and Crummy, A.B.: Essentials of Radiologic Imaging. Philadelphia: J.B. Lippincott, 1987.

Levy, R.C., Hawkins, H., and Barsan, W.G.: Radiology in Emergency Medicine. St. Louis: C.V. Mosby Co., 1986.

Mettler, F.A., and Guiberteau, M.J.: Essentials of Nuclear Medicine Imaging. 2nd Ed. New York: Grune and Stratton, Inc., 1986.

Toombs, B.D., and Sandler, C.M.: Computed Tomography in Trauma. Philadelphia: W.B. Saunders Co., 1987.

5

Genitourinary Tract

5.01 INTRAVENOUS PYELOGRAM (IVP)

A. Intravenous pyelography (IVP)
   1. Indications
      a. Obstructive uropathy
      b. Hematuria
      c. Abdominal mass
      d. Trauma
      e. Chronic pyelonephritis
   2. A "scout" film of the abdomen is obtained prior to administration of contrast (see Sec. 4.01).
   3. Following infusion of contrast, serial films may be obtained at 1-minute, 5-minute, and 15-minute intervals. There should be prompt bilateral excretion of contrast along with visible nephrograms. Always look for the presence of symmetry. Renal size, position, and configuration should be evaluated. Careful examination of both collecting systems, ureters, and bladder is included.
   4. Normally, the kidneys are between 11 and 15 cm in length and are located between L1 and L3. The right kidney is usually 2 cm lower than the left.
   5. Common renal variations
      a. Dromedary hump appears as a bulge on the midportion of the lateral aspect of the kidney.
      b. Fetal lobulation appears as well-defined indentations on the lateral aspect of the renal cortex.
   6. A common ureteral variation is the duplicated ureter. The duplication may be complete or incomplete. The superior ureter drains the upper third of the kidney and inserts into the bladder below the ureter draining the remainder of the kidney.
   7. Water-soluble contrast is filtered by the glomeruli and is not excreted or reabsorbed by the tubules. Contrast is nephrotoxic, and adequate renal function and an optimal state of hydration should exist prior to infusion. In the presence of renal failure, contrast is excreted by the liver and biliary systems. If superimposed liver failure is present, contrast is excreted by the intestinal mucosa. Alternative routes of excretion of contrast are known as vicarious excretion.
   8. Contraindications to contrast infusions
      a. Previous contrast allergy
      b. Known sensitivity to iodine
      c. Abnormal renal function
      d. History of multiple myeloma and sickle cell anemia in the presence of dehydration

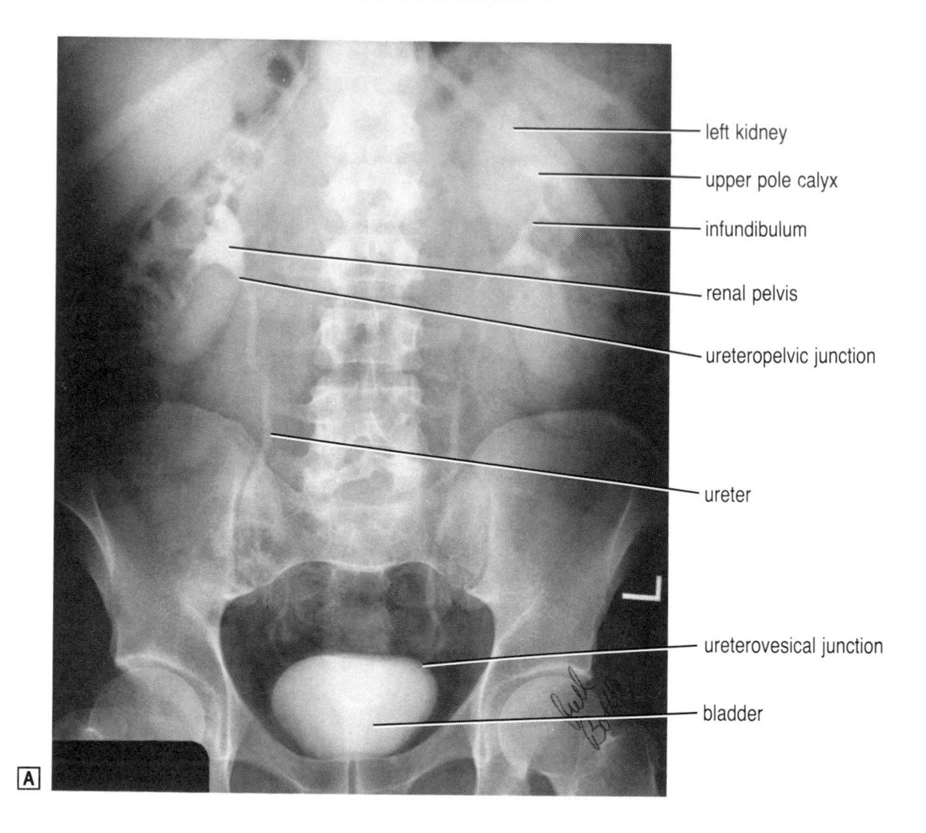

Figure 5.01. *A,* Intravenous pyelogram (IVP).

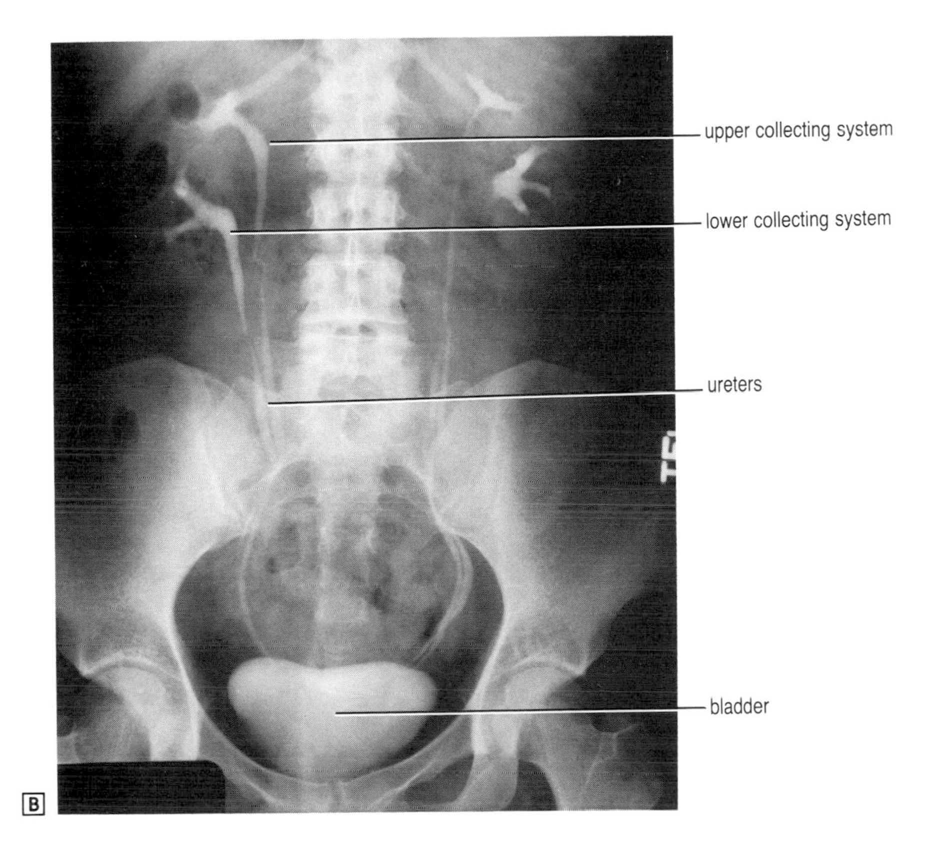

Figure 5.01. *B,* Intravenous pyelogram (IVP).

5.02 LARGE KIDNEY/SMALL KIDNEY

A. Unilateral large kidney
  1. Differential diagnosis
    a. Compensatory hypertrophy: congenital absence or disease of opposite kidney
    b. Obstruction resulting in hydronephrosis
    c. Neoplasm (renal cell carcinoma, transitional cell carcinoma, or Wilm's tumor)
    d. Metastatic disease
    e. Cysts
    f. Congenital conditions
    g. Trauma (see Secs. 5.15, and 5.16)
    h. Acute arterial infarction
    i. Xanthogranulomatous pyelonephritis
B. Bilateral large kidney
  1. Differential diagnosis
    a. Bilateral obstruction resulting in hydronephrosis
    b. Lymphoma
    c. Acute glomerulonephritis
    d. Acute pyelonephritis
    e. Polycystic kidney disease
    f. Sickle cell anemia
    g. Leukemia
    h. Goodpasture's disease
    i. Systemic lupus erythematosus
    j. Amyloidosis
C. Unilateral small kidney
  1. Differential diagnosis
    a. Chronic pyelonephritis: scarring may be unifocal or multifocal, visualized as loss of renal cortex with associated dilatation of adjacent calyx.
    b. Reflux atrophy due to chronic vesicoureteral reflux
    c. Renal ischemia, visualized as a small kidney with ureteral notching due to enlarged collateral vessels
    d. Lobar infarction
    e. Congenital hypoplastic kidney
    f. Tuberculosis
    g. Radiation nephritis
D. Bilateral small kidney
  1. Differential diagnosis
    a. Chronic glomerulonephritis associated with hypertension, renal failure, and nephrotic syndrome
    b. Arteriosclerosis
    c. Chronic bilateral obstructive uropathy
    d. Chronic amyloidosis
    e. Papillary necrosis (see Sec. 5.09)
    f. Arterial hypotension

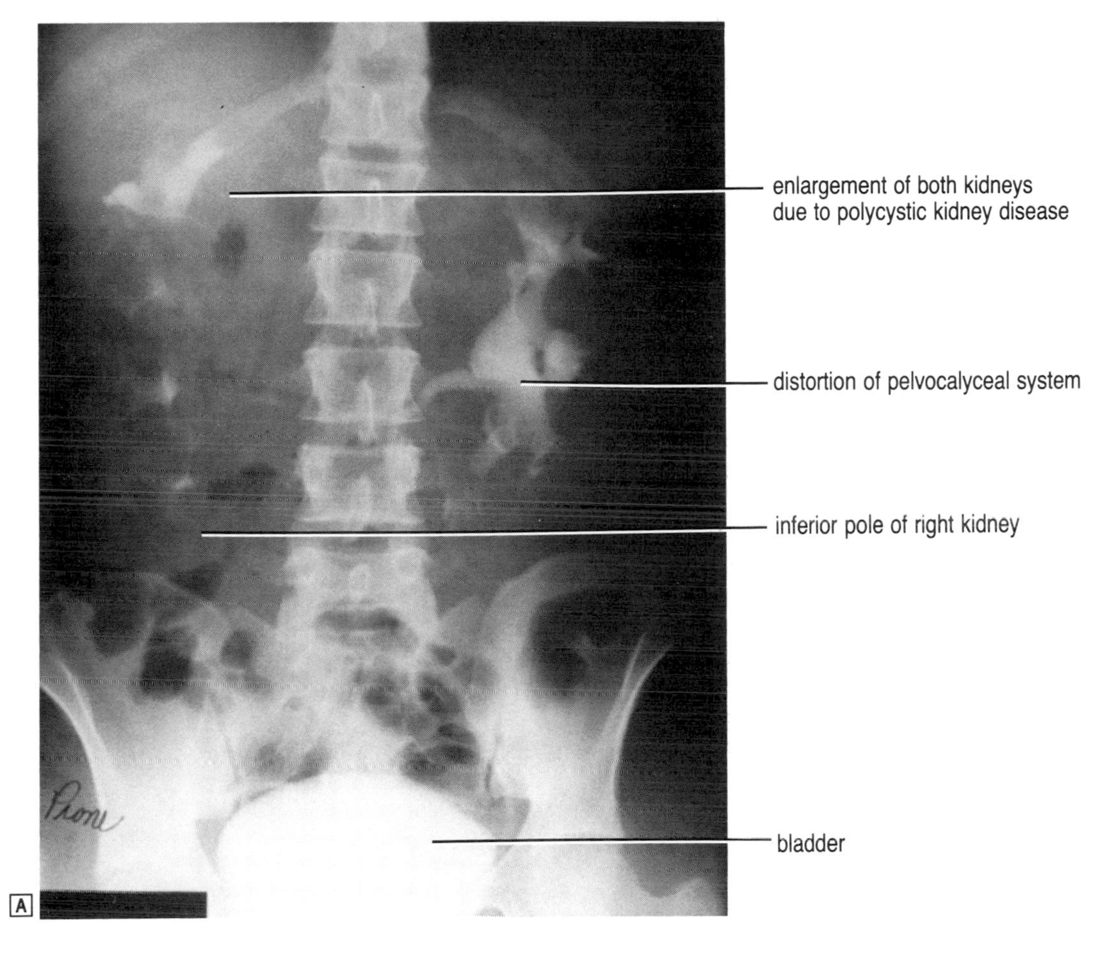

Figure 5.02. *A,* Large kidney/small kidney.

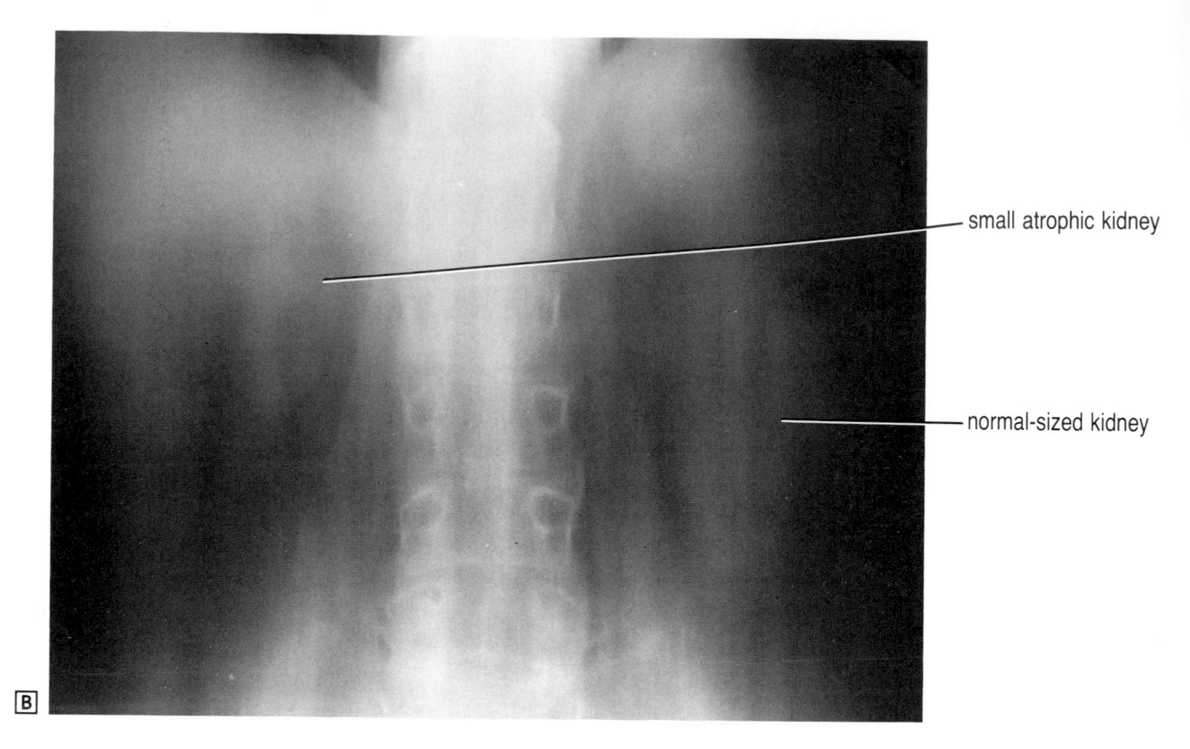

Figure 5.02. *B,* Large kidney/small kidney.

5.03 CALCULI AND HYDRONEPHROSIS

A. Approximately 90% of calculi are radiopaque owing to the presence of calcium salts.
B. Most radiopaque calculi are composed of calcium oxalate.
C. Differential diagnosis of calcium stones
  1. Urinary stasis
  2. Urinary tract infection
  3. Hyperparathyroidism
  4. Renal tubular acidosis
  5. Osteolytic metastases
  6. Inflammatory bowel disease
  7. Sarcoidosis
  8. Medullary sponge kidney
  9. Malignant tumor
  10. Multiple myeloma
  11. Hyperoxaluria
D. Radiolucent stones consist of uric acid, xanthine, and mucoprotein matrix.
E. Eighty percent of radiolucent stones are due to uric acid.
F. Radiolucent stones result from gout, polycythemia, leukemia, low urine pH, myeloproliferative disease, and Lesch-Nyhan syndrome.
G. Cystine calculi are mildly opaque and appear as a ground-glass density on plain film roentgenograms. Cystine calculi result from hereditary inability to reabsorb cystine.
H. Staghorn calculi form as a result of chronic urinary infection by a Proteus species (urea-splitting organism). The staghorn grows and may fill an entire calyx or renal pelvis. Staghorn calculi consist of magnesium ammonium phosphate. Eighty percent occur in females.
I. Nephrocalcinosis
  1. Represents multiple calcifications that become deposited in the renal parenchyma.
  2. Differential diagnosis
    a. Acute cortical necrosis—cortical distribution
    b. Chronic glomerulonephritis—cortical distribution
    c. Renal transplant rejection—cortical distribution
    d. Primary hyperparathyroidism—medullary distribution
    e. Renal tubular acidosis—medullary distribution
    f. Medullary sponge kidney—medullary distribution
    g. Neoplasm
    h. Hypercalcemic states
    i. Papillary necrosis
    j. Sarcoidosis
    k. Metastases
  3. Ureteral calculi
    a. Calculi may lodge at three sites of normal ureteral narrowing
      (1) Ureteropelvic junction (UPJ)
      (2) Ureterovesical junction (UVJ)
      (3) Distal third of the ureters as they cross the pelvic brim
    b. Presentation
      (1) Severe colicky flank pain that radiates to the groin
      (2) Hematuria
      (3) Nausea and vomiting
    c. Signs of ureteral obstruction on IVP
      (1) Delayed excretion by the affected kidney
      (2) Dilated renal collecting system and ureter
      (3) Increasingly dense nephrogram
      (4) Generalized renal enlargement
      (5) High-grade obstruction may result in rupture of a fornix of a calyx and may lead to contrast extravasation.
J. Approximately 40% of ureteral calculi are passed spontaneously, usually by 96 hours. Therapy includes rest, fluids, analgesia, and observation.

K. If the IVP fails to demonstrate a radiopaque calculi, then the differential diagnosis includes the following.
   1. Recently passed calculus with residual obstruction due to edema
   2. Radiolucent stone
   3. Obstruction due to blood clot
   4. Obstruction by stricture
L. Postobstructive renal atrophy
   1. Obstruction for 3 to 6 weeks results in irreversible renal parenchymal damage.
   2. Radiographic signs
      a. Calyceal clubbing
      b. Dilated pelvocalyceal system
      c. Generalized loss of renal parenchyma
M. In the presence of renal failure, contrast is excreted by alternative routes referred to as vicarious excretion. Contrast is excreted by hepatic and biliary routes and may result in opacification of the gallbladder. Contrast may also be visualized within the intestinal lumen.

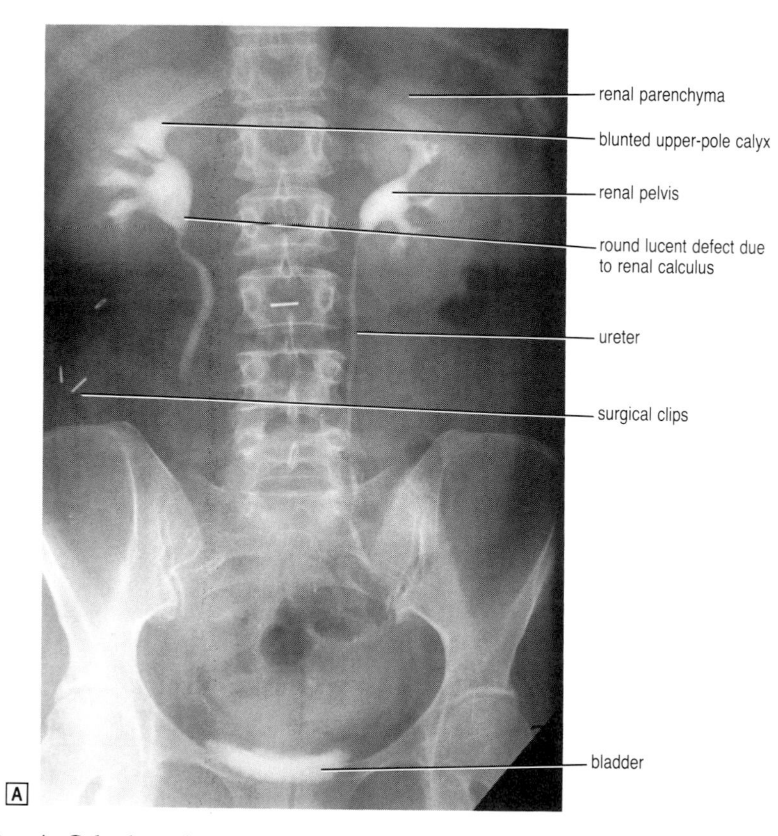

Figure 5.03. *A,* Calculi and hydronephrosis.

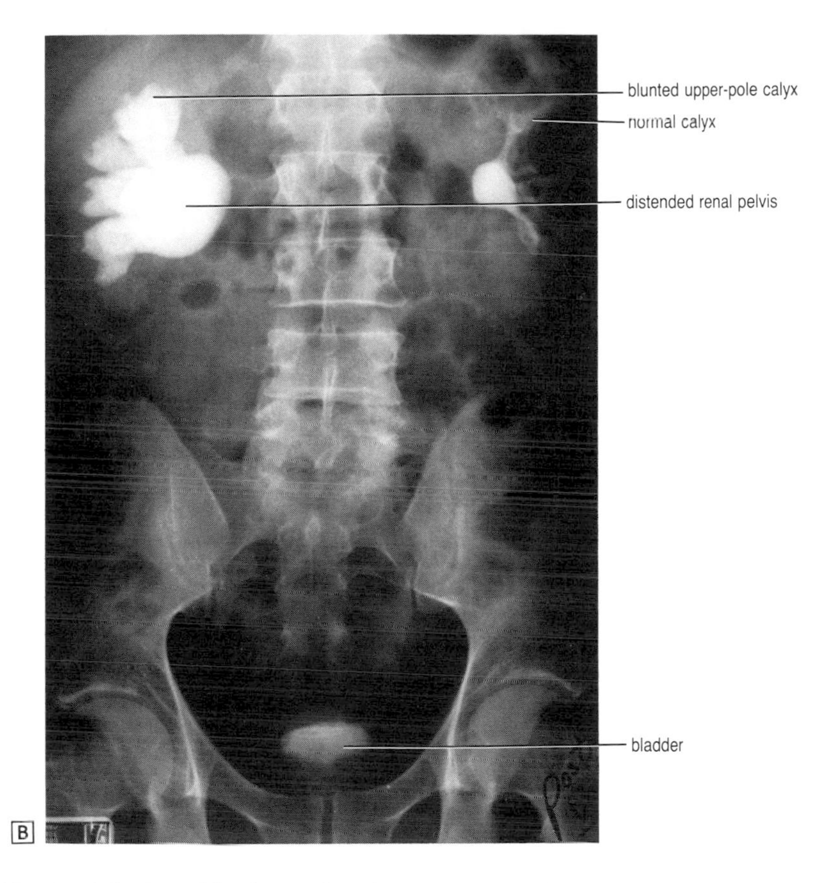

Figure 5.03. *B*, Calculi and hydronephrosis.

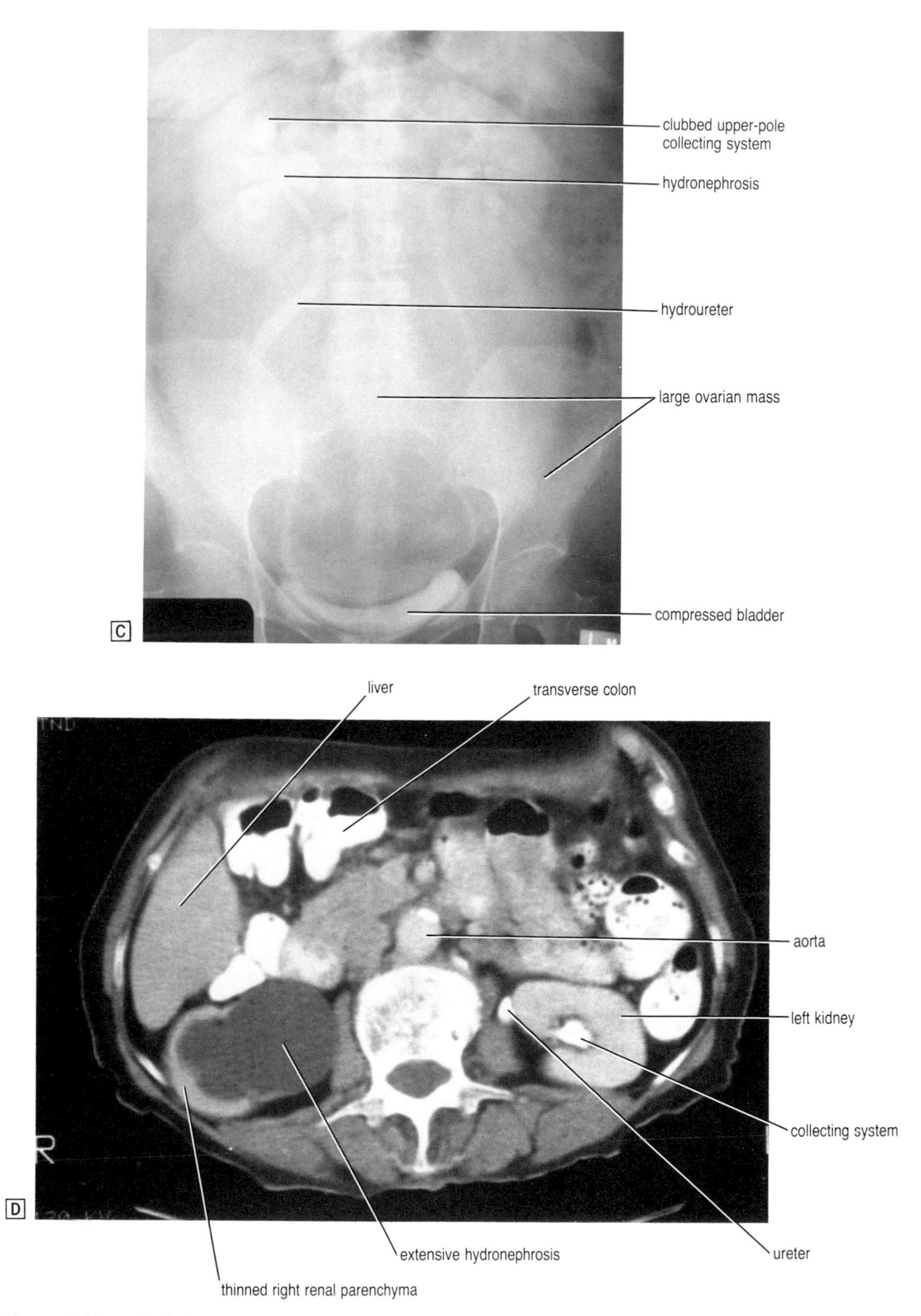

Figure 5.03. *C,* Calculi and hydronephrosis. *D,* Calculi and hydronephrosis.

5.04 DILATED URETER

A. Ureteral size varies considerably. One must appreciate a fairly marked degree of dilatation or narrowing before it is interpreted as such.

B. Differential diagnosis for dilated ureter

1. Calculus or edema due to calculus (see Sec. 5.03)
2. Blood clot: irregular filling defect usually causing incomplete obstruction. Common causes are trauma, tumor, instrumentation, and anticoagulation.
3. Ureterocele (see Sec. 5.13)
4. Inspissated pus from proximal infection
5. Sloughed papilla secondary to papillary necrosis (see Sec. 5.09)
6. Cystitis: unilateral or bilateral obstruction of distal ureter. In acute phase secondary to edema and inflammation; in chronic phase fibrosis and stricture.
7. Postoperative stricture: edema, ligature
8. Congenital ureteropelvic junction (UPJ) obstruction. Chief causes: extrinsic compression of UPJ by fibrous band or blood vessel and intrinsic stenosis of the ureter. Seen in patients with horseshoe and malrotated kidneys.
9. Vascular compression by normal vessel or aneurysm
10. Tuberculous stricture: late complication of renal tuberculosis. Renal calcification is more common than ureteral calcification. Early in the course of the disease, there is mild ureterectasis, ulcerations, and possibly reflux.
11. Schistosomiasis stricture of the distal ureter with bladder calcification
12. Postradiation stricture and fibrosis
13. Pregnancy and postpartum state, more common on the right
14. Invasion or compression by extrinsic malignant tumor: lymphoma, carcinoma of pancreas, cervix, colon, and other pelvic organs
15. Vesicoureteric reflux: most common in children, may result in renal scarring
16. Neurogenic bladder: "grossly trabeculated" bladder with unilateral or bilateral dilatation of the ureter and pelvocalyceal system. Disease or injury to bladder innervation may result from spinal cord trauma or tumor, spina bifida, myelomeningocele, sacral agenesis.
17. Retroperitoneal fibrosis: medial deviation of both ureters between L4 and S2. Proximal ureter dilatation with smooth narrowing. May be associated with methysergide, methyldopa, phenacetin, or ergot derivative ingestion.
18. Neoplasm: transitional cell carcinoma most common

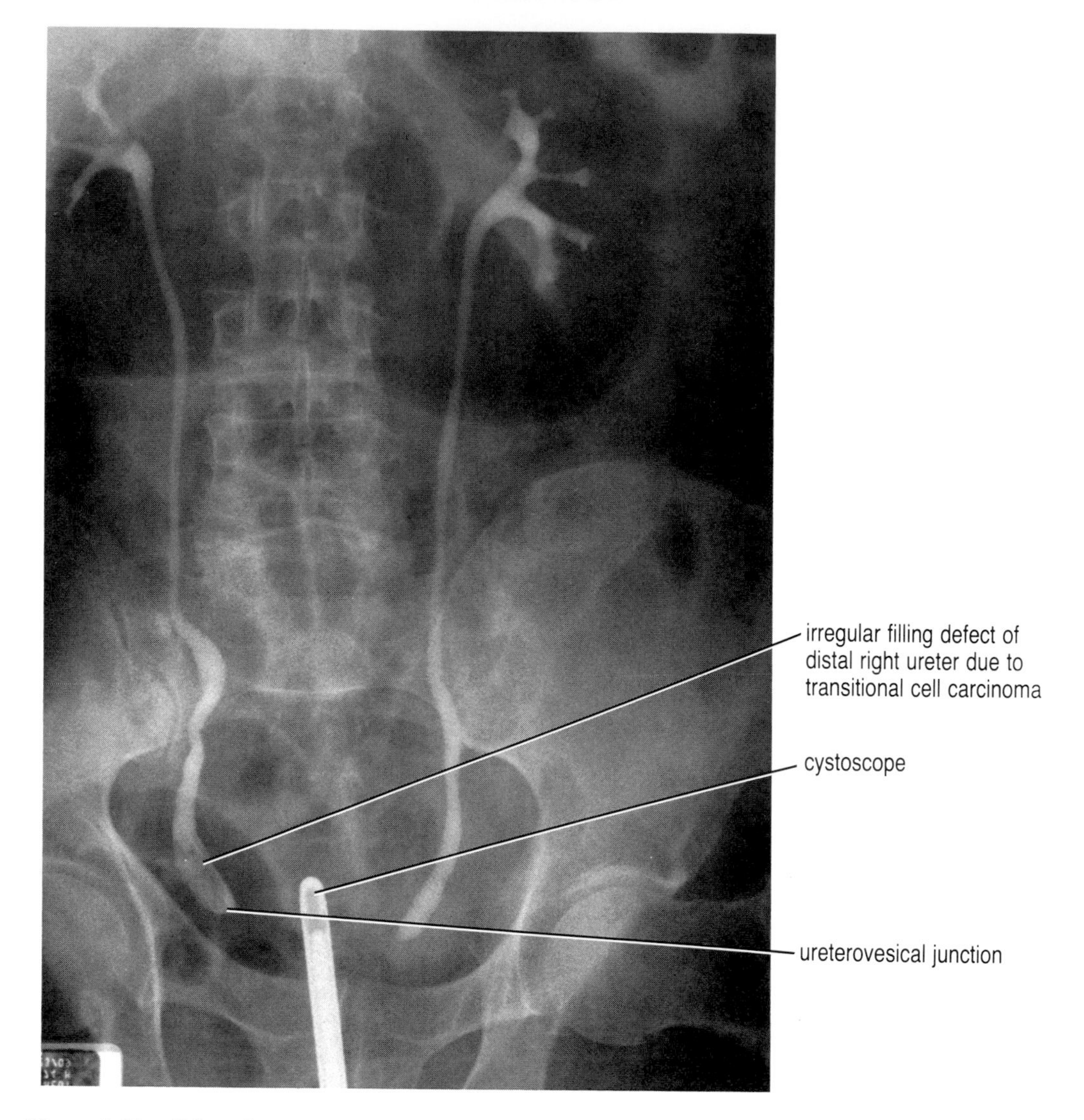

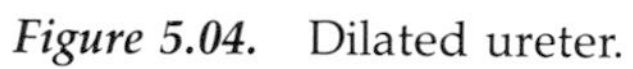
Figure 5.04. Dilated ureter.

5.05 RENAL MASS

A. Differential diagnosis
   1. Renal cyst
      a. Usually a unifocal mass, but may be multiple. IVP reveals smooth splaying of calyces with a thin well-defined wall that may have a "beak" appearance. Ultrasound or CT can confirm the diagnosis.
   2. Benign neoplasm
      a. Hamartoma (angiomyolipoma) is a benign lesion that has a high fat content. Association with tuberous sclerosis.
      b. Other benign tumors include adenoma, hemangioma, lipoma
   3. Malignant neoplasm
      a. Renal cell carcinoma (hypernephroma) is the most common malignant renal neoplasm. More common in middle-aged males. Results in mass effect and distortion of pelvocalyceal system. May contain calcification.
      b. Wilm's tumor (nephroblastoma) is the most common abdominal neoplasm in children. Most occur by age 3.
   4. Renal abscess
   5. Metastasis from stomach, lung, and breast
   6. Trauma: subcapsular hematoma
   7. Normal variants: fetal lobulation, dromedary hump, enlarged column of Bertin
   8. Hydronephrosis (see Sec. 5.03)

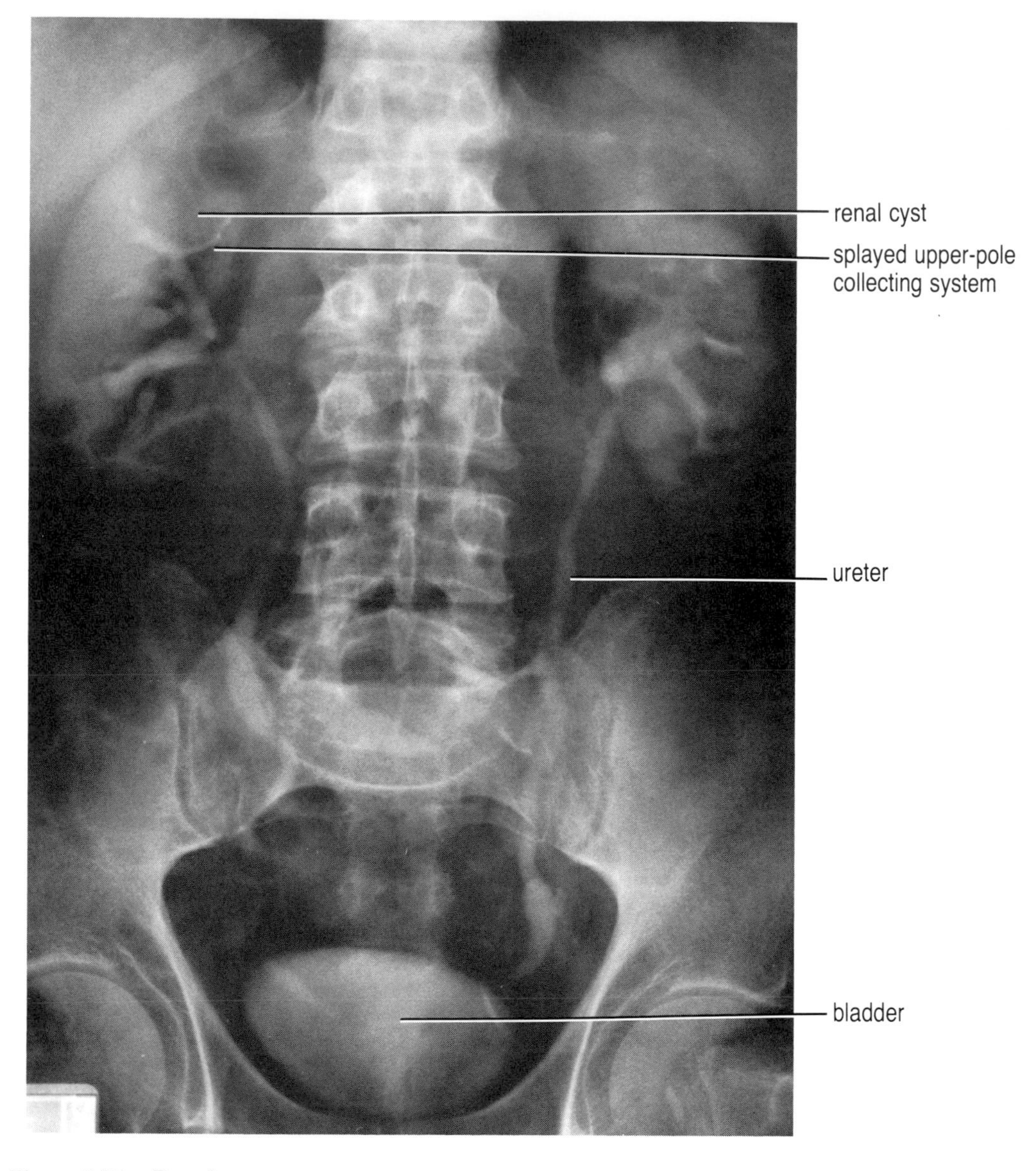

Figure 5.05. Renal mass.

5.06 FILLING DEFECT IN PELVOCALYCEAL SYSTEM

A. Differential diagnosis
   1. Malignant neoplasm
      a. Transitional cell carcinoma accounts for approximately 90% of malignant tumors in this region. Presentation includes hematuria and obstructive uropathy.
      b. Renal cell carcinoma
      c. Squamous cell carcinoma, associated with chronic infection
   2. Blood clot
      a. Trauma
      b. Bleeding disorder
      c. Tumor
      d. Instrumentation
      e. Nephritis
      f. Anticoagulation
   3. Calculi (see Sec. 5.03)
   4. Air: round movable collections result from instrumentation, surgery, or trauma
   5. Papillary necrosis (see Sec. 5.09)
   6. Pyelitis cystica: multiple small fixed submucosal cysts related to chronic infection
   7. Fraley's syndrome: impression of a vascular structure upon the collecting system resulting in an extrinsic defect
   8. Renal sinus lipomatosis: accumulation of excessive fat within the hilum
   9. Papilloma

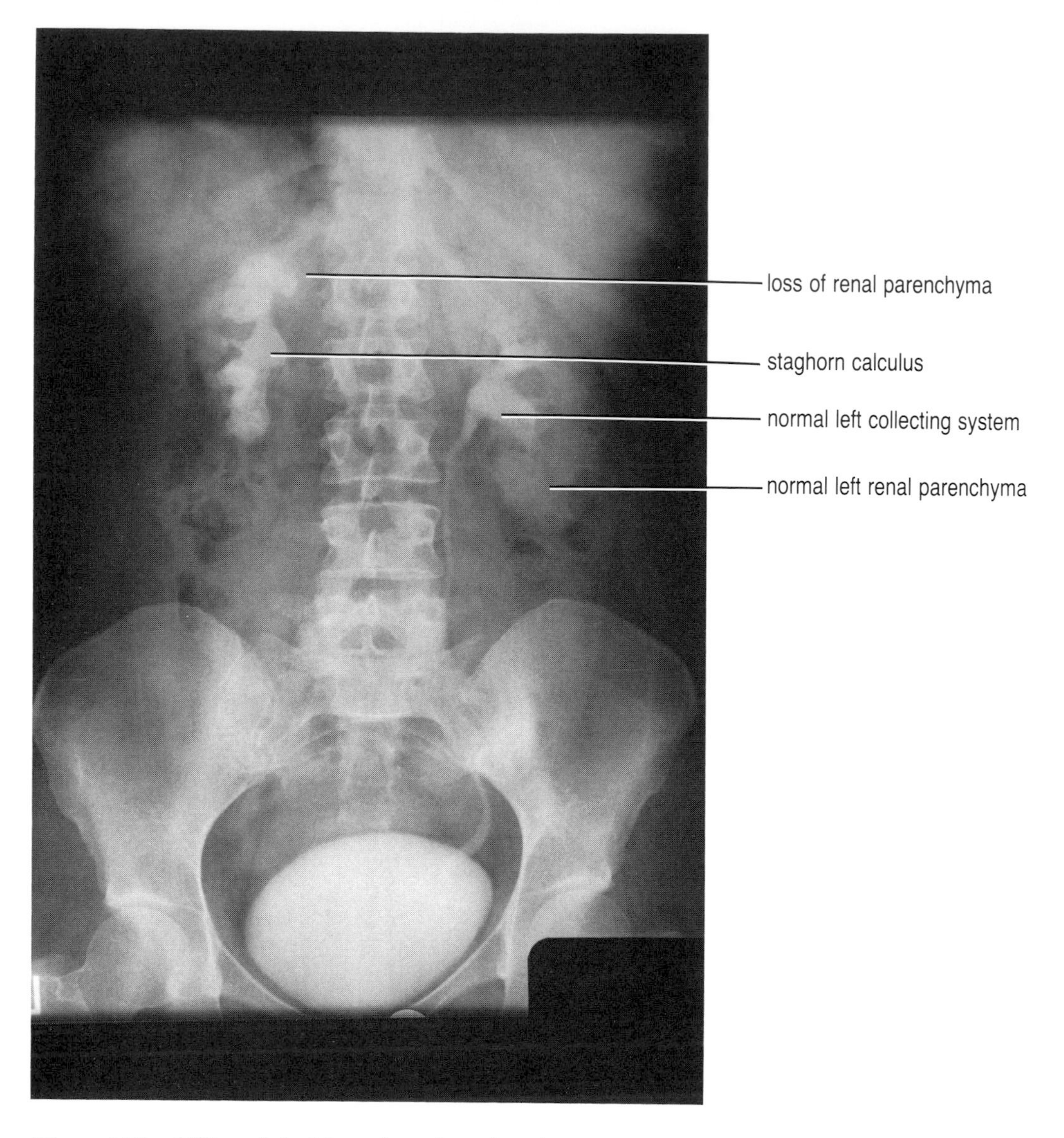

Figure 5.06. Filling defect in pelvocalyceal system.

5.07 ABSENT OR ECTOPIC KIDNEY

A. Ectopic kidney: may have abnormal rotation and abnormal location and origin of renal arteries
   1. Pelvic kidney results from abnormal embryologic ascent.
   2. Transplanted kidney is usually present in iliac fossa.
   3. Ptosis
   4. Horseshoe kidney is the most common type of fusion.
   5. Crossed fused ectopia: both kidneys located on the same side
   6. Malrotation
   7. Displacement by abdominal mass or organomegaly

B. Absence of kidney
   1. Unilateral renal agenesis
   2. Postnephrectomy: usually the twelfth rib has been resected
   3. Congenital absence
   4. Normal variant: is present but not visualized owing to fecal debris within bowel or little perinephric fat
   5. Ectopic or displaced kidney
   6. Hematoma
   7. Chronic atrophy due to obstruction, infection, or infarction

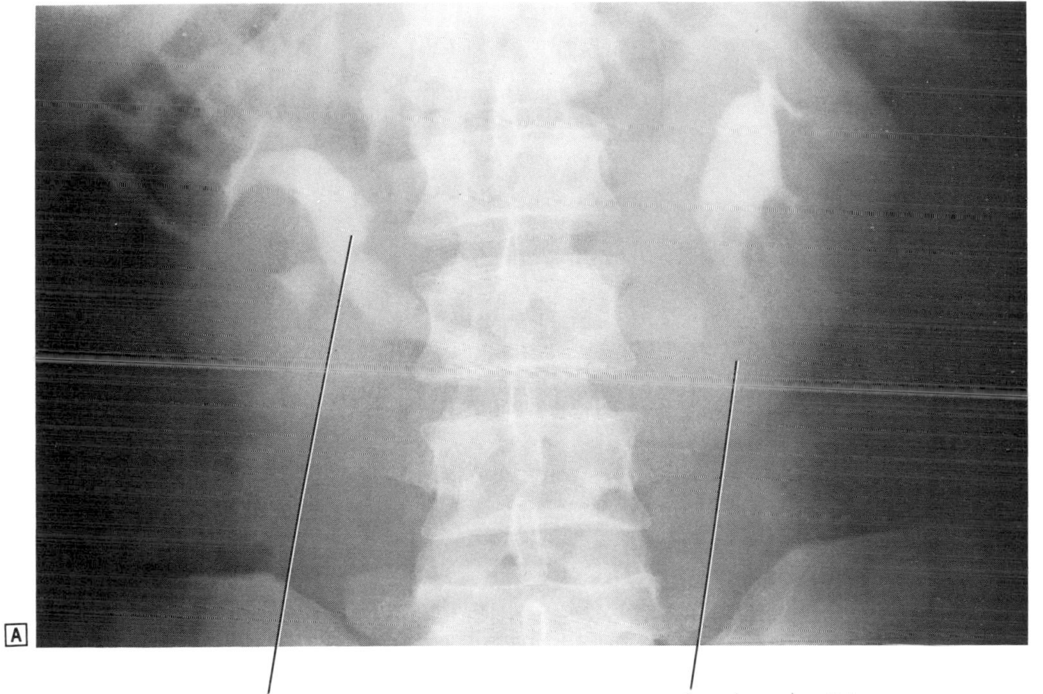

Figure 5.07. *A,* Absent or ectopic kidney.

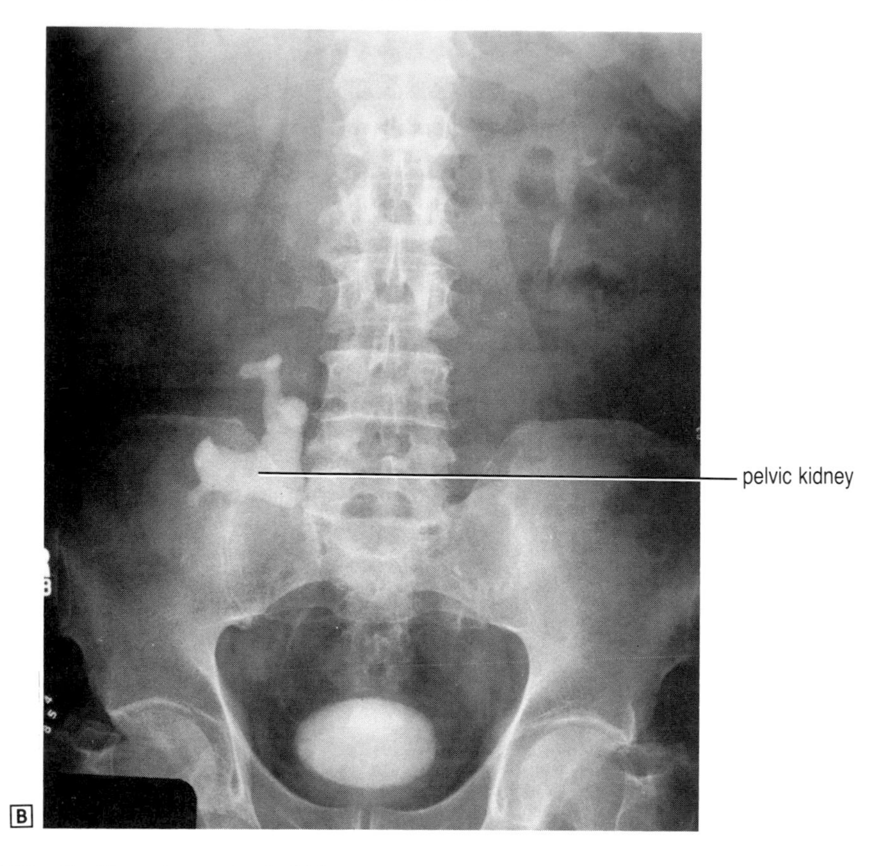

Figure 5.07. *B,* Absent or ectopic kidney.

5.08 ACUTE AND CHRONIC PYELONEPHRITIS

A. An inflammatory process of the kidney resulting from hematogenous or ascending bacterial infection from the bladder, ureter, or urethra
B. Acute pyelonephritis
   1. Usually a clinical diagnosis. Presentation includes the following.
      a. Sudden onset of flank pain
      b. Fever
      c. Bacteriuria
      d. Frequency
      e. CVA tenderness
   2. An IVP is usually normal.
   3. In approximately 25%
      a. Generalized renal enlargement
      b. Focal enlargement due to abscess
      c. Decreased density of the pelvocalyceal system
      d. Ultrasound may demonstrate renal enlargement with decreased echogenicity.
C. Chronic pyelonephritis
   1. A chronic inflammatory process due to recurrent urinary tract infections, ureteral reflux, or focal ischemia
   2. IVP findings
      a. Renal involvement may be unifocal, multifocal, unilateral, or bilateral.
      b. Decreased renal size
      c. Clubbing of the calyceal system, which appears rounded and blunt
      d. There may be normal or hypertrophied renal parenchyma between areas of involvement.
   3. CT demonstrates findings similar to those of the IVP.
   4. Ultrasound demonstrates small shrunken kidneys with increased echogenicity and ill-defined borders.
   5. Chronic pyelonephritis is differentiated from atrophy occurring as a result of long-standing hydronephrosis by the presence of focal scarring and a more irregular pattern in chronic pyelonephritis.

There is no Figure for 5.08

5.09 RENAL PAPILLARY NECROSIS

A. Papillary necrosis results from impairment of the blood supply to the medullary papillae.

B. Radiographically visualized as linear streaks extending through the renal papilla, fornix, and involved calyx. When the medullary tissue becomes completely separated from adjacent tissue, it may be visualized as a triangular lucent-filling defect within the calyx. The normal architecture of the calyx is disrupted and appears round or saccular.

C. The sloughed tissue may pass down the ureter and become lodged resulting in obstructive uropathy (see Secs. 5.03, 5.04).

D. The sloughed papilla may also remain in place within the pelvocalyceal system and become calcified.

1. Differential diagnosis
    a. Diabetes mellitus
    b. Analgesic abuse (phenacetin)
    c. Sickle cell anemia
    d. Pyelonephritis
    e. Urinary tract infection
    f. Obstructive uropathy
    g. Ethanol abuse

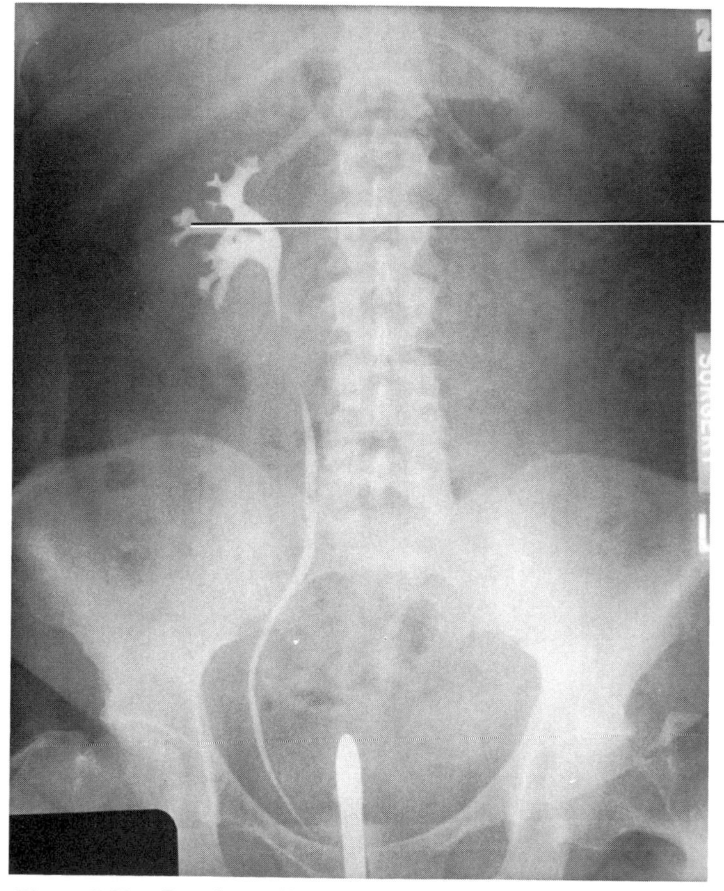

Figure 5.09. Renal papillary necrosis.

5.10 LARGE URINARY BLADDER

A. The shape and size of the urinary bladder vary considerably. The bladder parallels the pubic rami, and its dome appears rounded in men and concave or flat in women. Normal bladder wall is smooth.

B. Differential diagnosis

1. Benign prostatic hypertrophy is the most common cause. Elevation of the bladder floor with "fishhook" or "J"-shaped terminal ureters as they course toward the trigone. Typically produces smooth impression on bladder floor. May result in bladder outlet obstruction.
2. Prostatic carcinoma. If encapsulated, indistinguishable from benign prostatic hypertrophy. Bladder invasion or bony metastases suggests the diagnosis. Pulmonary metastases occurs in approximatley 25%.
3. Neurogenic bladder: result of disease or injury to spinal cord or peripheral nerves. Incontinence or urinary retention may result. Atonic, smooth-walled, dilated bladder suggests diabetes, tabes dorsalis, and syringomyelia. Alternatively, the small, spastic, grossly trabeculated and pyramidal bladder (pine-tree pattern) is the pathognomonic radiographic appearance of the neurogenic bladder.
4. Acquired urethral stricture: results from infection (e.g., gonorrhea), trauma (post-instrumentation or TURP) associated with pelvic fracture or straddle injury (see Sec. 5.16).
5. Posterior urethral valves: a thin membrane arising near verumontanum with varying degree of obstruction that leads to infection, vesicoureteral reflux, or hydronephrosis. Voiding cystourethrography is done to demonstrate this lesion.
6. Bladder prolapse: usually secondary to relaxation of bladder floor during pregnancy with descent of bladder below the superior aspect of pubic symphysis on an upright film. May result in stress incontinence
7. Chagas disease: Trypanosoma cruzi, a protozoa endemic to South America, causes dilatation of the bladder secondary to infection and destruction of the myenteric plexus. Also causes achalasia
8. Megacystitis syndrome: more frequent in females. Usually diagnosed in childhood. Large, smooth-walled bladder with associated severe vesicoureteral reflux, ureterectasis, and chronic urinary tract infection. Trigone larger than normal
9. Iatrogenic or drug-induced: tranquilizers or muscle relaxants
10. Diabetes insipidus: related to fluid overloading the urinary system with dilated bladder and ureter

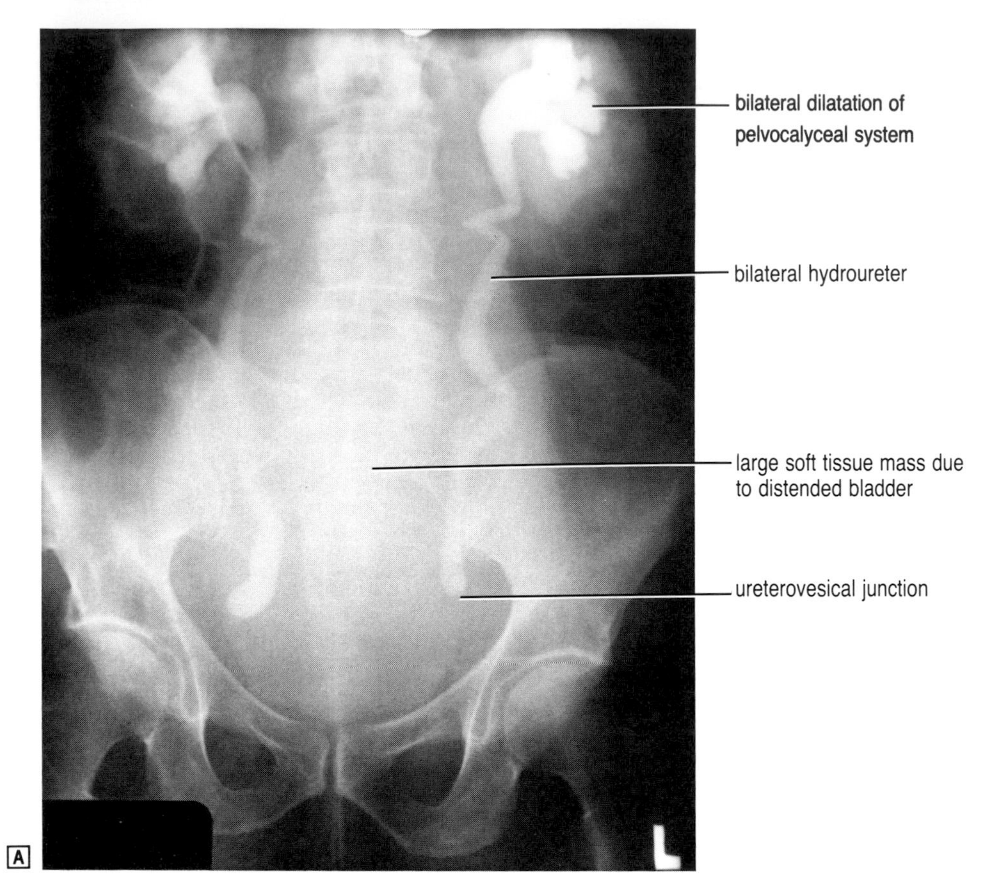

Figure 5.10. *A,* Large urinary bladder.

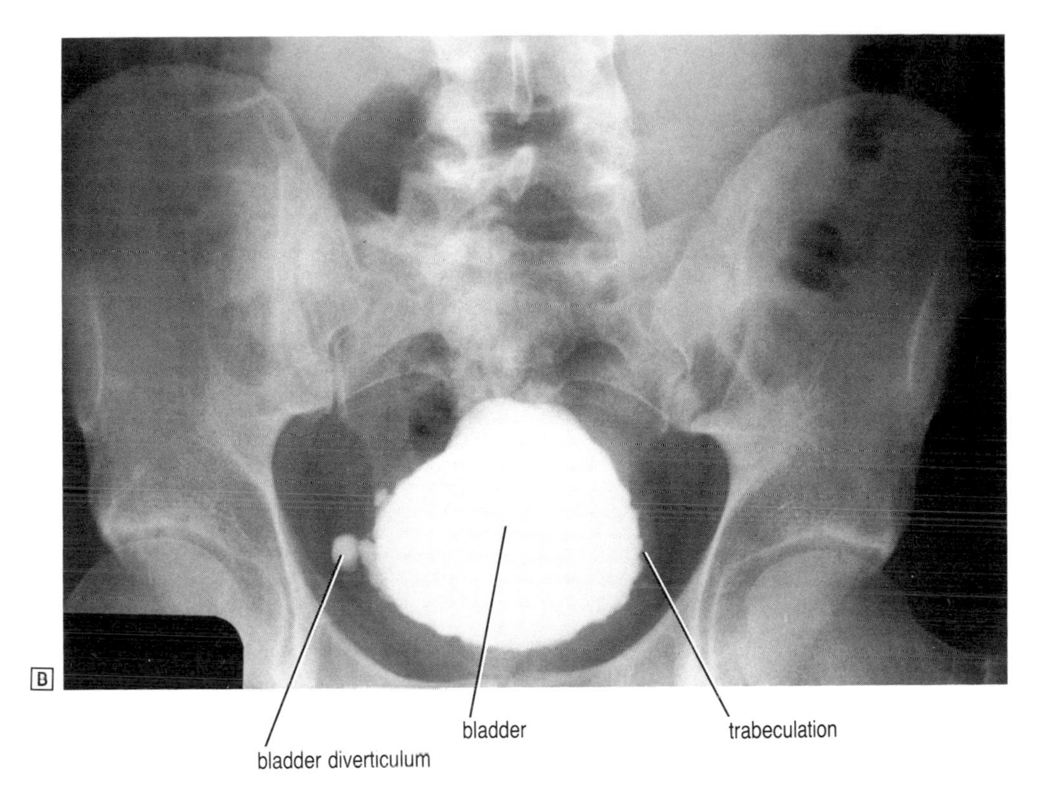

Figure 5.10. *B,* Large urinary bladder.

5.11 SMALL URINARY BLADDER

A. Differential diagnosis
  1. Neurogenic bladder (see Sec. 5.10)
  2. Infiltrating carcinoma
     a. Transitional cell carcinoma: most common type, demonstrated as an irregular filling defect or wall thickening
     b. Squamous cell carcinoma: fairly rare, nonpapillary, and aggressive bladder tumor
  3. Extrinsic compression: pelvic neoplasm, hematoma, inflammation, or uterine enlargement
  4. Chronic cystitis: wall may be serrated with contraction of the bladder dome producing the "Christmas tree or pine-shaped bladder" (see Sec. 5.10). Acute cystitis usually does not result in any cystographic abnormalities.
  5. Radiation cystitis: results in bladder wall necrosis and decreased bladder capacity
  6. Cyclophosphamide (Cytoxan) cystitis: used in treatment of leukemia and lymphoma, ultimately leads to bladder contracture

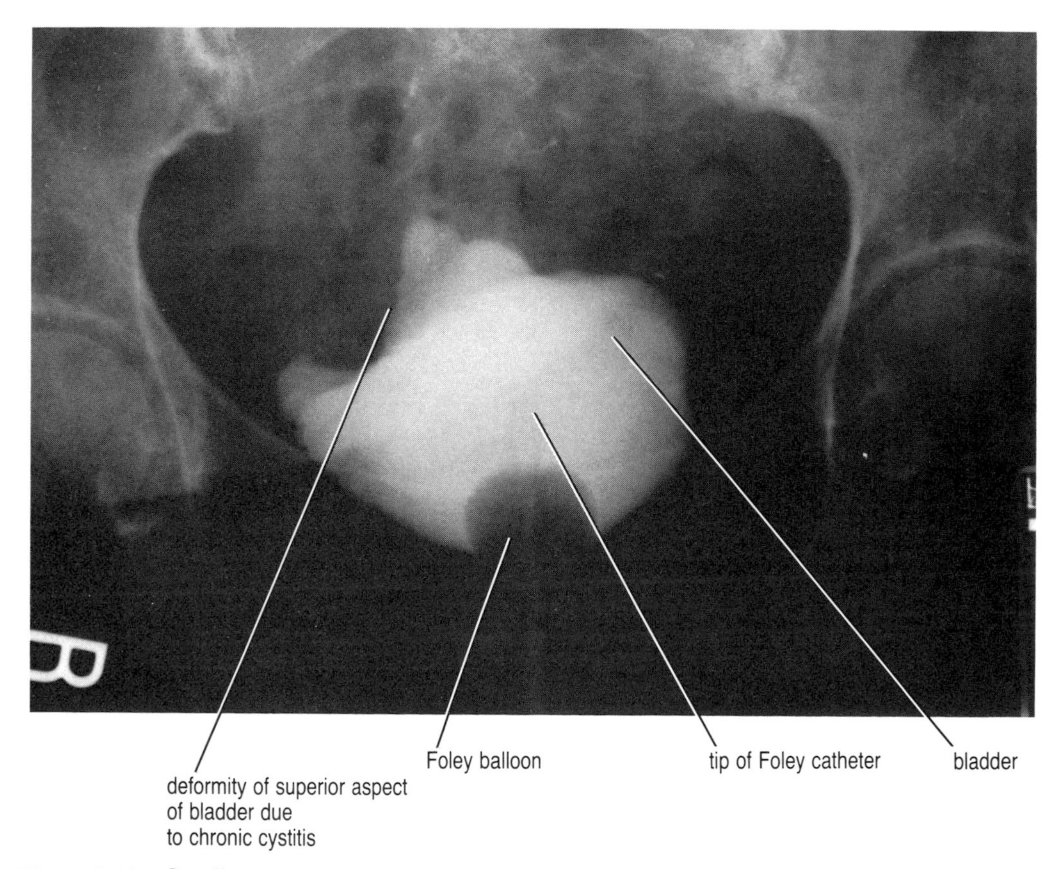

Figure 5.11. Small urinary bladder.

5.12 GAS IN URINARY BLADDER OR WALL

A. Differential diagnosis for intraluminal gas
   1. Iatrogenic: following trauma, cystoscopy instrumentation, surgery, or catheterization
   2. Emphysematous cystitis: usually in diabetes, caused by gas-forming bacteria, e.g., Escherichia coli
   3. Vesicovaginal or vesicointestinal fistula: occurs secondary to Crohn's disease, diverticulitis, carcinoma of pelvic structures (uterus, colon, cervix, bladder, and rectum), postsurgical or postpartum, trauma, inflammation, or congenital anomaly

B. Differential diagnosis for bladder wall gas
   1. Emphysematous cystitis
   2. Fistula tract and iatrogenic causes can also be responsible.

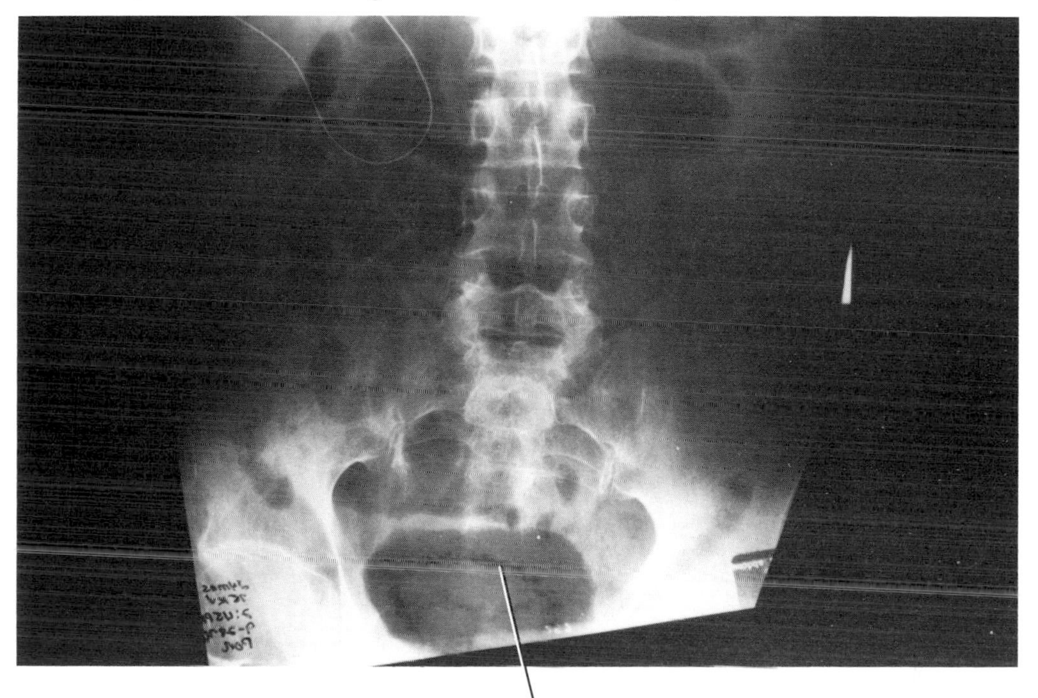

Figure 5.12. Gas in urinary bladder or wall.

5.13 BLADDER-FILLING DEFECTS

A. Differential diagnosis

1. Blood clot: often result of trauma, instrumentation, tumor, inflammatory process, or anticoagulation. Clots appear as irregular intraluminal filling defects and may move with positioning.
2. Calculus: obstruction with urinary stasis and chronic infection are common causes. Examples include neurogenic bladder, bladder outlet obstruction, bladder diverticuli, urethral obstruction/stricture, and cystocele. About half of the stones are radiopaque. May be single or multiple and vary in size from tiny concretions to a single large calculus filling the entire bladder. They tend to be midline in position, except when contained in bladder diverticuli. Usually amorphous or laminated. A foreign body within the bladder from previous instrumentation or therapy may act as a nidus for calculus formation. Must be differentiated (by position or with oblique views) from the following.
   a. Uterine fibroid: higher in position, mottled appearance
   b. Lymph node calcification: usually higher in pelvis
   c. Prostatic calcification: multiple irregular 1- to 10-mm calcifications found at the base of the bladder and within 3 cm of symphysis pubis. Stones are calcified concretions of prostatic fluid and increase with age.
   d. Fecalith: oblique view may show it to be outside bladder. Appears as particulate density.
   e. Seminal vesicle calcification
3. Prostatic enlargement: benign prostatic hypertrophy and carcinoma are the chief causes. Radiographically these cannot be differentiated unless osteoblastic bony metastases, bladder invasion, or pulmonary metastasis is seen. Severe prostatic hypertrophy elevates the entire bladder with characteristic fishhook appearance of the terminal ureter.
4. Iatrogenic: ureteral stents, Foley or suprapubic catheters
5. Neoplasm
   a. Benign lesions such as fibroma, neurofibroma, leiomyoma, hemangioma appear as a mass extending into or indenting the bladder wall. No radiographic characteristics to distinguish histology.
   b. Malignant lesions of bladder
      (1) Transitional cell carcinoma: usually an irregular polypoid filling defect of the bladder base with ureteral obstruction if near ureteral orifice. Calcifications may be present. Because 60% of symptomatic bladder carcinoma is seen by urography, it is best assessed by direct visualization cystoscopy.
      (2) Squamous cell carcinoma: nonpapillary, aggressive
      (3) Rhabdmyosarcoma (sarcoma botryoides): usually involves trigone with bladder obstruction. Comprises about 10% of malignant tumors of childhood.
      (4) Direct extension of metastases from rectum, uterus, cervix, or ovary
6. Ureterocele: may be acquired from ureteral meatus stenosis (inflammation, instrumentation) or may be congenital. Located at ureterovesical junction (UVJ) where the distal ureter prolapses into the bladder and causes "cobra head" or "spring onion" appearance. Ectopic ureteroceles occur in duplex kidneys, arising from the ureter and draining upper pole.
7. Hematoma: results from trauma, instrumentation, or surgery. Movable smooth or irregular defects.
8. Infection: e.g., cystitis, endometriosis, malacoplakia

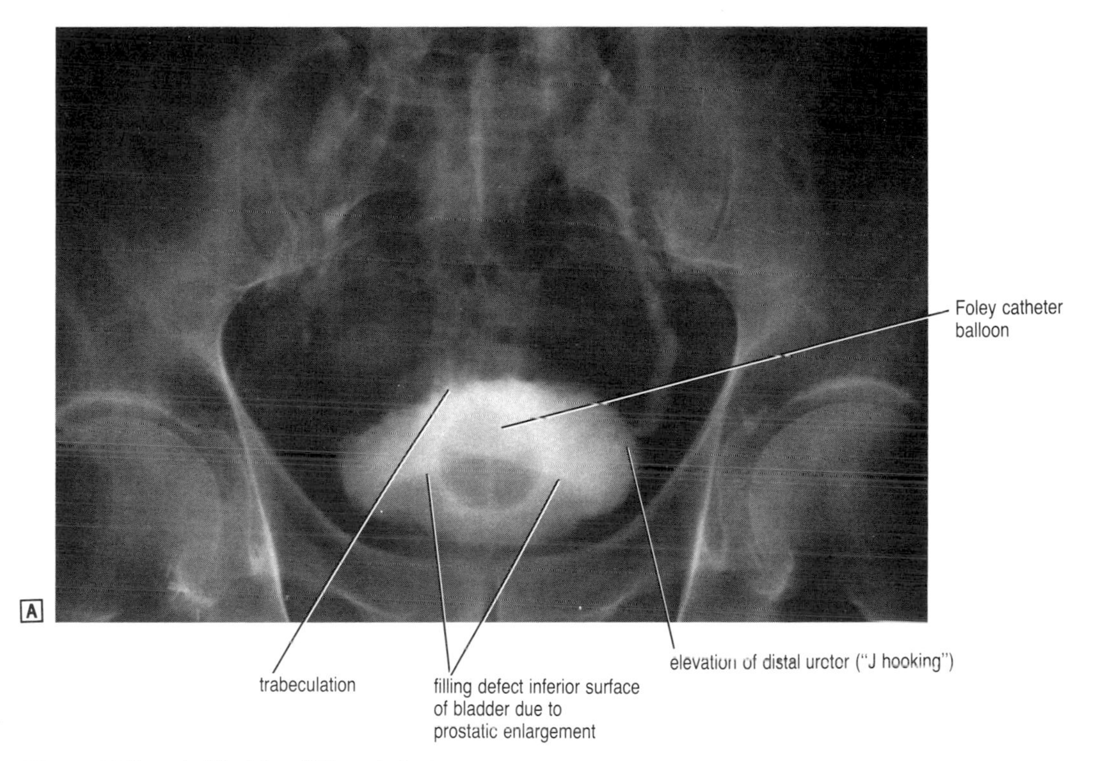

Figure 5.13. *A,* Bladder-filling defects.

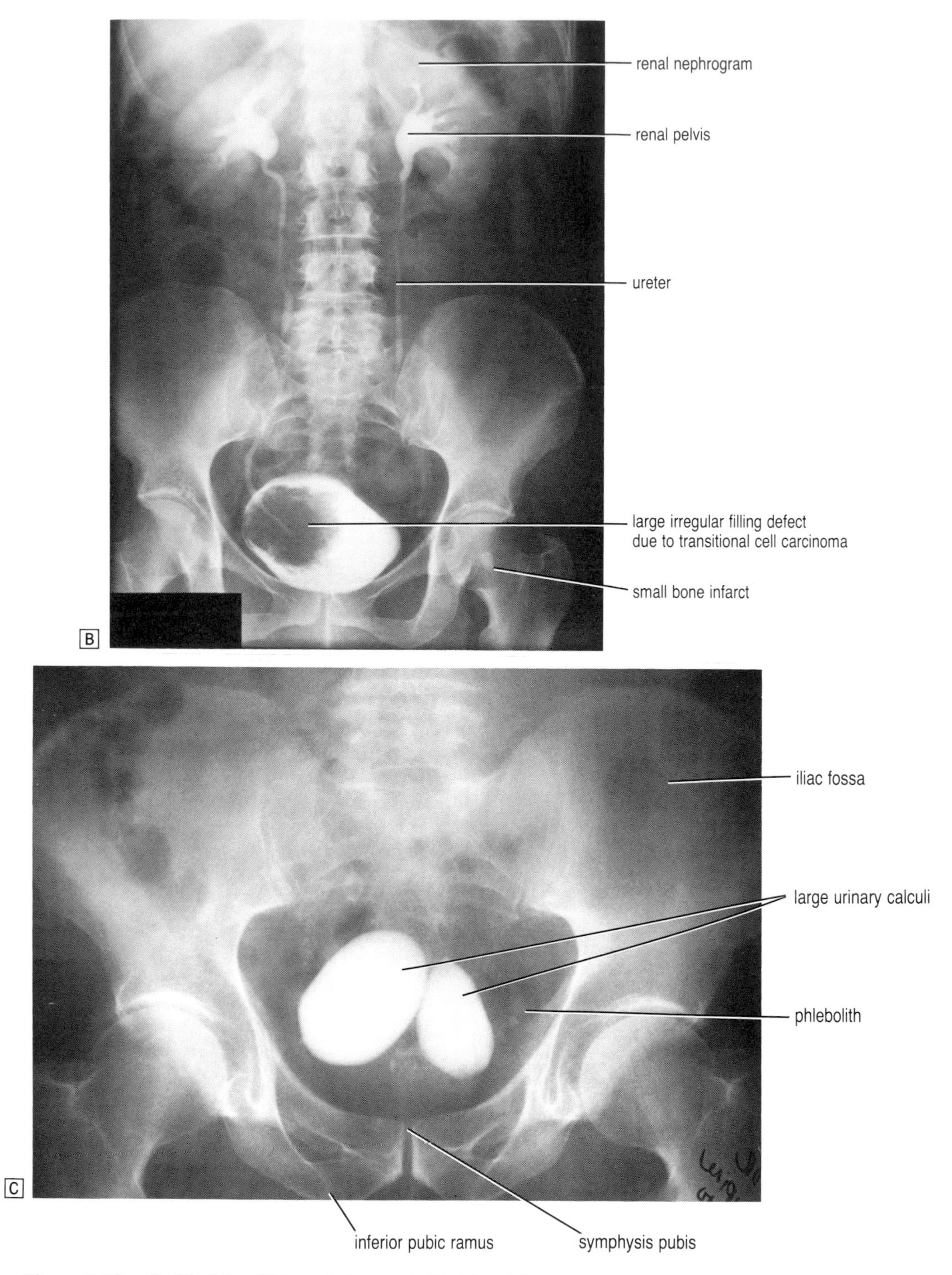

Figure 5.13. *B*, Bladder-filling defects. *C*, Bladder-filling defects.

5.14 CT OF RENAL CYSTS AND SOLID MASSES

A. Renal masses found on IVP may be further defined by the use of ultrasound (cystic versus solid) and CT
B. Simple renal cysts may be solitary or multiple with wide range in size.
  1. Found in 50% of population, they are the most common renal mass. Have no malignant potential and rarely are found in association with hypernephromas
C. Ultrasound (US) criteria of a simple renal cyst: diagnostic accuracy about 98%
  1. No internal echoes
  2. Good through wall transmission of the sound wave
  3. Well-defined far wall
  4. Circular or oval shape
D. Computed tomography criteria similar to those for ultrasound and include
  1. Near water CT attenuation coefficient (darker, water = 0, decreased density)
  2. Thin walls
  3. No enhancement with intravenous contrast
  4. Sharp interface with normal renal parenchyma
E. A hyperdense renal cyst has all the characteristic findings of a simple cyst with an increased CT attenuation coefficient due to hemorrhage or infection within it.
F. Solid-appearing masses on ultrasound are more adequately evaluated by CT because it evaluates tumor size, extension, adenopathy, invasion of inferior vena cava or renal vein, and presence of metastases (liver, brain), all of which are necessary to characterize and stage the tumor.
  1. CT findings of a solid mass
    a. Improved definition of the tumor from the normal surrounding parenchyma with postcontrast images
    b. Less contrast enhancement than surrounding normal renal parenchyma
    c. Areas of low attenuation within the mass usually represent necrosis or hemorrhage.
G. CT findings of an enhancing indistinct solid mass may be suggestive of a hypernephroma, which accounts for 85% of adult renal tumors. Because diagnostic accuracy by radiographic methods is approximately 50% in differentiating various tumors, a biopsy with CT or ultrasound guidance is required. Angiography is useful to define tumor blood supply and to differentiate vascular neoplasms such as hemangiomas and renal angiomyolipomas (hamartoma) from hypernephromas that may be hyper or hypovascular. The tumor vessels do not respond to epinephrine injected into the renal artery, producing a tumor blush.

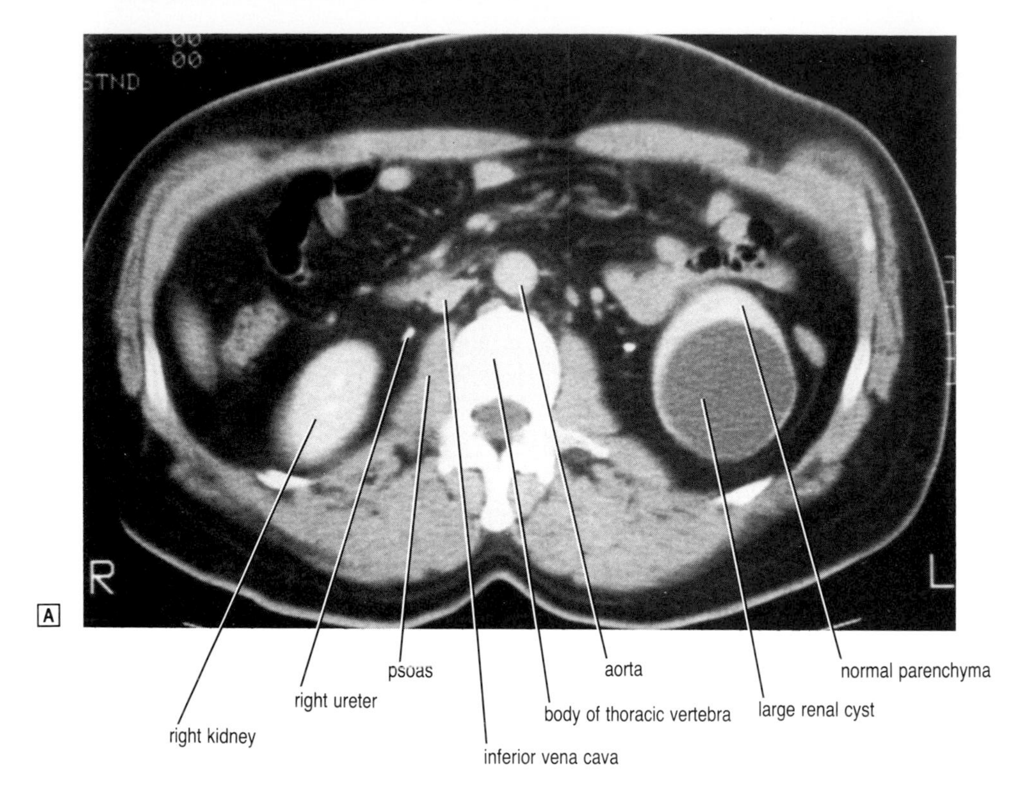

Figure 5.14. *A*, CT of renal cysts and solid masses.

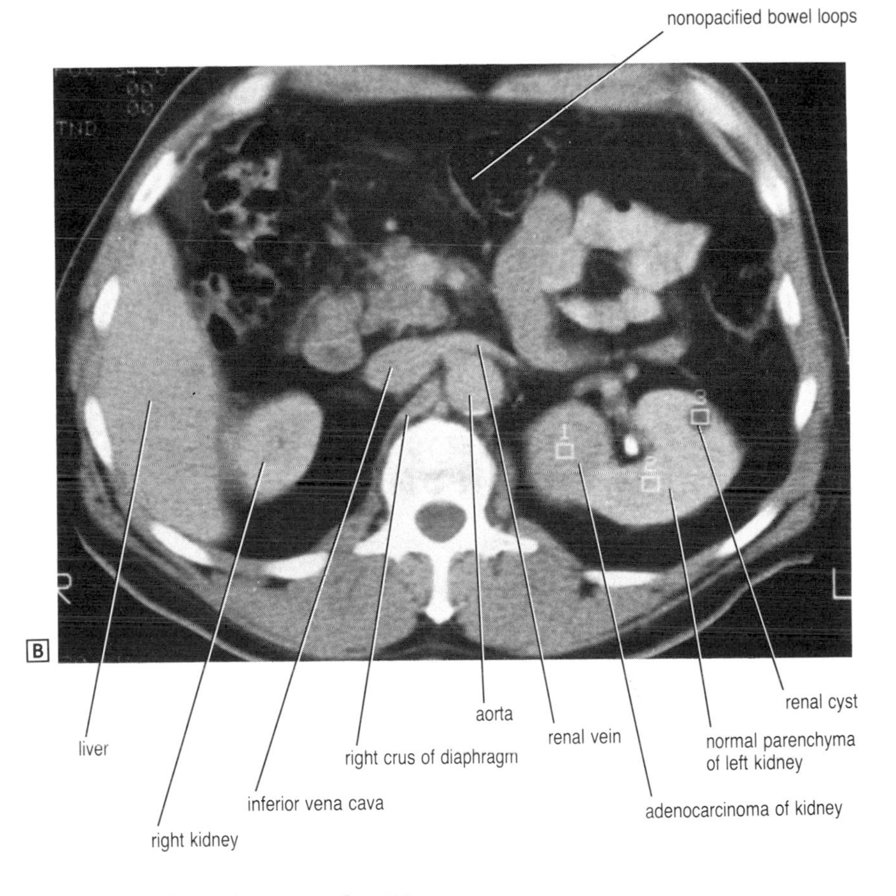

Figure 5.14. B, CT of renal cysts and solid masses.

5.15 RENAL TRAUMA AND LOWER GENITOURINARY TRAUMA

A. Blunt injury is the most common cause of renal trauma. Based on clinical history and a physical exam revealing flank tenderness, abrasions, penetrating wounds, and the presence of hematuria, the possibility of renal injury is suggested. Abdominal plain films obtained prior to an IVP may reveal fractures of either ribs or lumbar transverse processes, loss of renal function, and psoas outline secondary to hemorrhage.

B. Most important IVP findings
   1. Nonfunction (fractured kidney, renal artery avulsion due to deceleration injury or thrombosis, renal vein thrombosis secondary to blood clots, as well as conditions not related to trauma such as massive tumor involvement, renal agenesis, multicystic kidney, ureteral obstruction, or xanthogranulomatous pyelonephritis)
   2. Contrast extravasation (fractured/lacerated kidney, instrumentation, calculus, abdominal compression)
   3. Decreased or delayed function (large subcapsular hematoma decreases cortical perfusion, renal vessel spasm, postrenal obstruction)
   4. Renal displacement or distortion of renal contour and calyceal system (intrarenal hematoma, blood clot, and other nontraumatic causes)

C. CT demonstrates renal morphologic changes with higher sensitivity
   1. Intrarenal hematoma appears as an area without contrast enhancement with poorly defined margins.
   2. Subcapsular hematoma typically is a nonenhancing crescent-shaped defect within the normal enhancing renal contour.
   3. Perinephric hematomas appear as streaked densities within the perirenal fat.
   4. Urinomas: persistant extravasation of urine or blood into the perinephric space, a complication of renal trauma. Appears as a mass with a line separating it from the kidney. May opacify on IVP if contrast extravasates into it.
   5. Renal lacerations appear on dynamic flow images as areas lacking contrast enhancement and correlate with tissue viability and vascular compromise.
   6. Allows evaluation of other abdominal organs and spaces simultaneously

D. Arteriography is useful to assess bleeding site, vascular injury, tissue viability, arteriovenous fistulas, to map vascular supply prior to surgery, to stabilize the patient temporarily prior to surgery via catheter embolization.

E. Ultrasound may be used to assess renal contour and tissue, and retroperitoneal hemorrhage.

F. Traumatic injury to the urethra and bladder may result from compressive or decelerative forces, pelvic fractures, penetrating or straddle injuries, and instrumentation. Typical clinical findings: inability to void spontaneously, urinary retention, blood present on external meatus.

G. Bladder injury occurs in 5 to 10% of patients with pelvic fractures (usually ramus fracture or widening of the symphysis pubis), and urethral injury usually occurs at the membranous urethra in 5 to 15% (almost exclusively in men). Blunt trauma is the most common cause of urethral injury.

H. Extraperitoneal bladder rupture occurs as the result of laceration by a bony fragment in 70 to 80% of cases. Intraperitoneal rupture occurs in patients with a distended bladder with traumatic compression or deceleration injury 20 to 30% of the time. Intraperitoneal rupture is more common in children because the bladder is located intra-abdominally. Retrograde urethrogram is used to initially evaluate urethral integrity for laceration, transection, or extravasation and is done prior to an excretory urogram if urethral injury is suspected. Extraluminal extravasation of contrast media may represent urethral laceration or transection. Urethral disruption appears as an abrupt termination of the contrast column. The posterior urethra is the most common site for disruption. Once urethral abnormality is excluded, a retrograde cystogram may be performed via cannulization of the bladder and filling with contrast.

I. Extraperitoneal bladder rupture demonstrates extravasated contrast material outlining the pelvic floor, whereas intraperitoneal bladder rupture fills the paracolic gutters and outlines the pelvic recesses and loops of bowel.

J. Spontaneous rupture of the bladder rarely occurs secondary to severe cystitis, neoplasm, or outlet obstruction (neurogenic bladder and mechanical outlet obstruction).

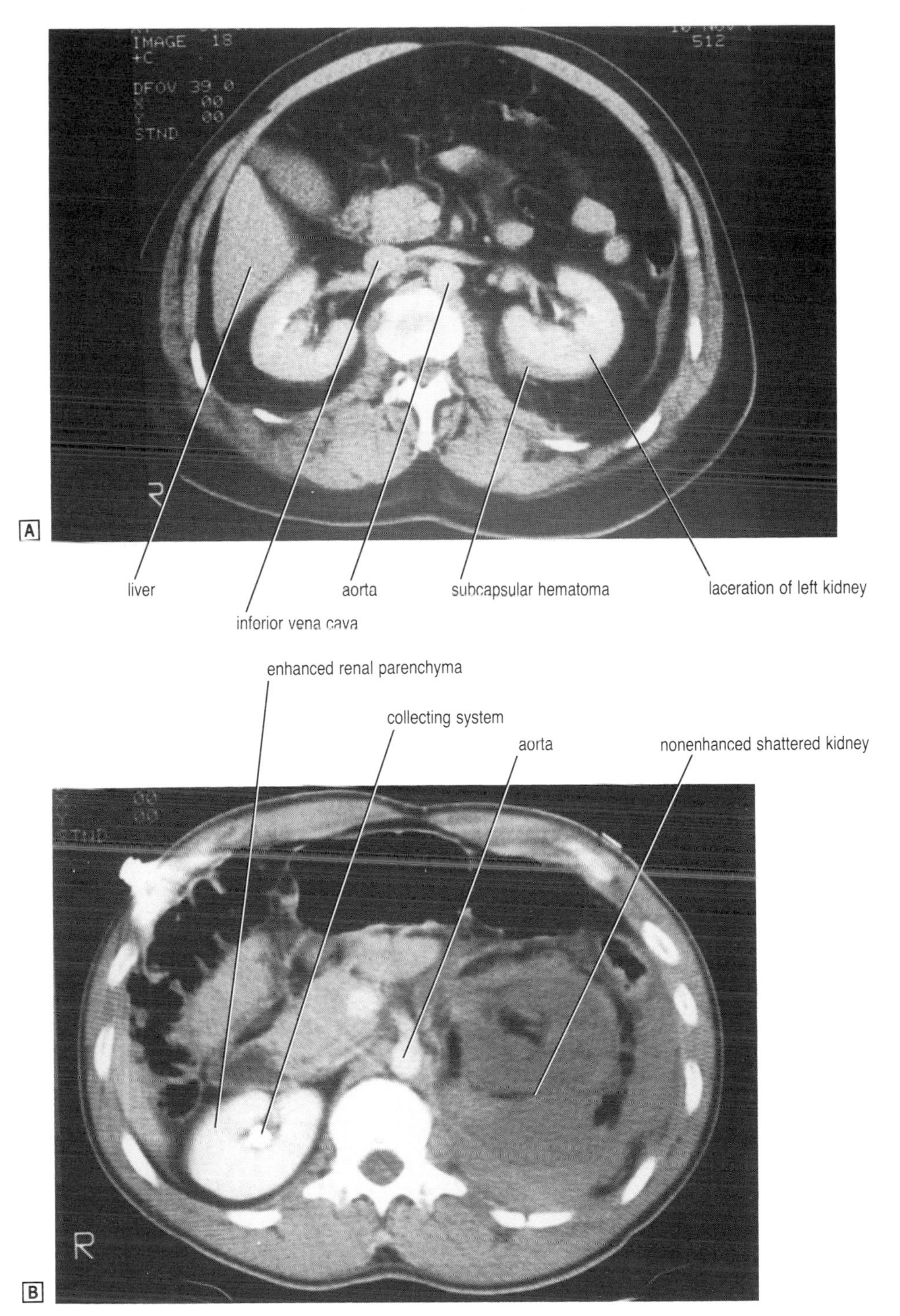

Figure 5.15. *A,* Renal trauma and lower genitourinary trauma. *B,* Renal trauma and lower genitourinary trauma.

References

Bartrum, R.J., and Crow, H.C.: Real-time Ultrasound—A Manual for Physicians and Technical Personnel. Philadelphia: W.B. Saunders Co., 1983.

Eisenberg, R.L.: Diagnostic Imaging in Internal Medicine. New York: McGraw-Hill Book Co., 1985.

Harris, J.H., and Harris, W.H.: The Radiology of Emergency Medicine. 2nd Ed. Baltimore: Williams & Wilkins, 1981.

Juhl, J.H., and Crummy, A.B.: Essentials of Radiologic Imaging. Philadelphia: J.B. Lippincott, 1987.

Lang, E.K.: Current concepts in the diagnosis of renal trauma. In: Contemporary Diagnostic Radiology, Vol. 6. Baltimore: Williams & Wilkins, 1983.

Lang, E.K.: Radiologic diagnosis of lesions of the ureter. In: Contemporary Diagnostic Radiology, Vol. 3. Baltimore: Williams & Wilkins, 1980.

Levy, R.C., Hawkins, H., and Barsan, W.G.: Radiology in Emergency Medicine. St. Louis: C.V. Mosby Co., 1986.

Toombs, B.D., and Sandler, C.M.: Computed Tomography in Trauma. Philadelphia: W.B. Saunders Co., 1987.

6

Osseous System

6.01 NORMAL APPENDICULAR ANATOMY

A. Roentgenographic evaluation of the osseous system is important in assessing skeletal abnormalities that result from trauma or bone disease.

B. Evaluation should include:
   1. Correlation with clinical history, mechanism of injury, if relevant, age, and physical findings
   2. Anatomic alignment and position of the involved bones
   3. Assessment of the entire bone or involved joint including the articular surface, cortex, medullary canal and, in children, the epiphyseal growth plate regions for fracture or bony changes that may indicate skeletal disease.
   4. In equivocal cases, a comparison view of the contralateral bone or extremity is often helpful.

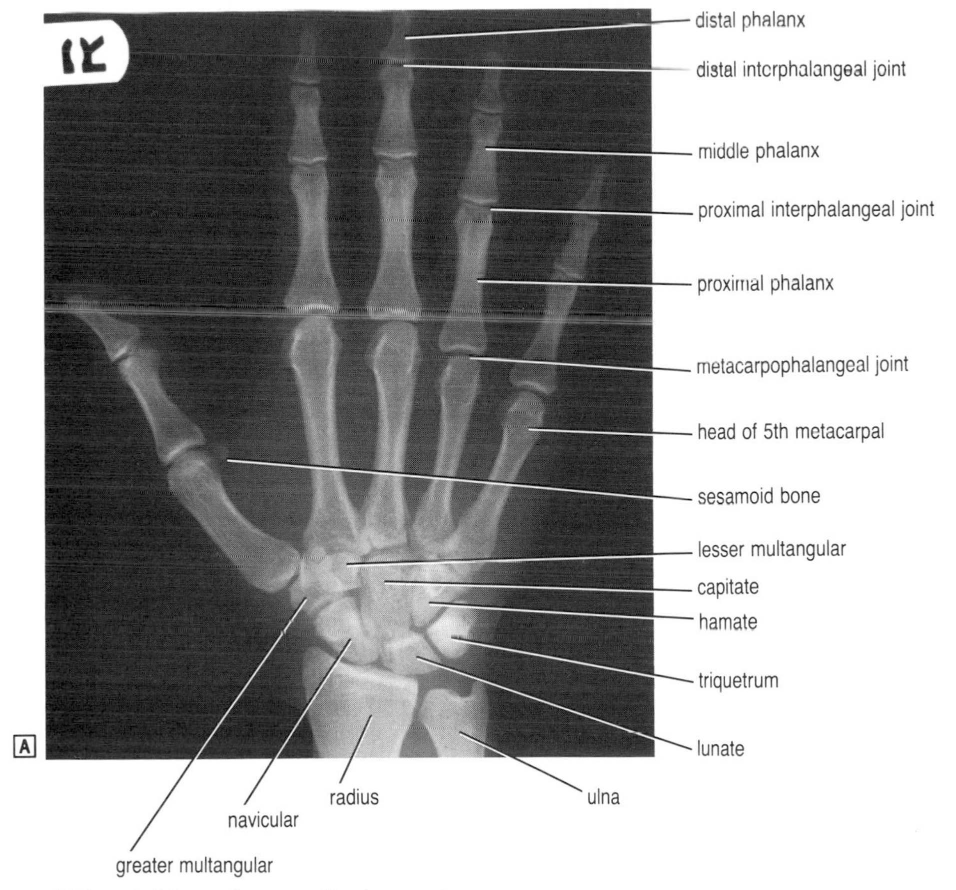

Figure 6.01. *A,* Normal appendicular anatomy.

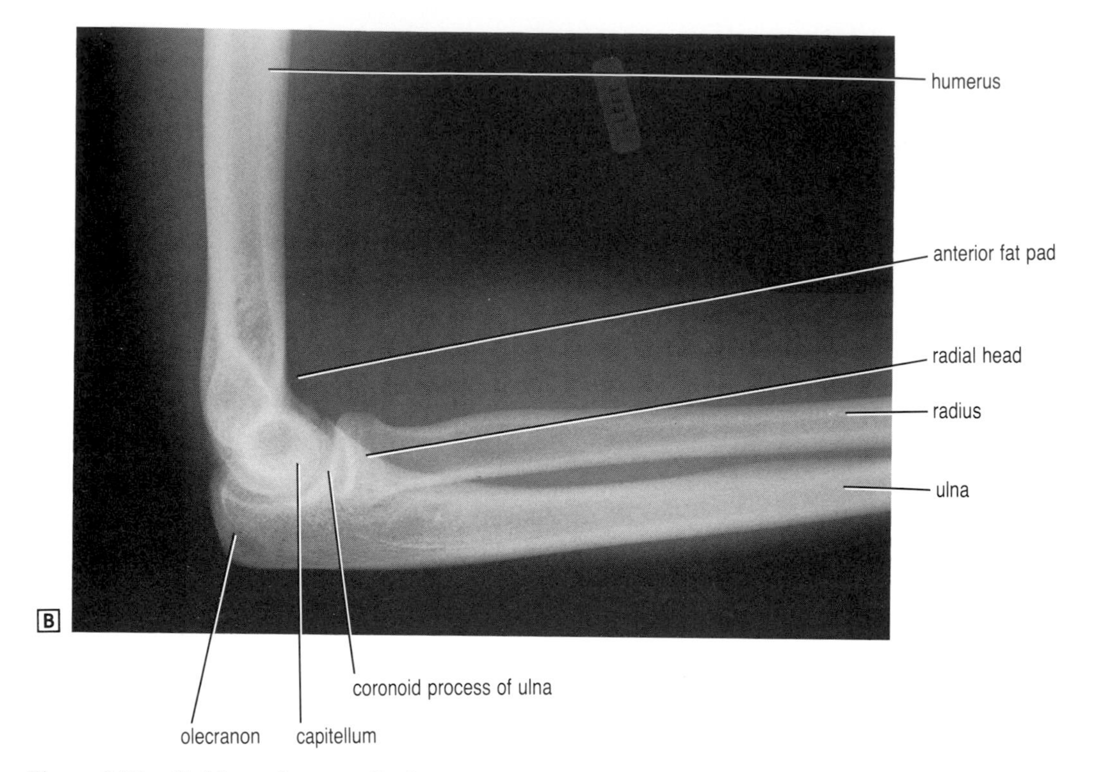

Figure 6.01. *B,* Normal appendicular anatomy.

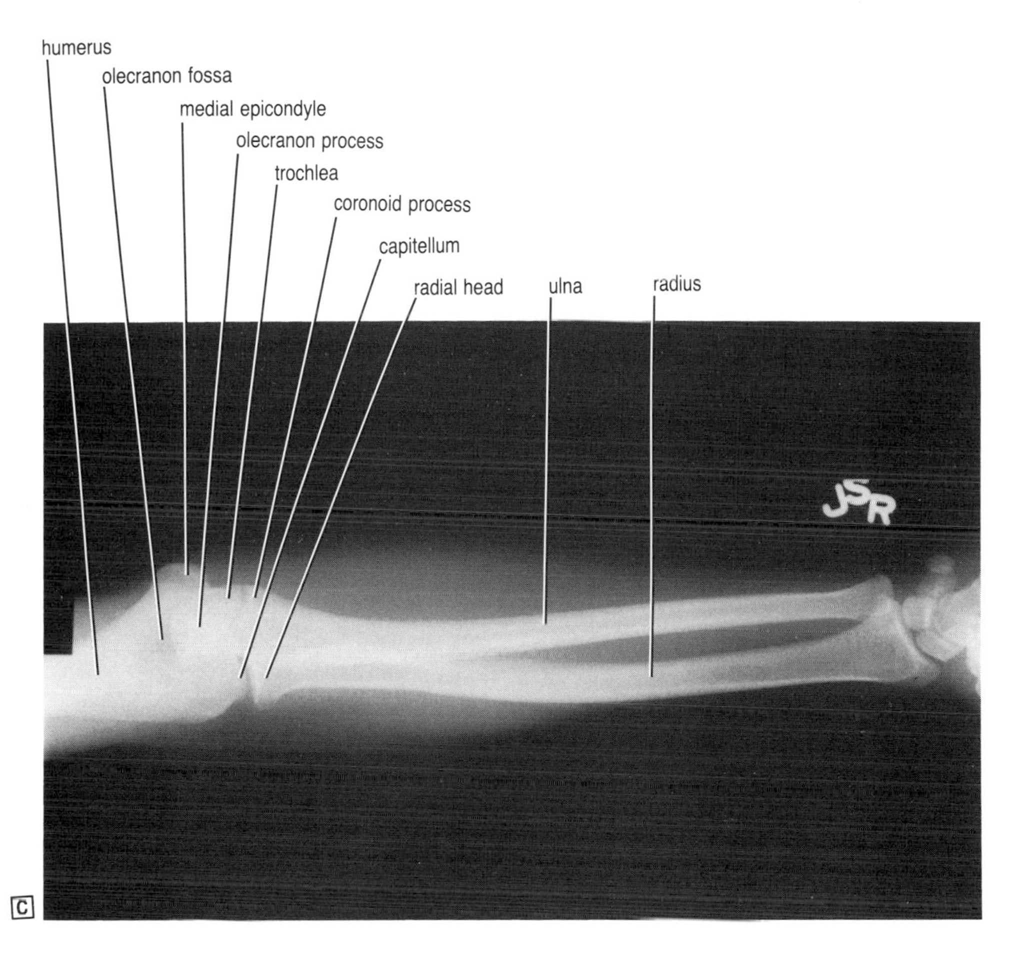

Figure 6.01. C, Normal appendicular anatomy.

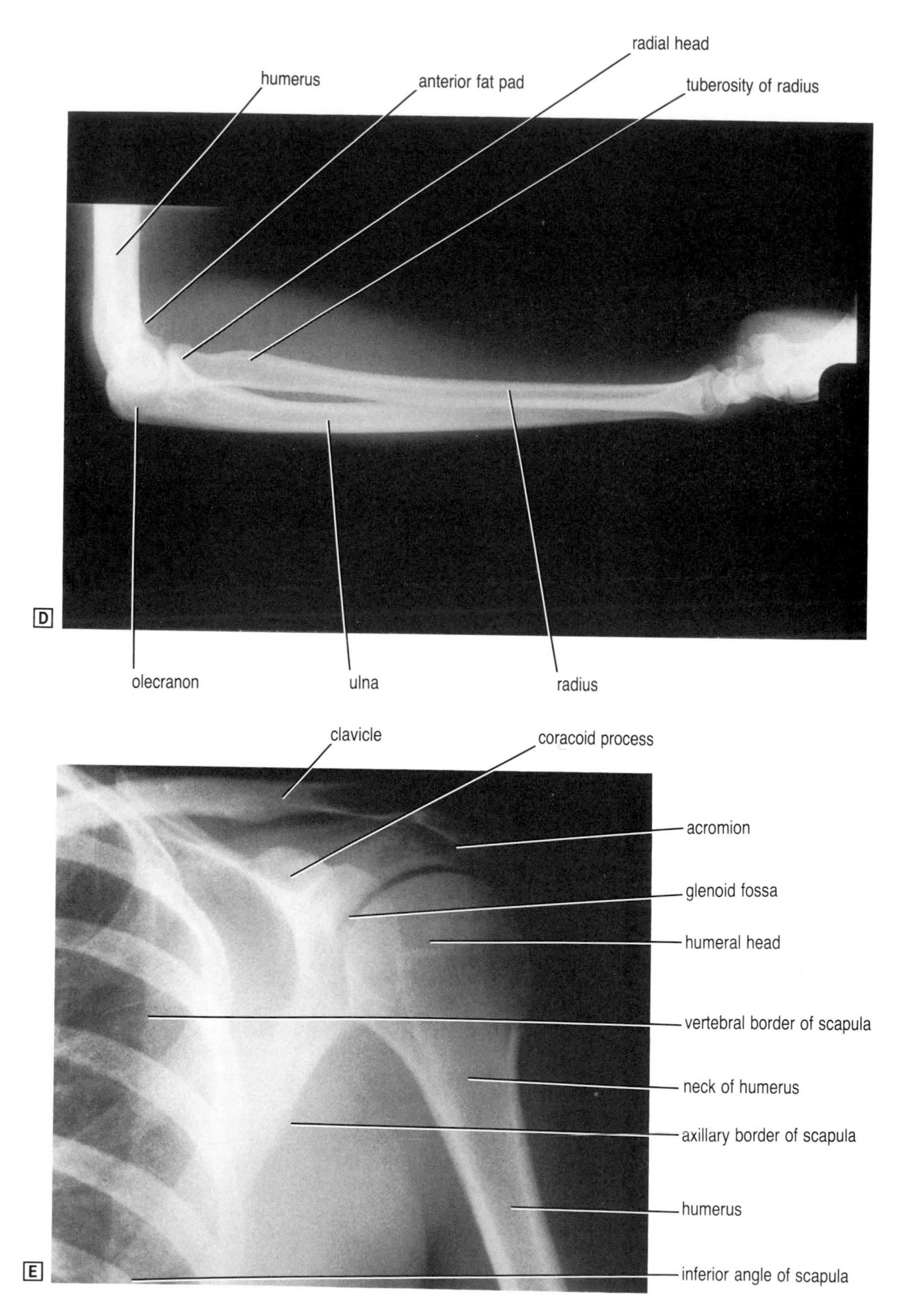

Figure 6.01. *D,* Normal appendicular anatomy. *E,* Normal appendicular anatomy.

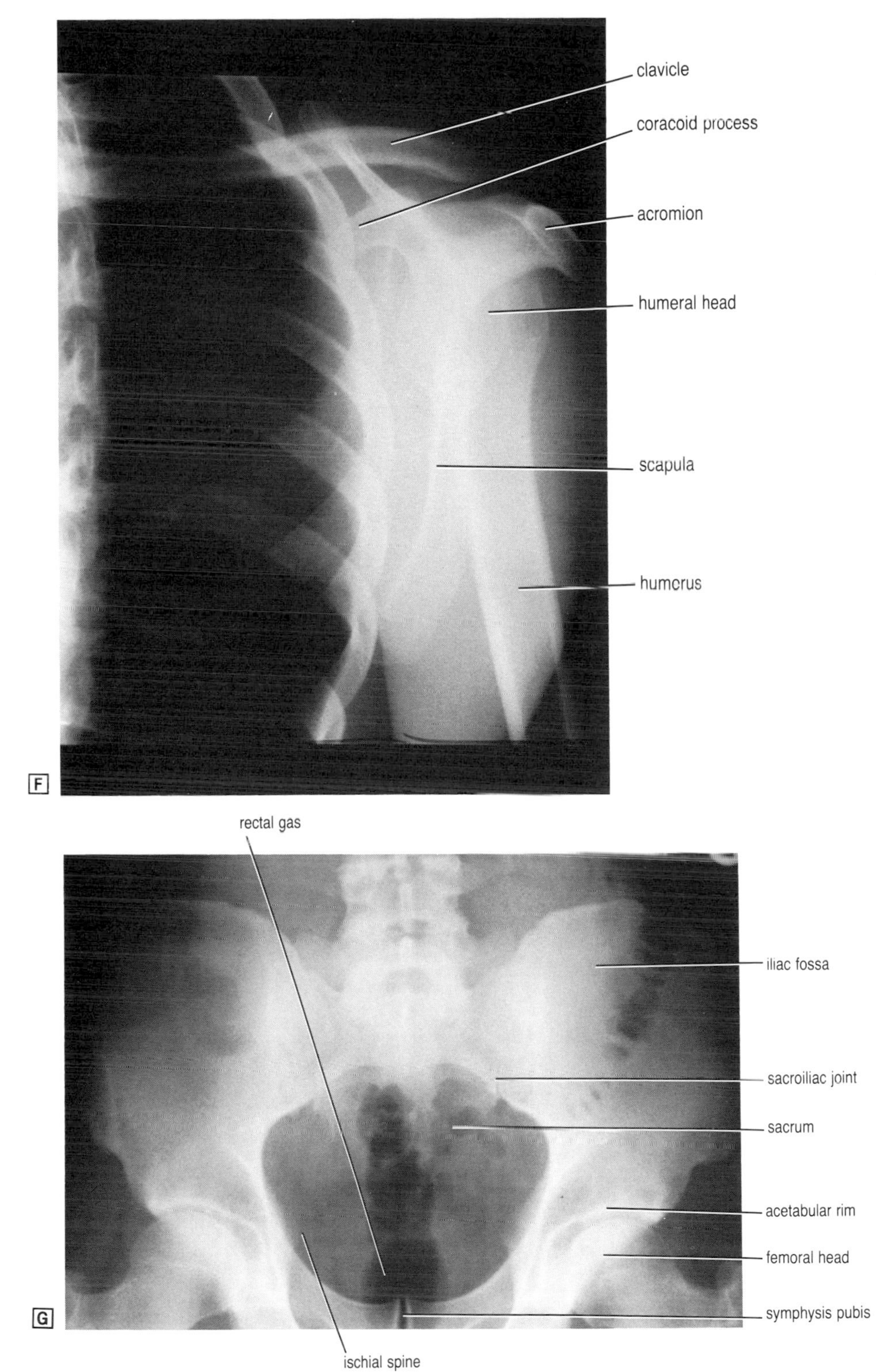

Figure 6.01. *F,* Normal appendicular anatomy. *G,* Normal appendicular anatomy.

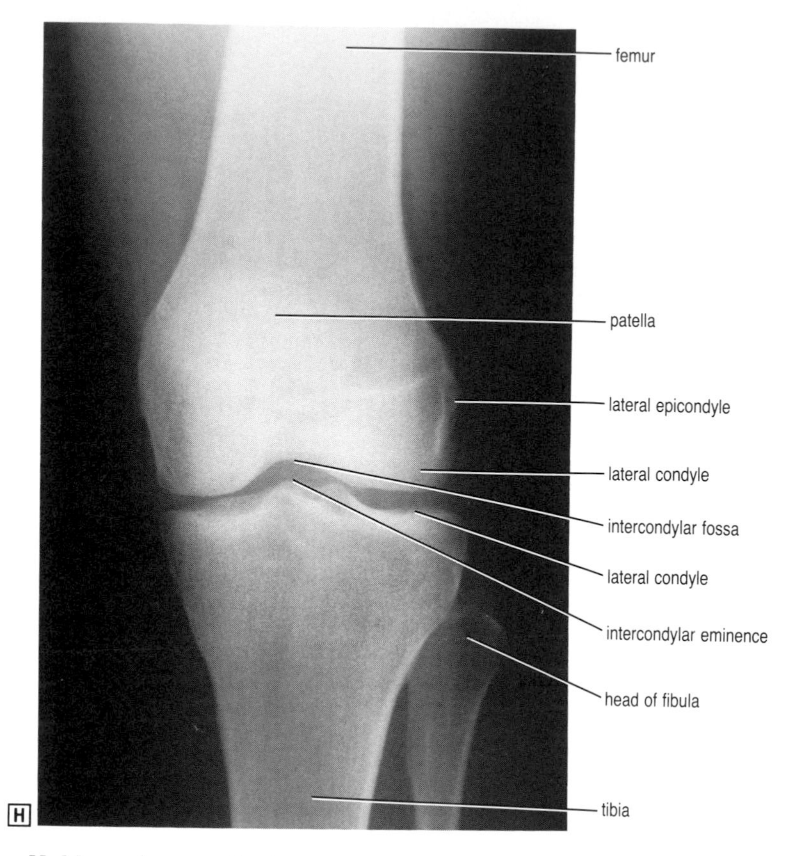

Figure 6.01. *H,* Normal appendicular anatomy.

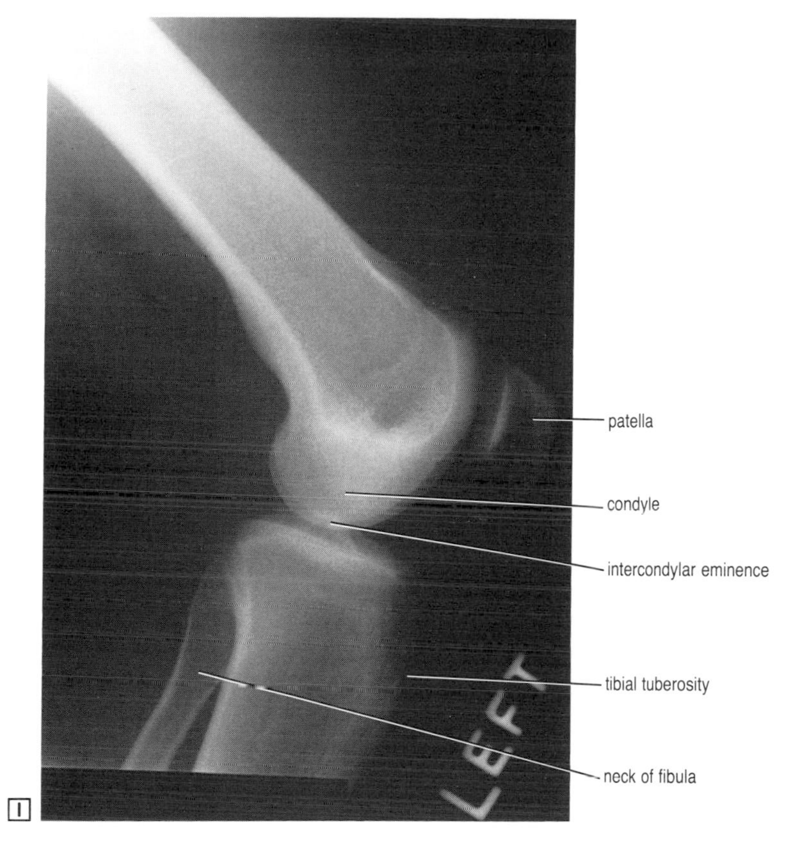

Figure 6.01. *I,* Normal appendicular anatomy.

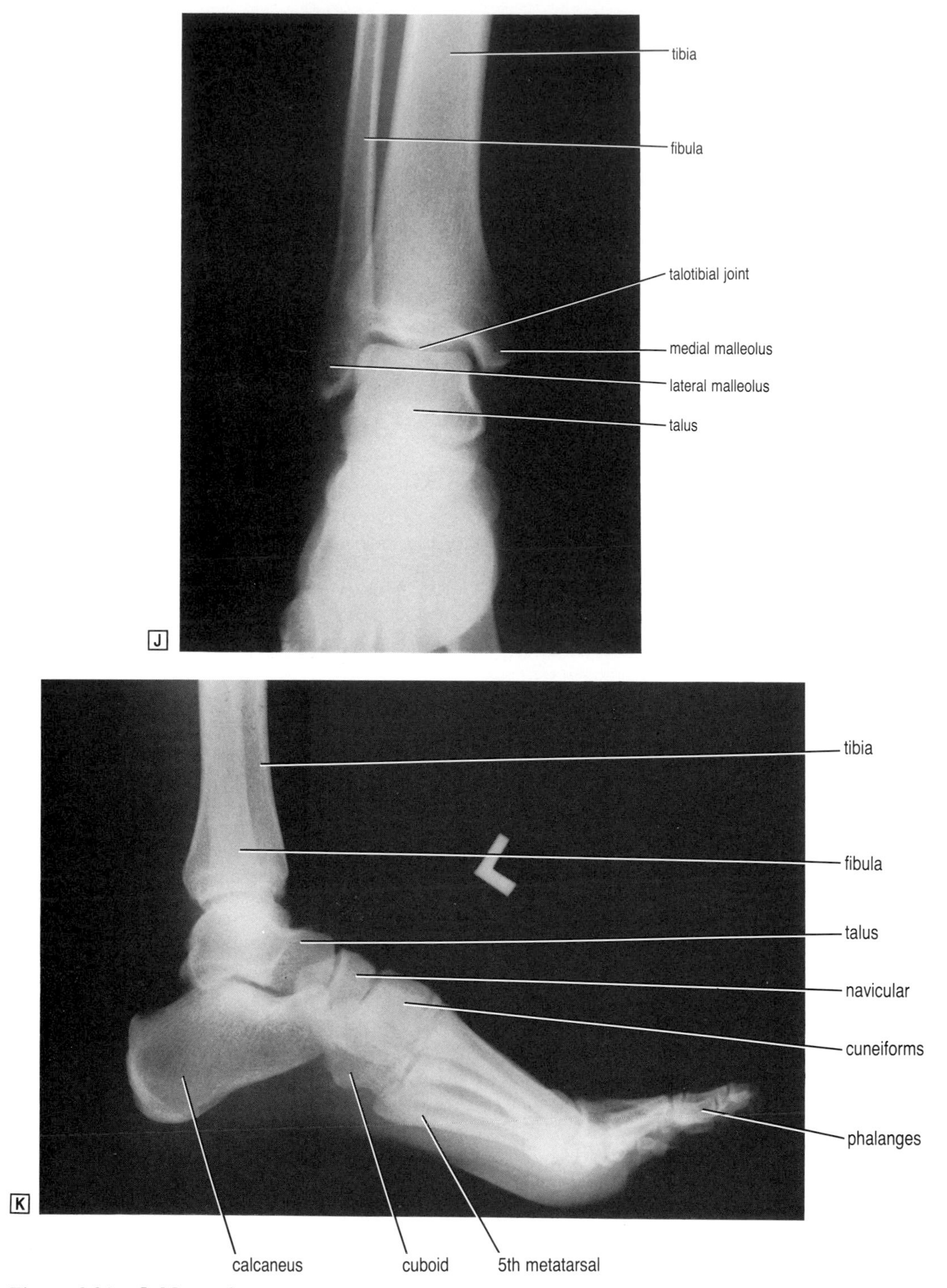

Figure 6.01. *J,* Normal appendicular anatomy. *K,* Normal appendicular anatomy.

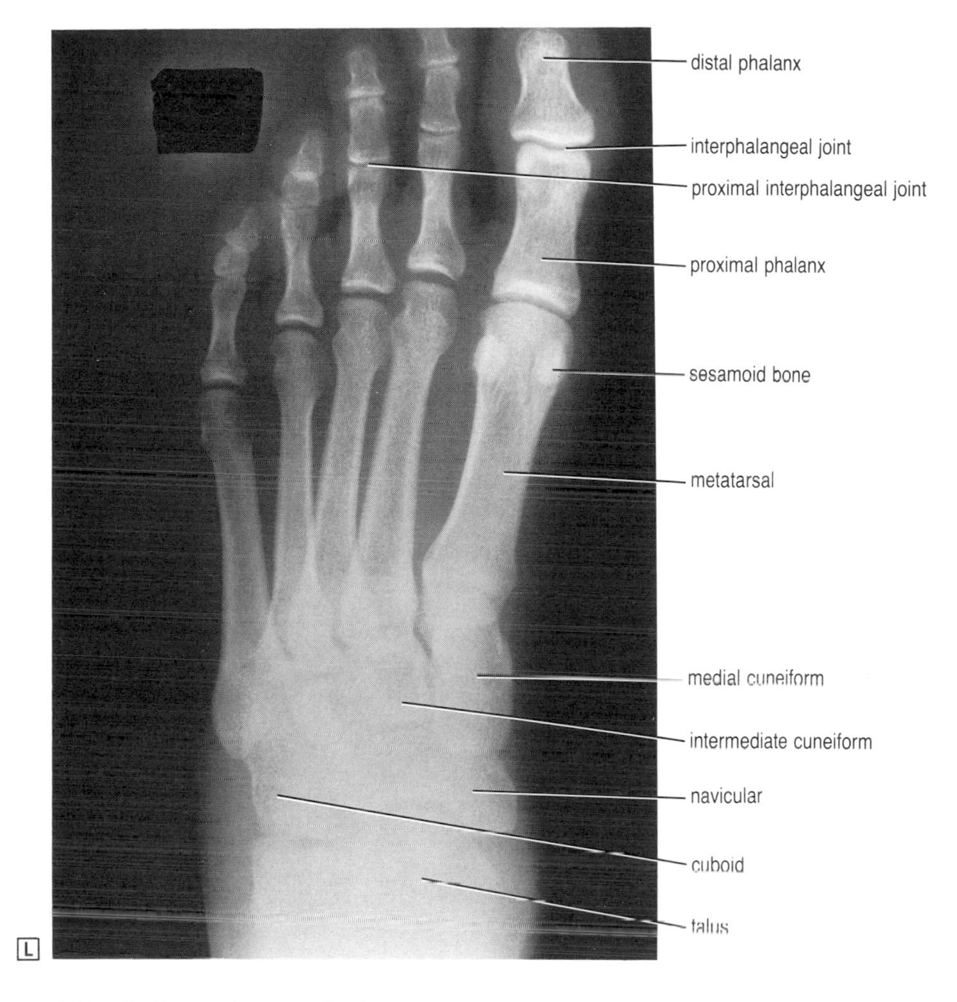

Figure 6.01. *L,* Normal appendicular anatomy.

6.02 SALTER-HARRIS CLASSIFICATION OF EPIPHYSEAL PLATE INJURIES

A. Used to categorize epiphyseal and metaphyseal fractures that occur commonly and exclusively in childhood
B. Distal radius is involved in 50% of epiphyseal injuries.
C. Approximately 85% of epiphyseal injuries have no growth disturbance. Those that cross the epiphyseal plate (type IV) or crush injury (type V) disrupt the blood supply and produce growth retardation and angular deformity.
   1. Type I
      a. Complete separation of epiphysis from metaphysis without bony fracture.
      b. The epiphyseal line appears widened with or without displacement. Comparison with the opposite side is often helpful.
      c. Prognosis is excellent
   2. Type II
      a. Most common type of epiphyseal injury: approximately 75%
      b. Fracture through a portion of metaphysis with associated epiphyseal widening
      c. Characteristic triangular metaphyseal fragment
      d. Prognosis is good
      e. Treatment: closed reduction
   3. Type III
      a. Uncommon injury, usually involves proximal and distal tibial epiphyses
      b. Fracture extends through epiphysis from articular surface to growth plate with or without displacement of fragments.
      c. Prognosis: good assuming the epiphyseal fracture is reduced with smooth articular surface margins
   4. Type IV
      a. Most frequently occurs at lateral condyle of the humerus
      b. Fracture extends from articular surface of epiphysis through growth plate and into the metaphysis, with or without displacement.
      c. Prognosis: guarded to good assuming perfect anatomic reduction; otherwise, growth arrest or joint deformity results. Long-term follow-up is required.
   5. Type V
      a. Rare, often involves knee or ankle, difficult to detect
      b. Result of crushing force to the epiphysis
      c. No radiographic findings initially except for swelling near epiphyseal and metaphyseal junction.
      d. Premature closure of epiphyseal plate with resultant angular deformity and decreased growth are potential complications.
      e. Treatment: resection of impacted portion or surgical fusion of the growth plate. Long-term follow-up is required.

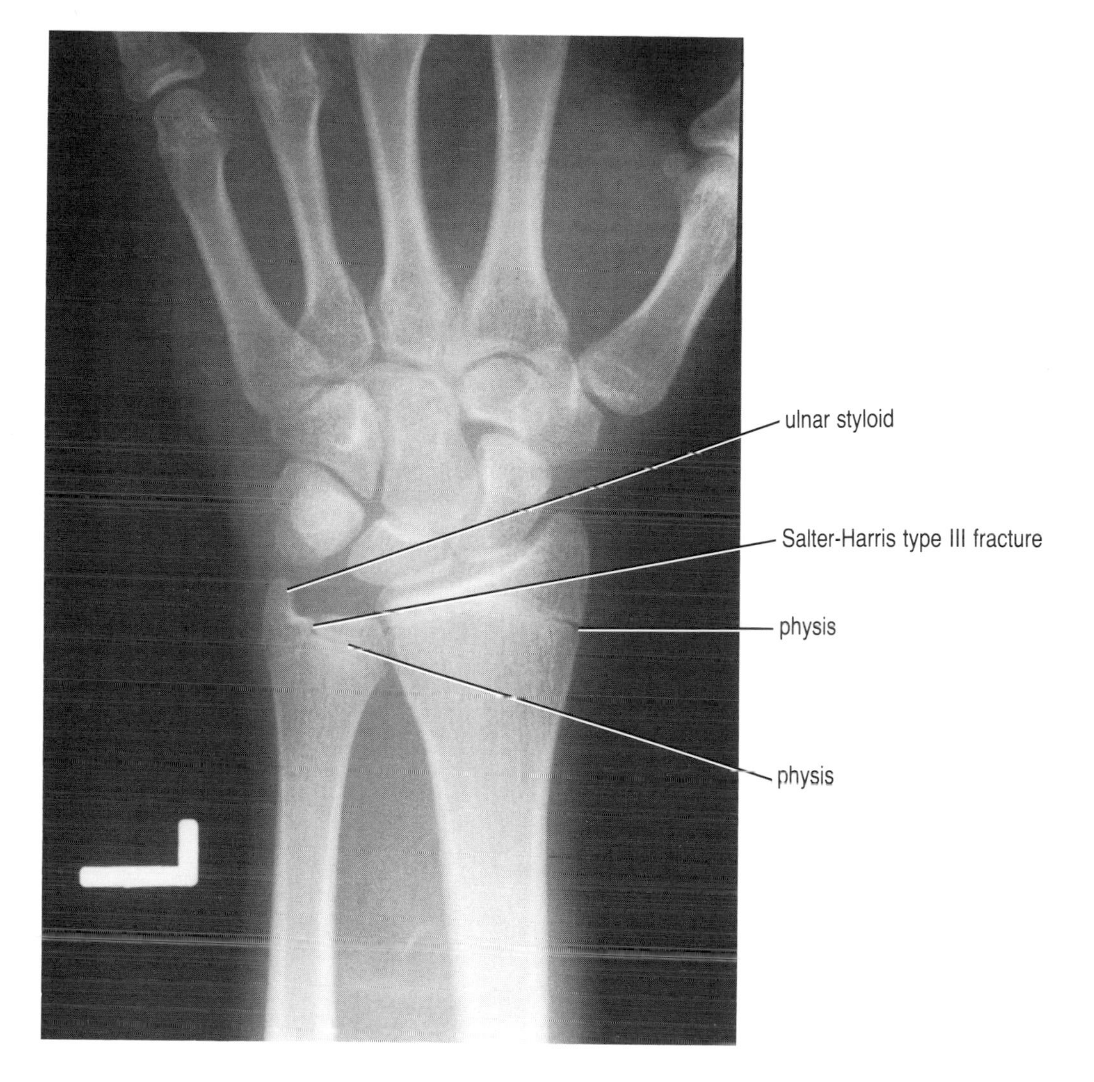

Figure 6.02. Salter-Harris classification of epiphyseal plate injuries.

6.03 ACROMIOCLAVICULAR LIGAMENT INJURY

A. Subluxation and dislocation of the acromioclavicular (AC) joint are common injuries. Also called shoulder or AC separation. Incomplete dislocation is called a subluxation. The AC and coracoclavicular (CC) ligaments together play a role in the appearance of the shoulder.
B. Mechanism of injury: a blow or fall upon the point of the shoulder
C. Physical exam: tenderness of AC region, internally rotated adducted arm
D. Injury classification (of AC and coracoclavicular ligaments)
   1. Grade I: sprain, consists of stretching or tearing a few ligamentous fibers
      a. Detected by comparing stress views (15-pound sandbags) of injured and non-injured shoulders, revealing minor widening of the AC joint
   2. Grade II: subluxation; partial or complete disruption of AC ligament with intact CC ligament. May require stress films to reveal widening
   3. Grade III: dislocation; disrupted AC and CC ligaments: scapula and acromion displaced downward and medially; widening usually evident without stressing the shoulder
E. Normal AC joint measures 3 to 5 mm in width.
F. Inferior surfaces of the clavicle and acromion lie on the same plane. Useful in evaluating the presence of a subluxation
G. Comparison with opposite shoulder and additional stressed films is required in AC joint injuries. AC joint separation is accentuated by weight bearing.

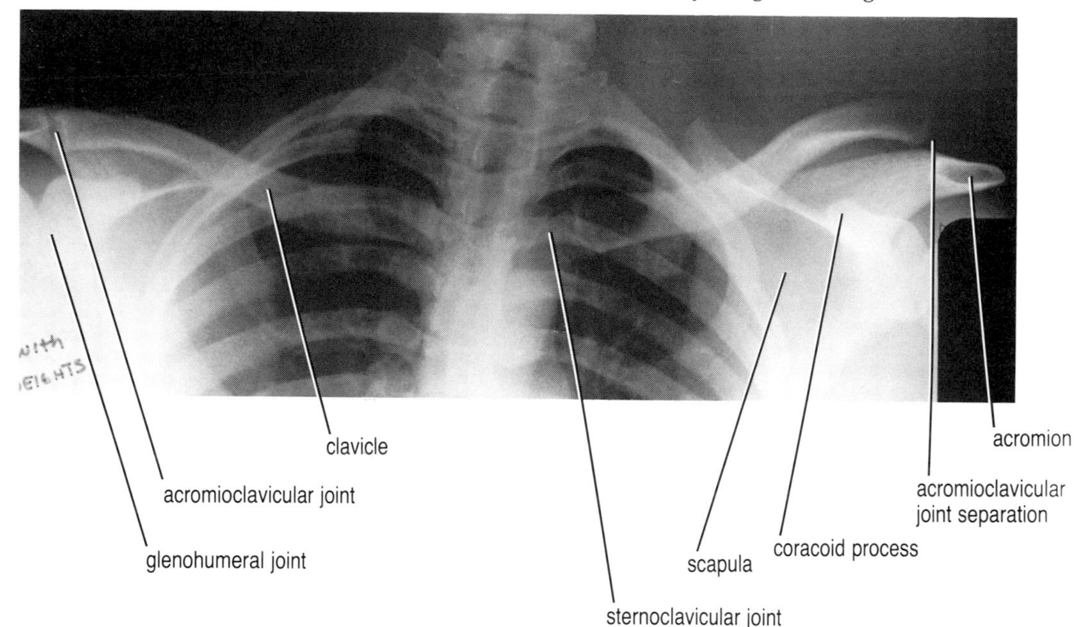

Figure 6.03. Acromioclavicular ligament injury.

6.04 SHOULDER DISLOCATIONS

A. Of all dislocations, 50% occur at the shoulder; of these, 90% are anterior dislocations with the humeral head lying beneath the coracoid process of the scapula. This represents a subcoracoid dislocation, the most common type.

B. Anterior inferior dislocation is commonly associated with Hill-Sachs deformity. This is a humeral head compression fracture with resulting notch indentation along the posterolateral humeral head due to recurrent dislocations as occur in young individuals.

1. History and physical exam: Result of excessive abduction, pain, arm held in abduction, humeral head palpated inferior to glenoid, neurovascular compromise secondary to brachial plexus compression
2. Common complication of a shoulder dislocation is a fracture of anterior inferior rim of glenoid fossa (Bankhart fracture).
3. Roentgenographic findings: anterior oblique "Y" view demonstrates humeral head anterior to the glenoid.

C. Posterior shoulder dislocations comprise approximately 2 to 4% of the cases.

1. Approximately 40 to 50% of the cases are missed because the AP view appears relatively normal.
2. Associated signs indicating dislocation
   a. The humeral head is locked in internal rotation with posterior displacement. Owing to severe internal rotation, superimposition of the humeral head and humeral neck produces the "light bulb" sign.
   b. "Positive rim sign": widening of the space between anterior glenoid rim and articulating surface of the humeral head. Normally, this space is 6 mm or less.
   c. "Trough" line: refers to an associated impaction fracture of the medial aspect of the humeral head with a curvilinear cortical bone density that parallels the articular surface of the humeral head.
3. Avulsion of lesser tuberosity is a common complication.
4. History and physical exam: direct blow or fall to the anterior shoulder while internally rotated and flexed. Posterior shoulder fullness on palpation, inability to externally rotate or abduct the arm, axillary nerve compression.
5. Fifty percent of posterior dislocations are result of epileptic seizures.
6. Roentgenographic findings: "Y" view: humeral head posteriorly and below acromion

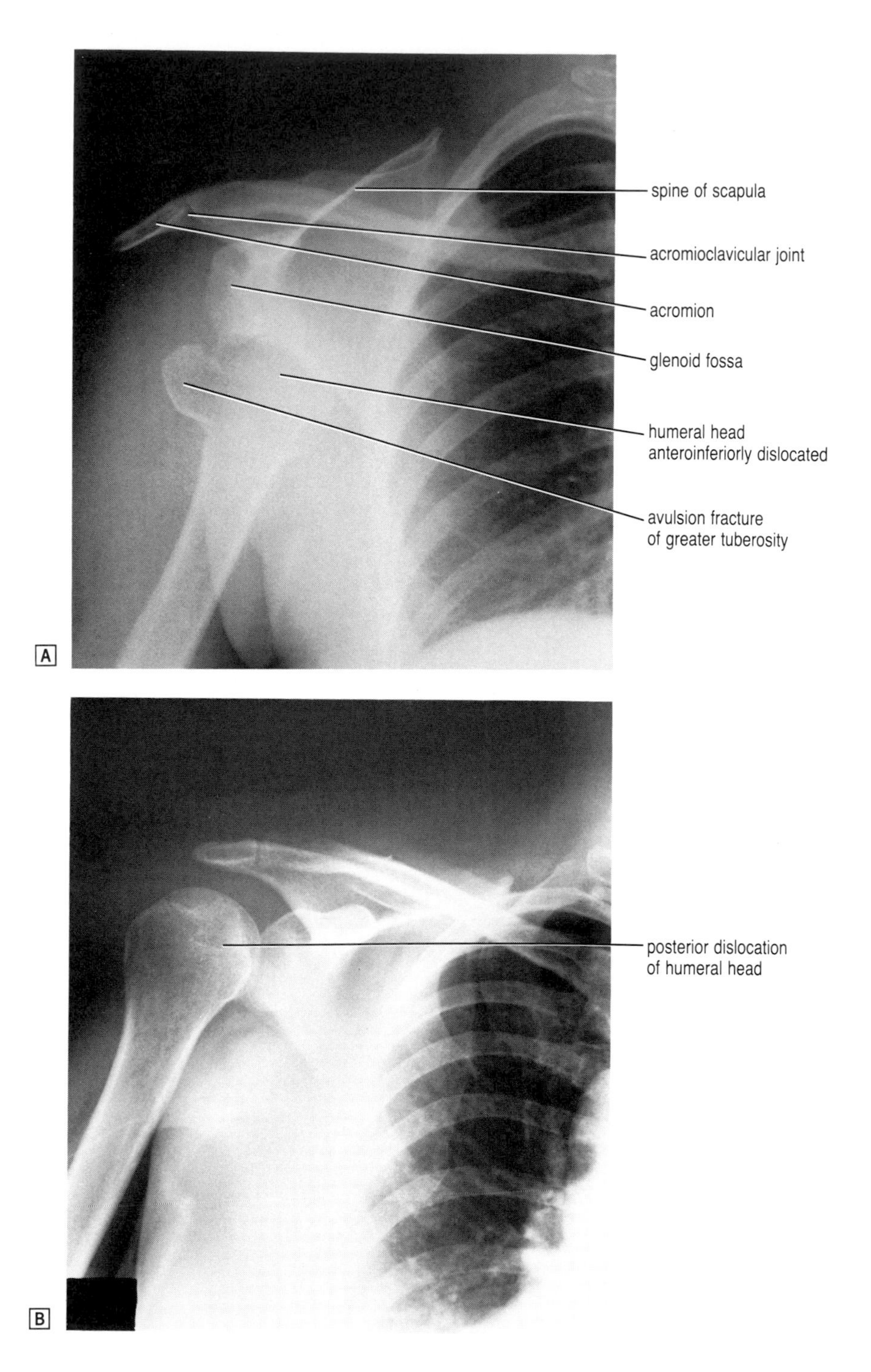

Figure 6.04. *A*, Shoulder dislocations. *B*, Shoulder dislocations.

6.05 SCAPULA FRACTURES

A. Fractures of the scapula are infrequent and usually the result of crushing injuries from motor vehicle accidents, direct trauma, or shoulder dislocation.

B. Fractures may involve:
   1. Body of the scapula
   2. Infraspinous portion
   3. Coracoid process
   4. Glenoid fossa
   5. Acromion process: associated with superior shoulder dislocations or direct trauma

C. Brachial plexus and acromioclavicular joint injury are common complications.

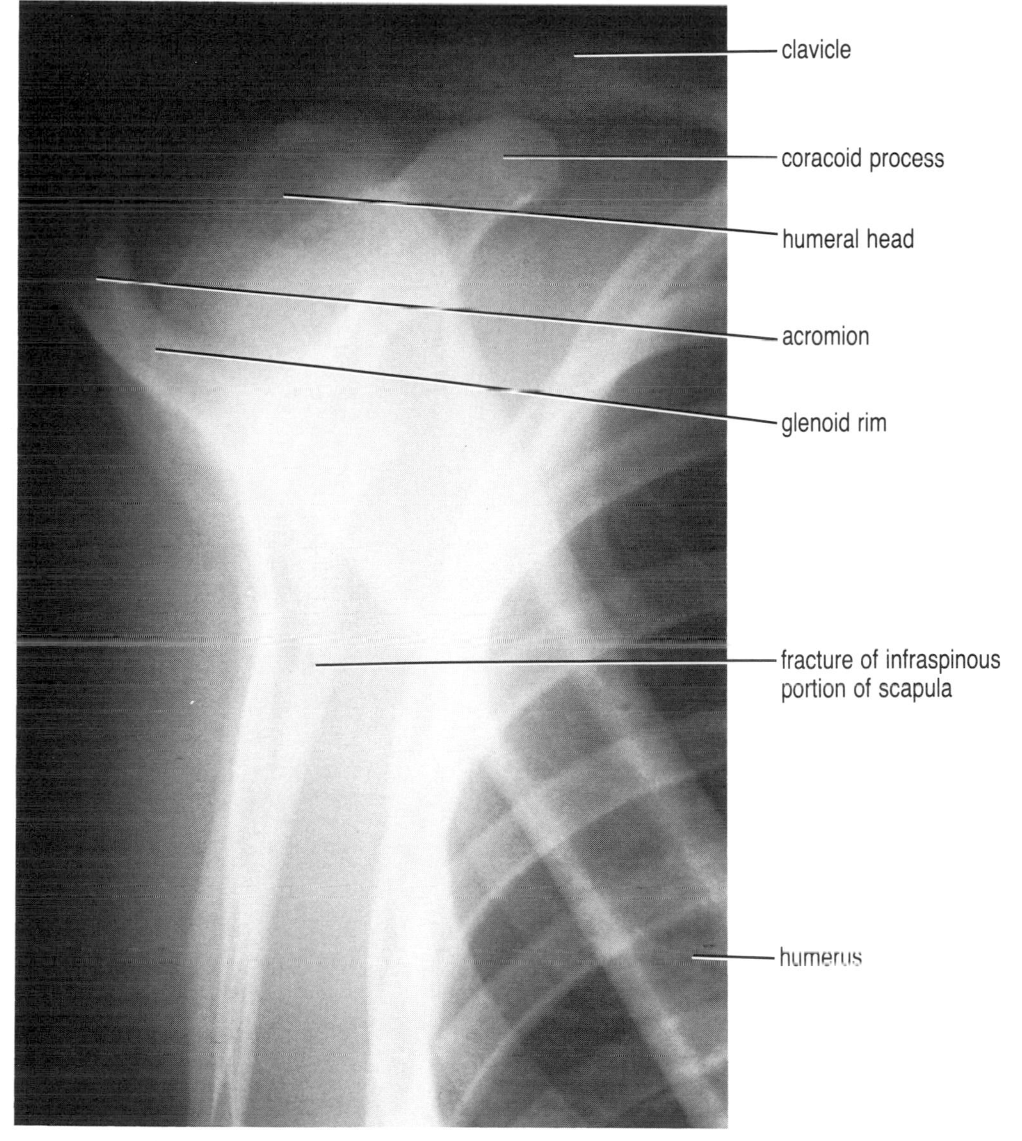

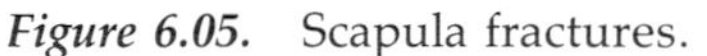

Figure 6.05. Scapula fractures.

6.06 CLAVICULAR FRACTURES

A. Classified with regard to position, i.e., distal third, mid-third, or proximal third, and the degree of displacement.
B. Mid-third fracture is the most common. Typical deformity: proximal fragment displaced superiorly and distal fragment inferiorly as a result of the pectoralis minor muscle and weight of the extremity.
C. Distal third fractures are less common and usually nondisplaced because the distal and medial fragments are secured by the acromioclavicular (AC) and coracoclavicular (CC) ligaments, respectively. Elevation of the proximal end indicates CC ligamentous disruption.
D. Proximal third fractures are much less common, usually caused by severe force with associated intrathoracic injuries.
E. History and physical: fall or blow to shoulder or clavicle, pain, tenderness, brachial plexus injury, inability to abduct

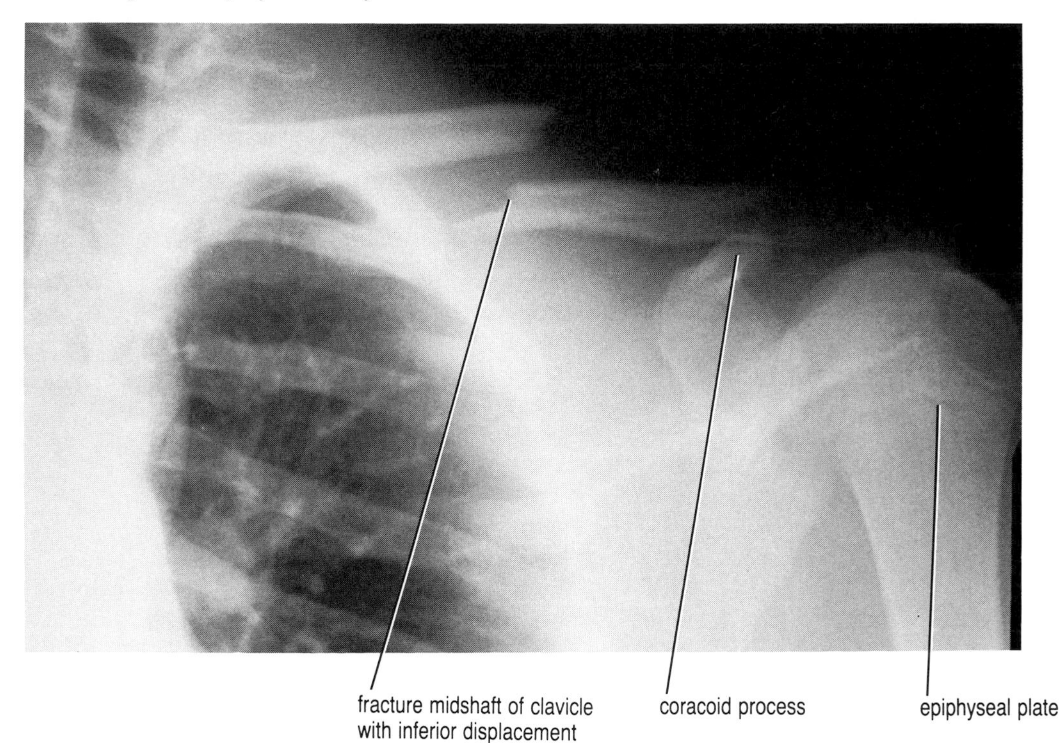

Figure 6.06. Clavicular fractures.

6.07 ELBOW: OLECRANON FAT PAD SIGN

A. Fat pad sign: soft tissue sign indicating high probability (greater than 90%) of intra-articular fracture of the elbow
B. The normal anterior fat pad appears as a small thin radiolucent area anterior to the coronoid fossa, or may not be visualized.
C. Posterior fat pad is hidden in the olecranon fossa, and is normally not seen.
D. Positive fat pad sign indicates the presence of intra-articular hemorrhage that distends the joint capsule producing triangular lucencies anteriorly and posteriorly. These may also appear elevated.
E. May also occur in nontraumatic intra-articular fluid collections such as the synovitis of rheumatoid arthritis

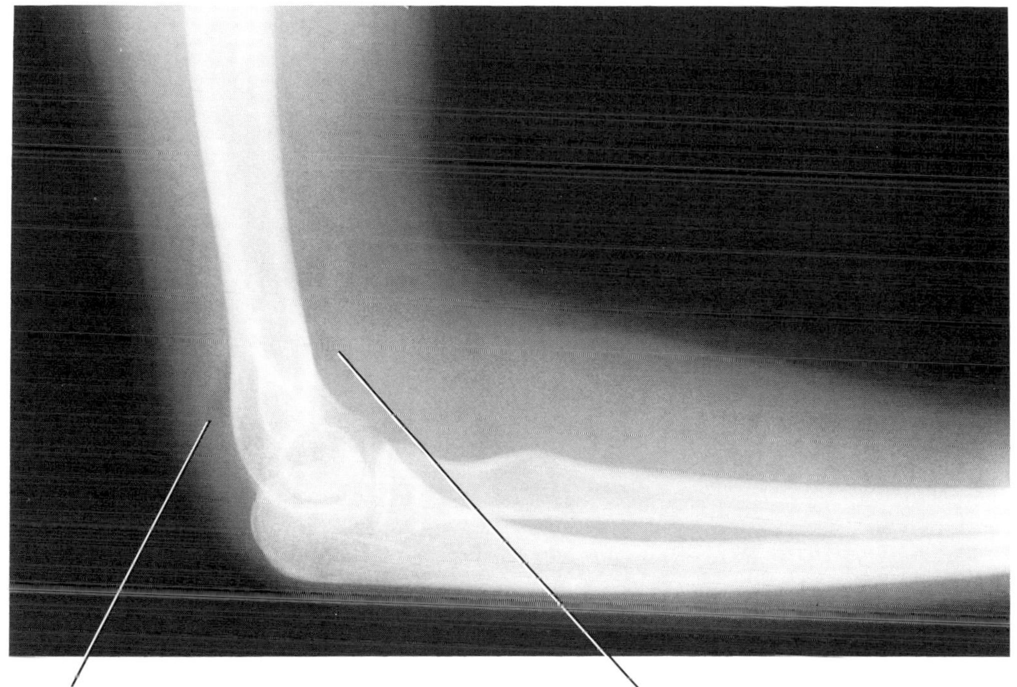

Figure 6.07. Elbow: olecranon fat pad sign.

6.08 ELBOW DISLOCATIONS

A. Elbow dislocation is the second most common site after shoulder dislocations.
B. Most common type of elbow dislocation is a posterior dislocation that results from a fall onto an outstretched or semiflexed hand. Radiographically there is posterior displacement of the radius and ulna.
C. Anterior elbow dislocations usually have an associated olecranon fracture.
D. Radial head subluxation, or "nursemaid's elbow," occurs in children ages 2 to 4 years when traction is placed on the elbow by swinging or lifting a child by the wrist. Diagnosis is made clinically, i.e., painful elbow held pronated and flexed with limited supination. Radiographic findings are limited because the subluxation is not evident as the epiphysis is not ossified.

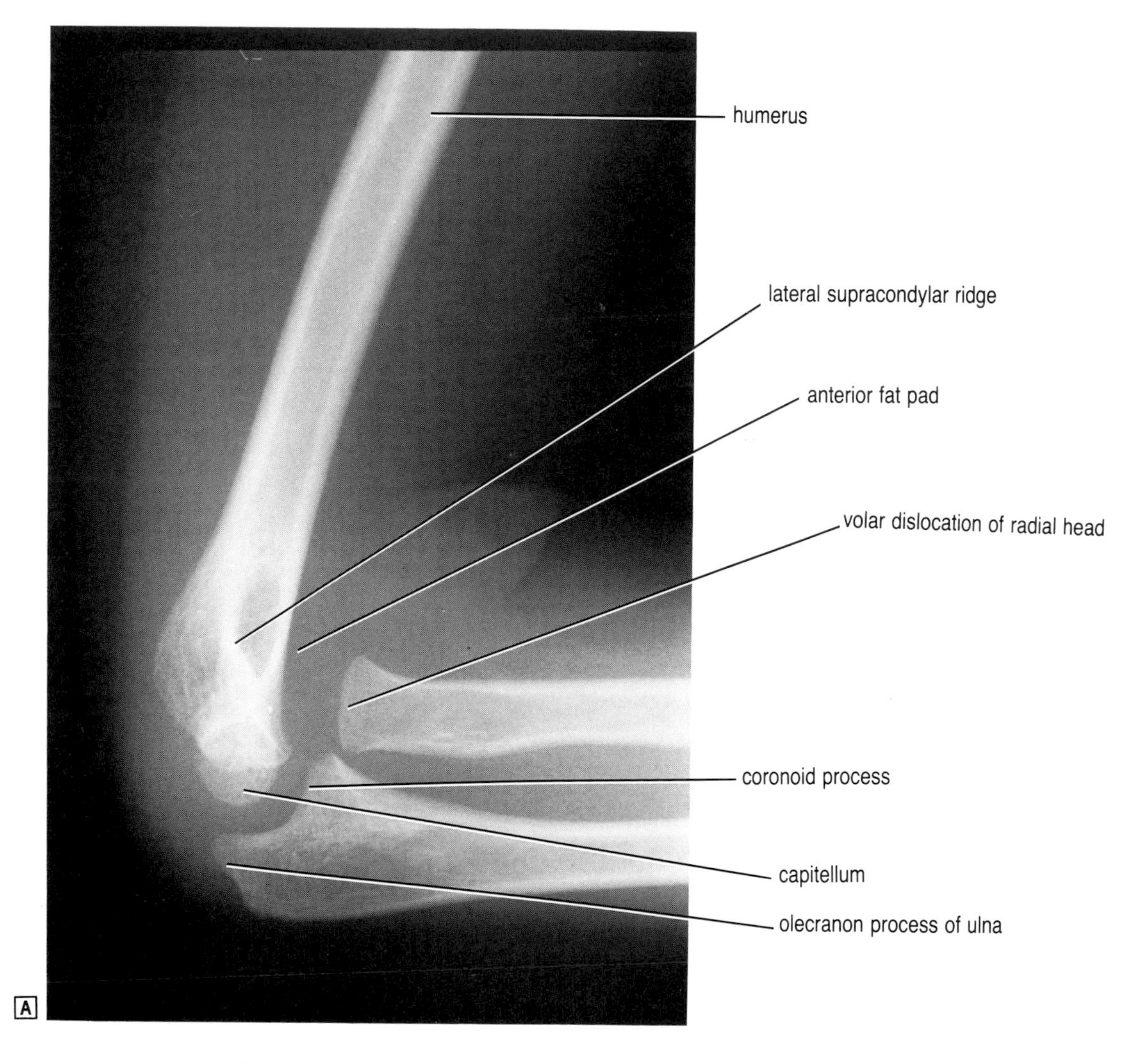

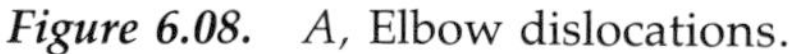

Figure 6.08. *A*, Elbow dislocations.

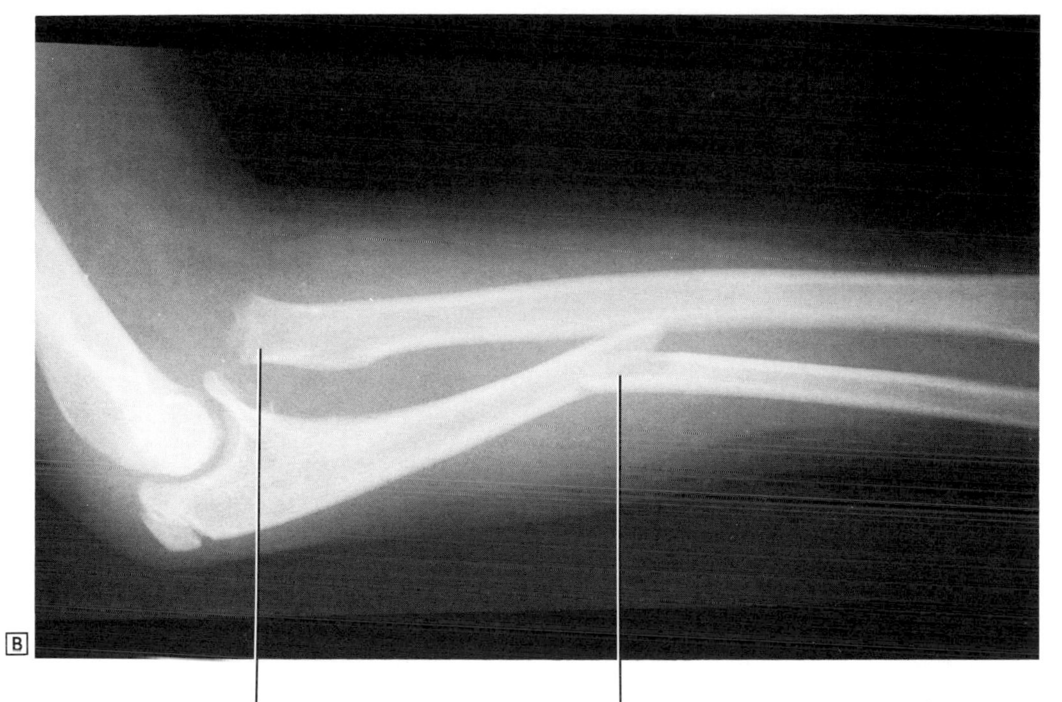

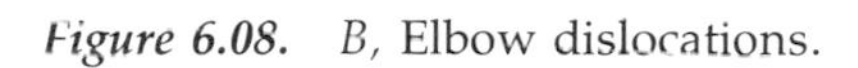

Figure 6.08. *B,* Elbow dislocations.

6.09 ELBOW FRACTURES

A. Distal humeral fracture usually results from a fall onto an outstretched hand.
B. "Little Leaguer's elbow" refers to separation of the apophysis of the medial epicondyle in adolescents. Often occurs while child is playing baseball.
C. Supracondylar fractures of the humerus may be subtle and nondisplaced with the only positive finding of an olecranon fat pad sign (see Sec. 6.07).
D. Falls onto an outstretched supinated hand may result in a radial head or radial neck fracture, and are associated with pain, swelling, and joint effusion. Fat pad sign is frequently seen in nondisplaced fractures.
E. Olecranon fractures result from a direct blow or fall onto a flexed elbow.
F. Usually intra-articular; patients have severe pain and difficulty extending the elbow.
G. Monteggia fracture: of the proximal ulna with volar angulation and volar dislocation of the proximal radius.

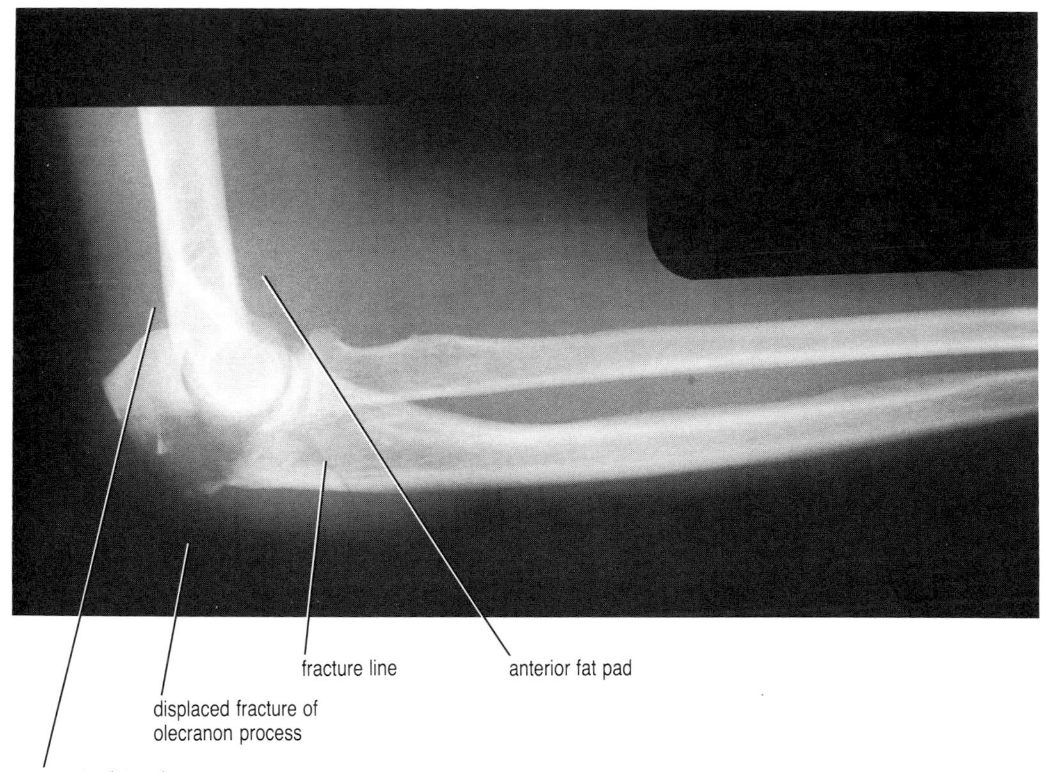

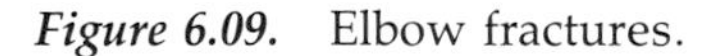

Figure 6.09. Elbow fractures.

6.10 DISTAL FOREARM FRACTURES

A. Usually caused by a fall onto an outstretched hand or direct trauma
B. Colles' fracture is the most common wrist fracture.
   1. It is a fracture of the distal radius with dorsal (posterior) angulation of the wrist.
   2. Associated ulnar styloid fracture often seen
   3. Navicular fracture also occurs in association with Colles' fracture.
C. Smith or reverse Colles' fracture: distal radius fracture with volar (anterior) displacement. May also have ulnar styloid fracture
D. Galeazzi fracture: constitutes a distal third radial fracture with distal ulnar dislocation.
E. Greenstick, torus, or buckling fractures are common in children under the age of 10 and frequently involve the radius and ulna.
   1. Fracture line does not extend across the entire bone shaft.

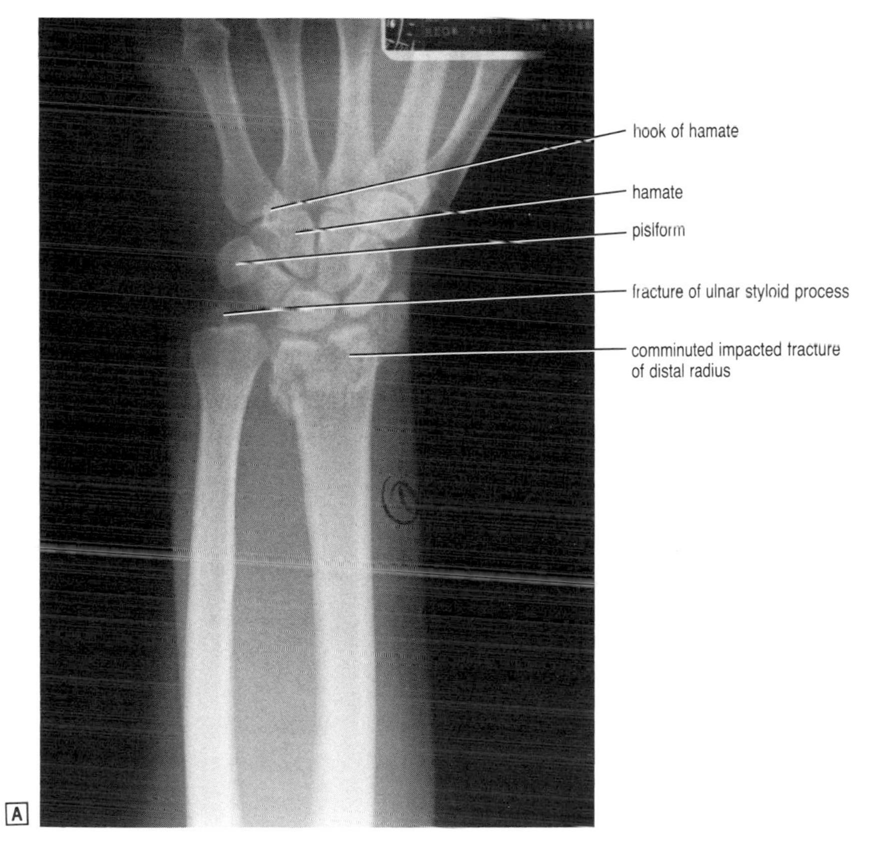

Figure 6.10. *A*, Distal forearm fractures.

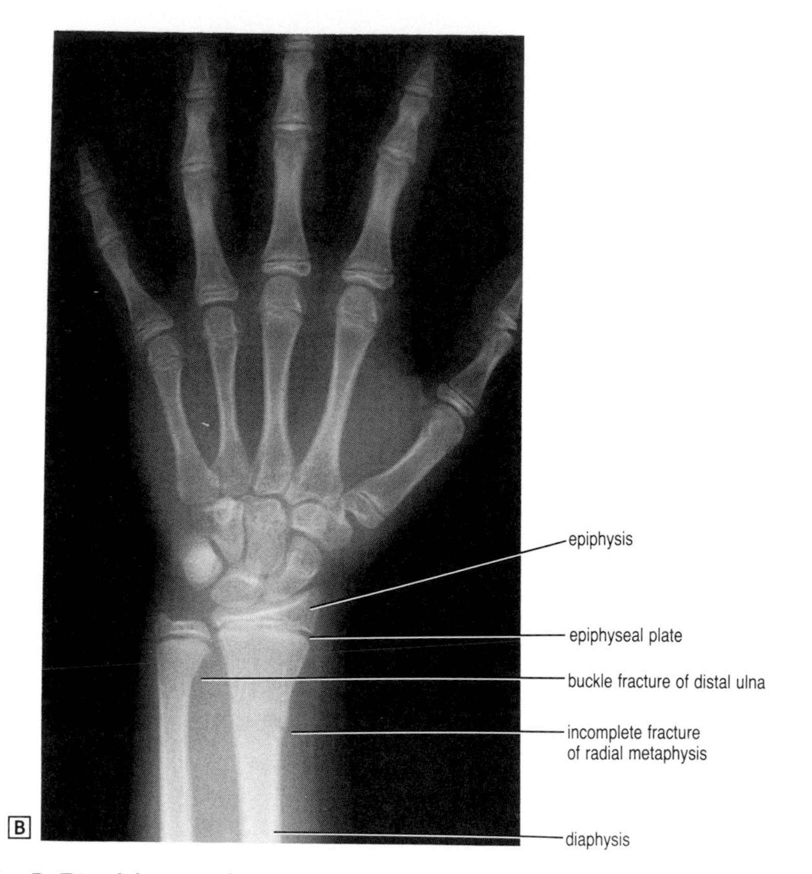

Figure 6.10. *B,* Distal forearm fractures.

6.11 WRIST DISLOCATIONS

A. Most common are lunate and perilunate, the result of a fall on extended fingers and hand
   1. Anterior lunate dislocation: lunate dislocated anteriorly from radius and carpal bones
      a. Associated with median nerve injury
      b. Indicates disrupted posterior radiolunar ligaments
      c. On AP view lunate appears triangular, and overlaps the base of the capitate
   2. Perilunate dislocation is more common than anterior lunate dislocation
      a. Distal row of carpal bones dislocated posteriorly relative to lunate and on AP view appears superimposed. Lateral view, lunate articulates normally with radius; carpal bones (distal row) displaced posteriorly
      b. Associated with fractured waist of the scaphoid (carpal navicular)
      c. Intact radiolunar ligaments and disrupted ligaments between lunate and capitate
      d. May be anteriorly (volar) or posteriorly (dorsal) dislocated
B. Rotary subluxation of scaphoid: rare, in AP view, increased space between scaphoid and lunate measuring greater than 4 mm.
   1. Scaphoid appears foreshortened.
C. Metacarpocarpal joint dislocation usually involves fourth and fifth metacarpals.
D. Normally in lateral view, radius, lunate, capitate, and metacarpals form straight line.
E. Soft tissue swelling the most obvious finding in subtle bony injury
F. Radiocarpal dislocations are rare.

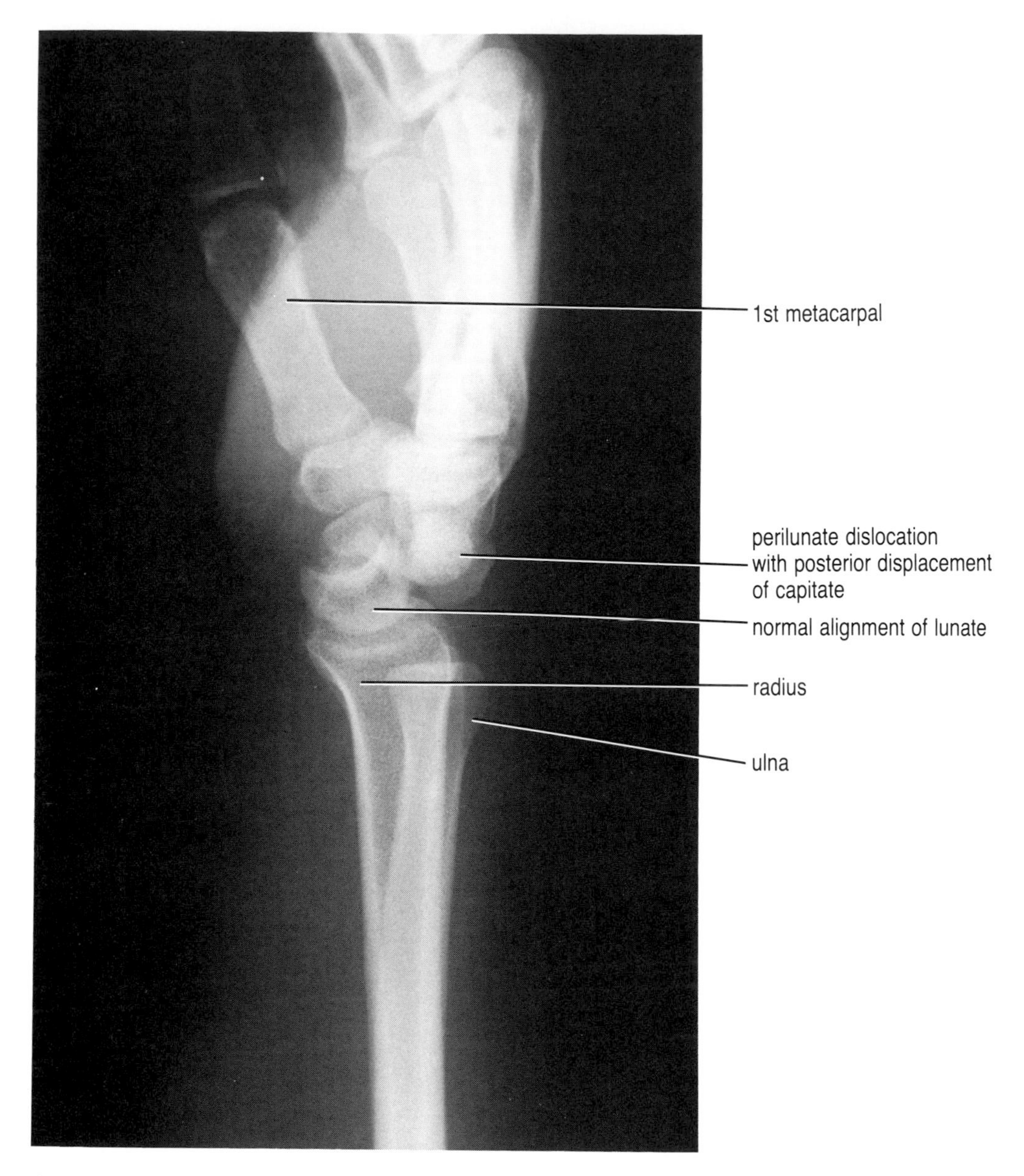

Figure 6.11. Wrist dislocations.

6.12 WRIST FRACTURES

A. Navicular (scaphoid) fractures: most common (75%) of the carpal fractures
   1. Usually occur at waist or central part, usually in men
   2. Navicular blood supply enters at distal end. After fracture, the proximal fragment may become avascular and frequently complicated by ischemic necrosis and nonunion. Proximal avascular fragment remains of normal bone density, i.e., more dense than surrounding viable bone, because the surrounding bone undergoes disuse osteoporosis (and demineralization) and proximal segment cannot.
   3. Significant displacement of navicular fragments increases probability of ischemic necrosis of proximal fragment to almost 100%; in nondisplaced ones it is 50%.
   4. Initially, fractures may not be visualized; if symptoms persist, repeat exam in 7 to 10 days. May reveal a fracture line due to bony resorption associated with healing
   5. The more proximal the fracture line, the greater the incidence of avascular necrosis.
   6. They usually occur as an isolated injury or are associated with perilunate dislocation.

B. Triquetral fracture: 15% of carpal fractures
   1. Commonly is small cortical avulsion fracture on posterior surface

C. Greater multiangular fracture: usually posterior surface with associated dislocation of metacarpohamate joint
   1. Associated with ulnar artery injury

D. Remainder of carpal bones may be fractured but are rare.

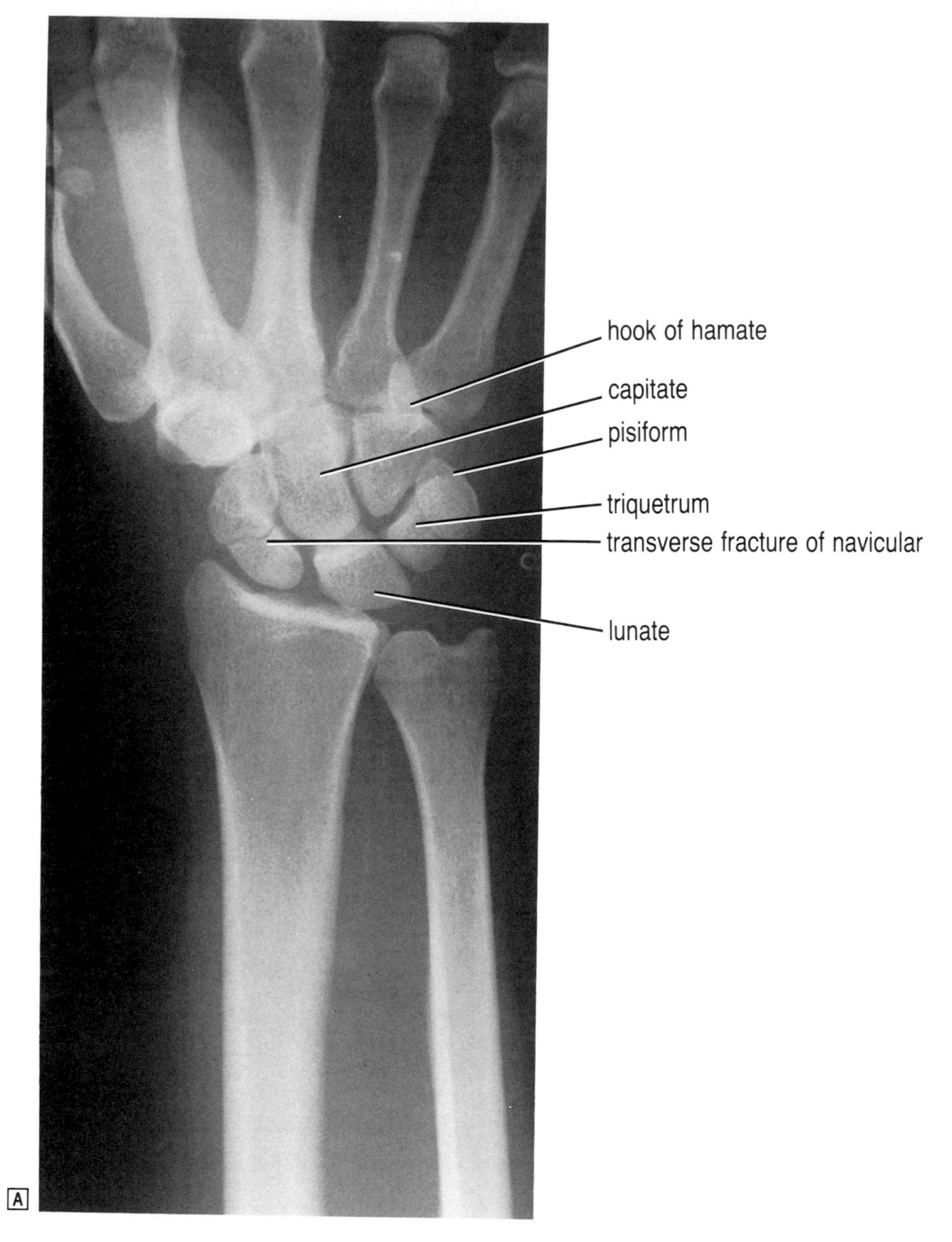

Figure 6.12. *A*, Wrist fractures.

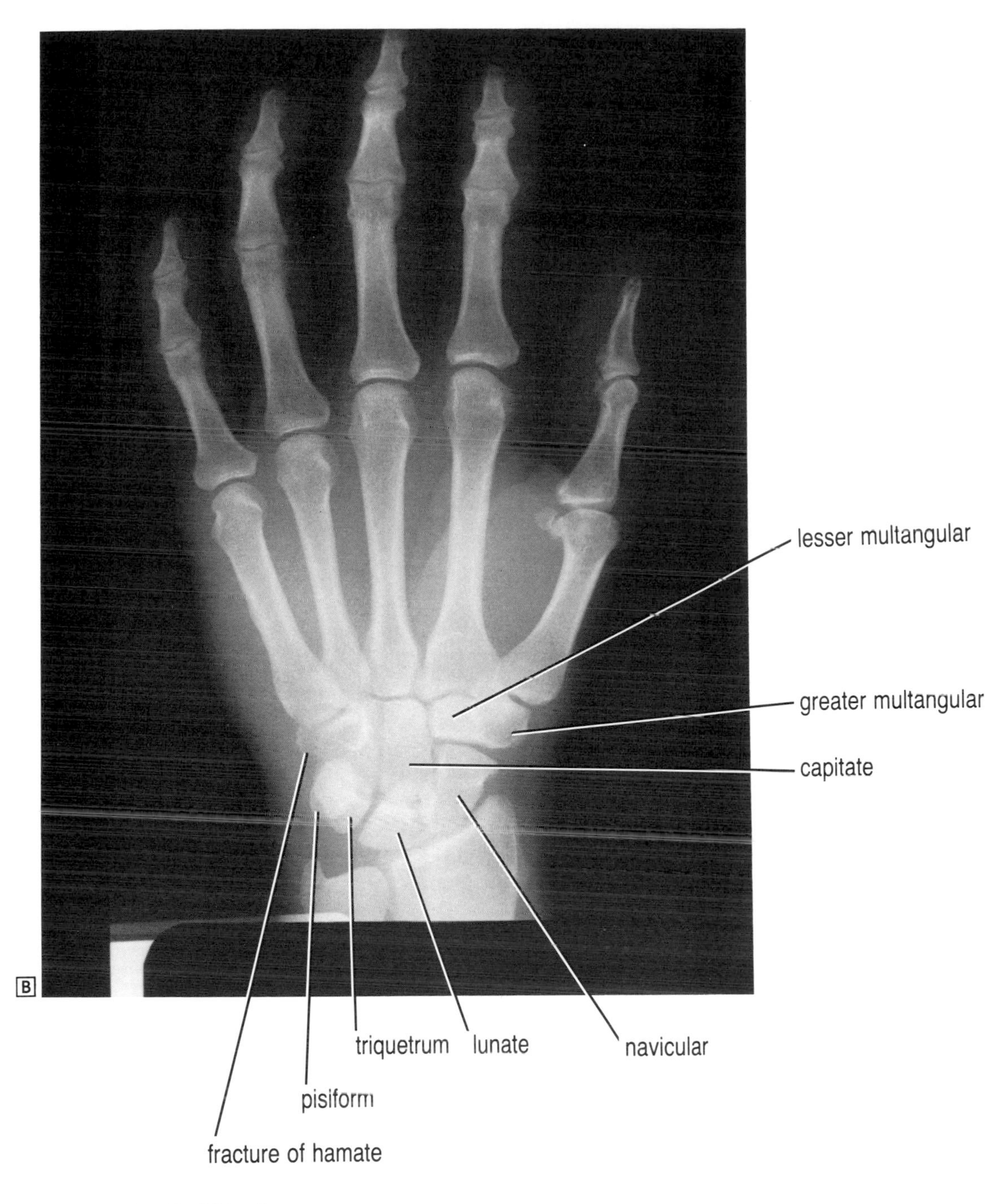

Figure 6.12. *B,* Wrist fractures.

6.13 HAND: METACARPAL FRACTURES

A. Boxer's fracture: involves neck of fourth or fifth metacarpal, with volar angulation
B. Bennett's fracture: oblique fracture through the base of the first metacarpal and proximal articulating surface with associated proximal dislocation of the distal fragment
C. Metacarpal shaft fractures more commonly are spiral than transverse. Those occurring prior to fusion of the epiphyses usually involve the metaphysis.
D. Always check for associated soft tissue swelling.
E. Physical exam of involved part: swelling, point tenderness, ecchymosis, visible deformity

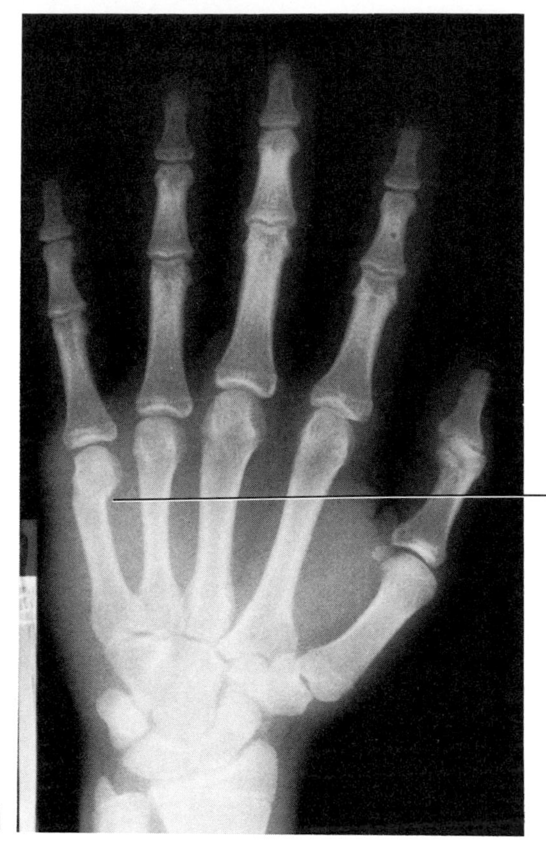

Figure 6.13. *A,* Hand: metacarpal fractures.

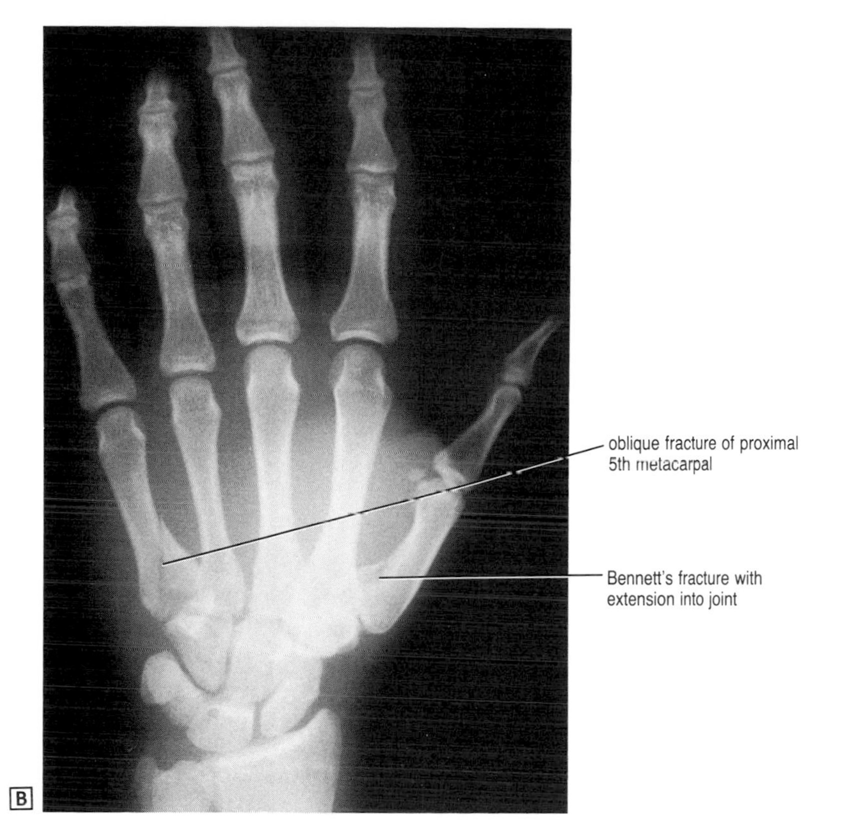

Figure 6.13. *B*, Hand: metacarpal fractures.

6.14 PHALANGEAL FRACTURES/DISLOCATIONS

A. Interphalangeal and metacarpophalangeal dislocations are common, the result of force on the volar aspect of the digit with resultant dorsal dislocation. Postreduction films are used to assess the presence of associated fracture or epiphyseal injury.
B. Epiphyseal injuries occur commonly (see Sec. 6.02).
C. Subungual tuft fractures are common, usually minimally displaced and comminuted, from a crushing injury.
D. Baseball or mallet finger: dorsal avulsion fractures of the base of the distal phalanx, with associated common extensor tendon injury (avulsion or small triangular bony fragment containing its insertion may be torn off). Flexion deformity results.

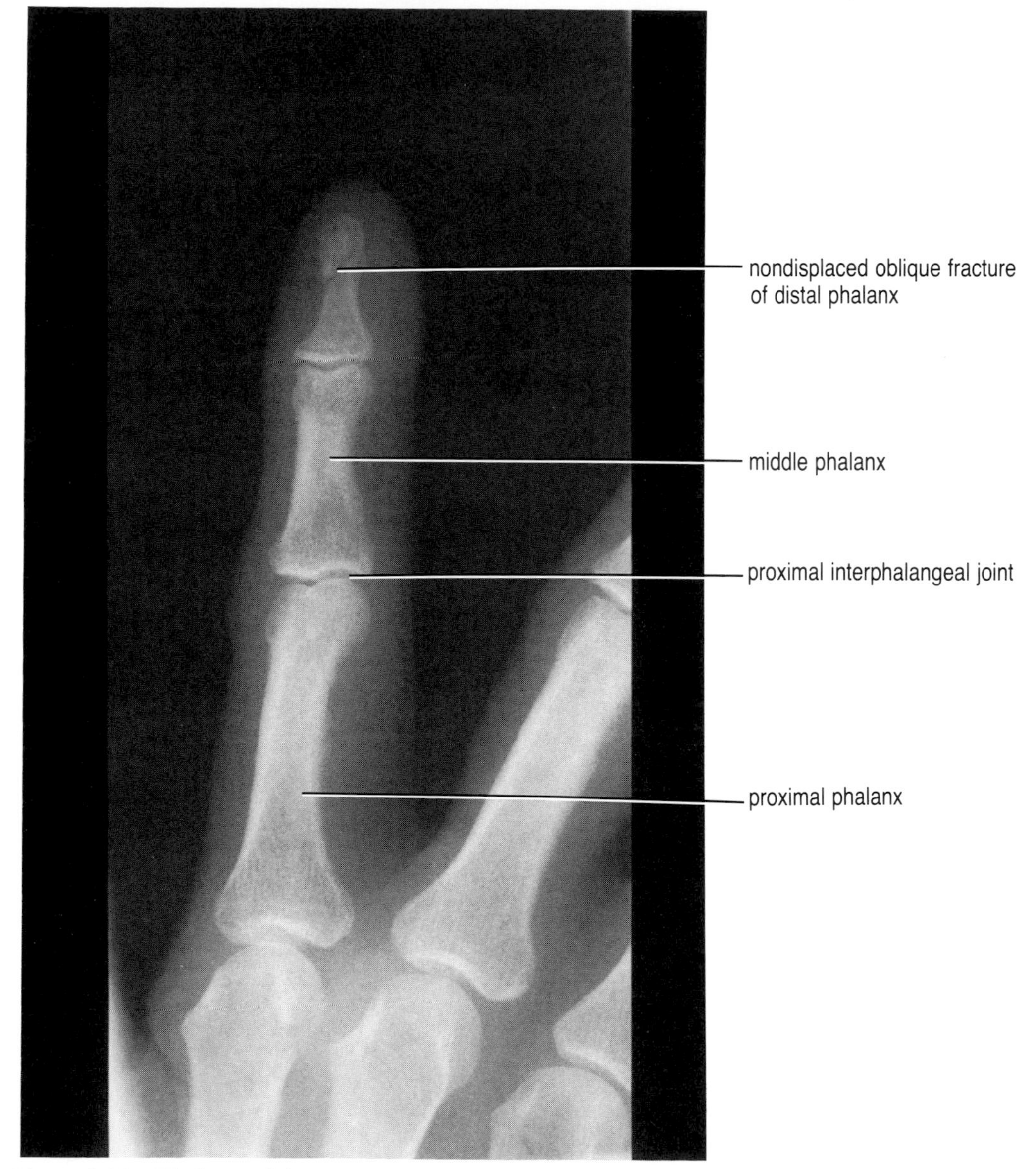

Figure 6.14. Phalangeal fractures/dislocations.

6.15 PELVIC/FEMORAL NECK FRACTURES

A. 1. Pelvic fracture classification
   a. Type 1: crush injury, unstable, result of severe force, high morbidity and mortality, associated with hemorrhage and soft tissue injury
      (1) Involves three or more pubic ring components (sacrum, ischium, ilium, pubic rami, acetabulum, sacroiliac joint, and symphysis pubis)
   b. Type 2: unstable fracture, Malgaigne fracture
      (1) Composed of ipsilateral superior and inferior pubic rami fractures with an oblique sacral fracture on the same side
      (2) Usually results from a motor vehicle accident
   c. Type 3: stable fracture
      (1) Involves pubic rami only
      (2) Usually results from a fall or recreational activity
2. Separation of the symphysis pubic results from anterior compressive forces.
3. Anterior superior and anterior inferior iliac spine avulsion fractures result from the muscular pull of the sartorius and rectus femoris muscles, respectively.
4. Fracture of the acetabulum may occur with or without hip dislocation. Occasionally CT evaluation is used to assess fragment position and extent of the injury.

B. Femoral neck fractures
1. In young patients, due to severe trauma, i.e., motor vehicle accident
2. In elderly, often the result of a simple fall and decreased bone strength due to osteoporosis. Frequently associated with simultaneous distal forearm and humerus fractures
3. The affected leg is usually shortened and externally rotated.
4. Most frequent types of femoral neck fractures
   a. Subcapital: may be impacted or displaced (leg in external rotation)
   b. Intertrochanteric: often comminuted
5. Subtrochanteric fractures are frequently pathologic—seen in patients with Paget's disease or metastatic disease.
6. Displaced subcapital fractures frequently disrupt the femoral head blood supply that enters laterally to the head and neck, with resultant nonunion. Treatment: prosthetic replacement of femoral head
7. Impacted and intertrochanteric fractures do not affect the blood supply.
8. Impacted fractures may be stable, and often patient may ambulate for several days prior to seeking help.
9. Typical findings of impacted fracture: shortened femoral neck, disrupted cortical margin along inferior neck to femoral head, disrupted cortical margin along superior surface, increased sclerosis across femoral neck caused by fragment impaction

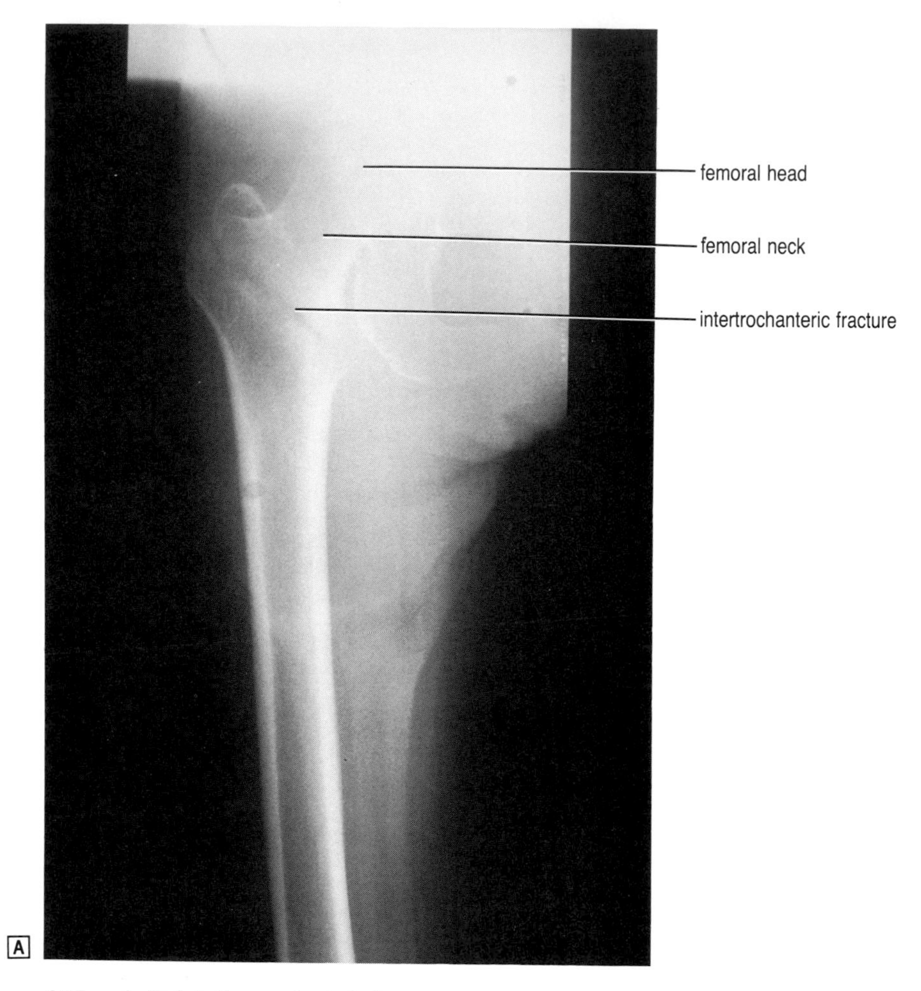

Figure 6.15. *A,* Pelvic/femoral neck fractures.

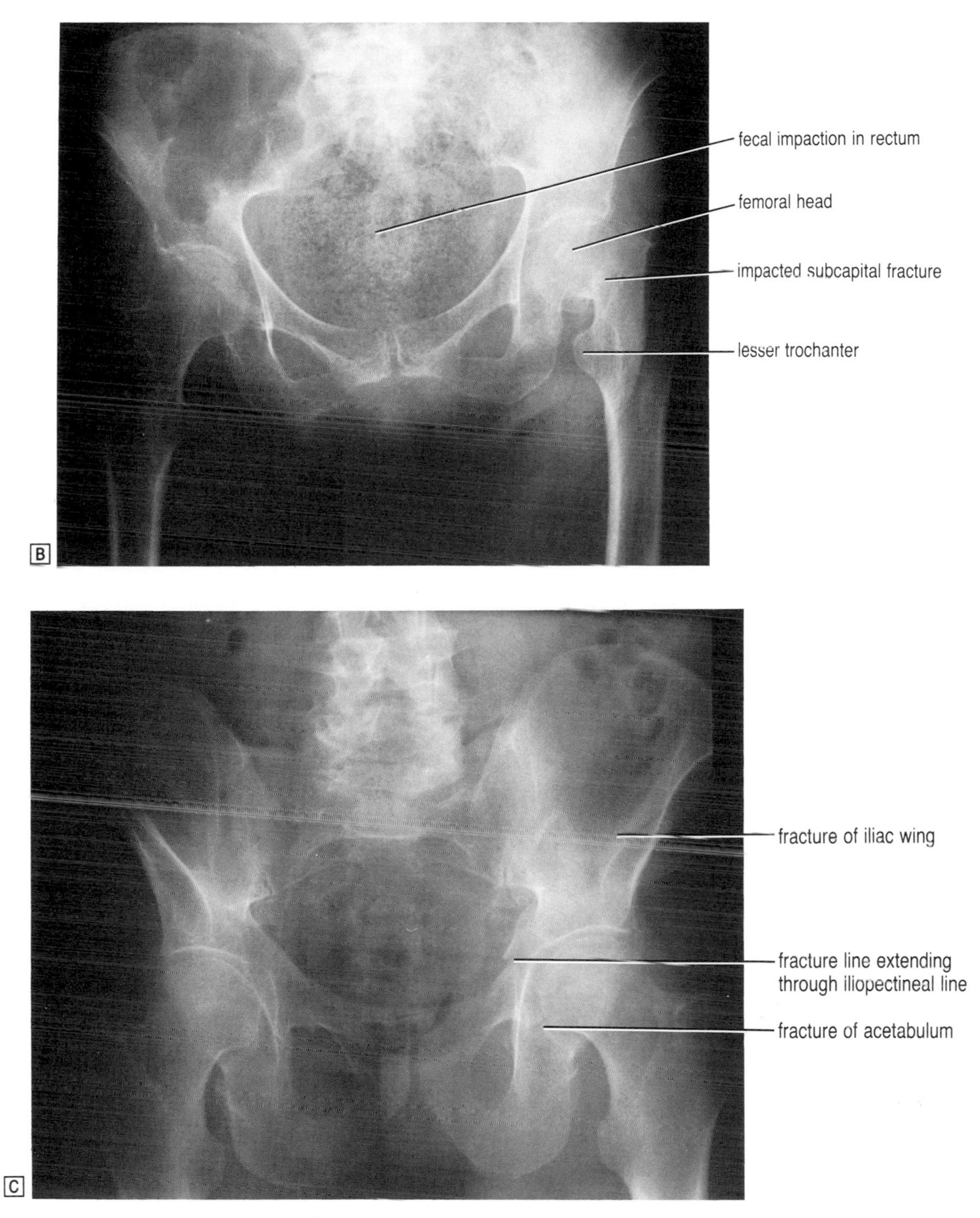

Figure 6.15. *B,* Pelvic/femoral neck fractures. *C,* Pelvic/femoral neck fractures.

6.16 FEMORAL HEAD DISLOCATION

A. Severe forces are necessary to produce hip dislocation. Often associated with neurovascular and other organ system injuries
B. Posterior dislocation is most common, the result of severe force, such as the knee striking a dashboard in a motor vehicle accident. Often associated with fracture of posterior rim of acetabulum (50%). Femoral head is displaced superiorly. May also be associated with sciatic nerve injury.
C. Anterior dislocation is less common. Femoral head is displaced inferior to acetabulum and into obturator foramen.
D. Femoral head irregularity or joint space widening may indicate associated fracture fragments entrapped within the hip joint. CT is indicated (see Sec. 6.15).
E. Anterior dislocation may occur when hip is flexed with resultant obturator dislocation (leg flexed, abducted, and externally rotated) or when hip is extended with resultant iliac dislocation (leg extended, abducted, and externally rotated).
F. Fractures of acetabulum are commonly associated with hip dislocations. Patient's legs are flexed, adducted, and internally rotated in posterior dislocations.
G. Risk of avascular necrosis and sciatic nerve compression and ischemia occurs with hip dislocation. Rapid reduction reduces the morbidity.
H. Usually posterior acetabular hip fracture fragments are displaced in same direction as femoral head
I. Femoral head epiphyseal separation may be secondary to violent trauma and may be complete (metaphysis of femoral neck articulates with acetabulum and capital femoral epiphysis displaced posteriorly) or a slipped capital femoral epiphysis (widened hip joint space, femoral head epiphysis no longer sits squarely atop femoral neck metaphysis).

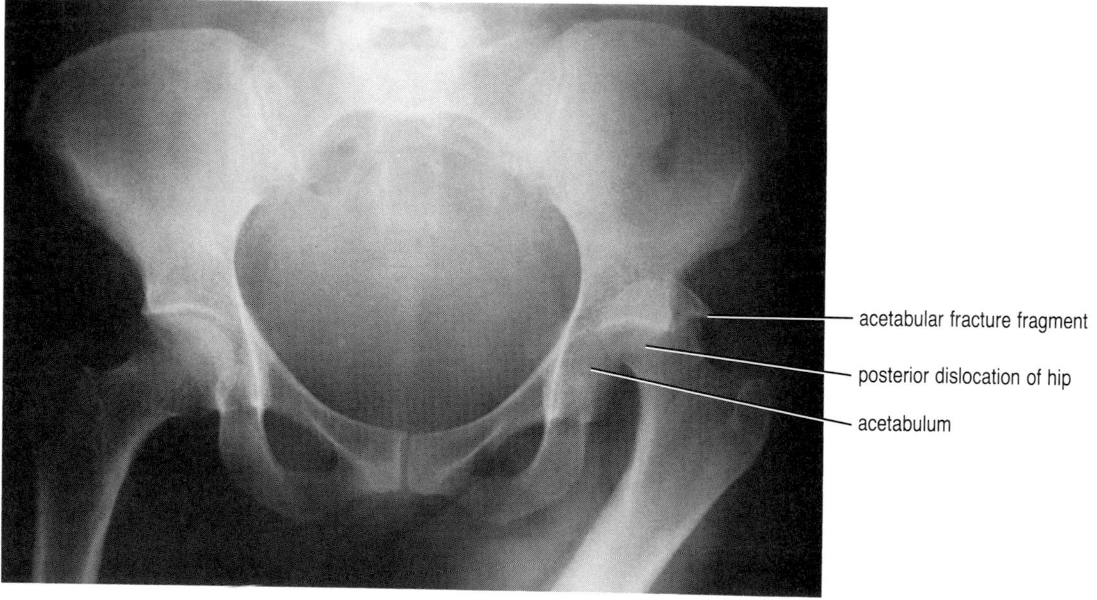

Figure 6.16. Femoral head dislocation.

6.17 TIBIAL PLATEAU FRACTURES

A. Physical exam reveals swollen knee joint, pain, and ligamentous injury. Important to check the neurovascular status and assess for common involvement of the peroneal nerve or popliteal artery, or development of a compartment syndrome. Femoral arteriogram may be indicated if peripheral pulses are decreased.
B. Usually associated with fat-fluid levels in suprapatellar bursa and ligamentous and meniscal injury. The fat-fluid sign, seen only in the lateral view, is associated with proximal tibial fractures that involve the articular surfaces with resultant blood and fat from the medullary cavity.
C. Fractures may involve tibial condyles, tibial spine, or intercondylar eminence.
D. Usually result of a fall, or auto-pedestrian accident.
E. Fracture typically appears as a separation or depression of the joint surface.

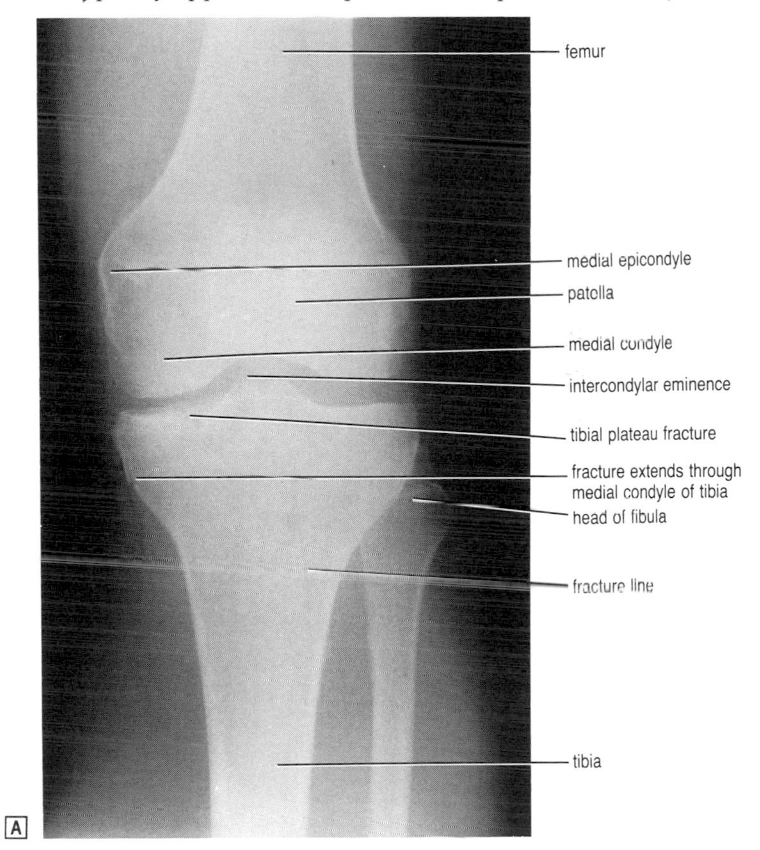

Figure 6.17. A, Tibial plateau fractures.

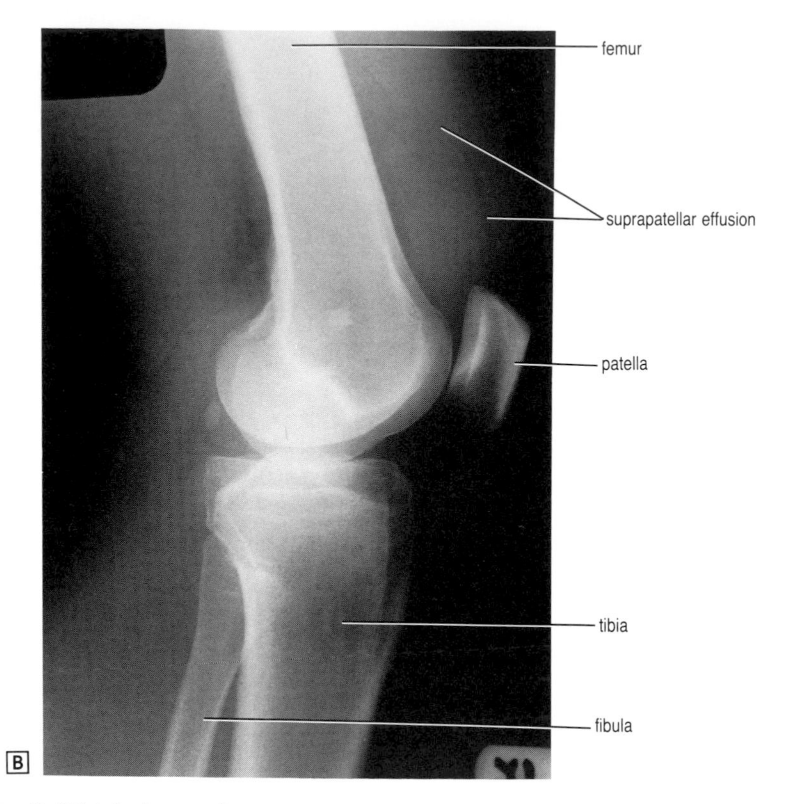

Figure 6.17. *B,* Tibial plateau fractures.

6.18 PATELLAR DISLOCATION/FRACTURE

A. Most patellar fractures are transverse and result from a direct blow or sudden contraction of the quadriceps muscle with the knee in flexion.

B. Patellar dislocations usually occur laterally. May be incomplete or complete (patella comes to rest parallel to the lateral condyle).

C. Patellar dislocations may be associated with an osteochondral fracture (a thin curved cortical bone fragment and its associated cartilage), as the medial patellar surface impacts the lateral condyle. Additional oblique or axial (sunrise) views may be needed to visualize the injury.

D. Anatomic variants such as bipartite or tripartite patellas should not be misdiagnosed as fractures. These occur bilaterally in 80% of cases, and have smooth cortical margins with rounded corners.

E. History and physical exam: pain, tenderness, decreased extension at the knee, physical deformity

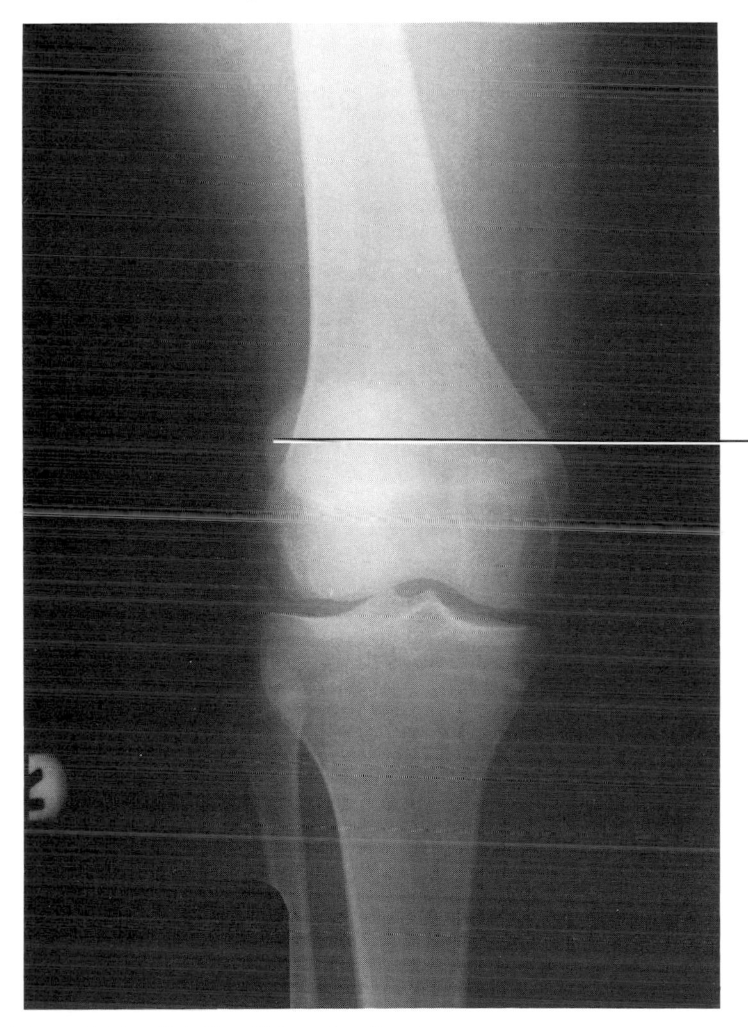

Figure 6.18. Patellar dislocation/fracture.

6.19 ANKLE FRACTURE/DISLOCATION

A. Most common is an oblique or spiral fracture of the lateral malleolus of the distal fibula. This represents an inversion injury.
B. All types of epiphyseal injuries occur at the ankle. Salter-Harris type III and IV epiphyseal injuries occur most commonly at the ankle (see Sec. 6.02).
C. Ankle sprain, an eversion injury, appears radiologically as soft tissue swelling around the medial malleolus, with intact bones and ankle mortise joint.
D. Avulsion injury of an ankle ligament may be associated with a cortical fracture of the medial and lateral malleolus.
E. Ligamentous injury may occur without bony injury, and is inferred from the relative bony positions of the ankle. Signs include soft tissue swelling, widening of the ankle mortise (normally 3 to 4 mm over the entire surface). Deltoid ligament rupture is represented by a distance of 6 mm or more between the medial talar and lateral medial malleolar surfaces. Stressed views will exaggerate the bony relationships.
F. Inversion or eversion injury may result in bi- or trimalleolar fractures (medial and lateral malleolar fracture with additional posterior tibial fracture).
G. Tibiofibular ligament rupture results in an unstable joint.
H. Ankle (or talus) dislocation occurs infrequently. A posterior dislocation is most frequent and is usually associated with a fracture of one of the ankle mortise components.
   1. Treatment: short leg cast, open reduction as needed. Dislocations require immediate reduction to restore circulation.

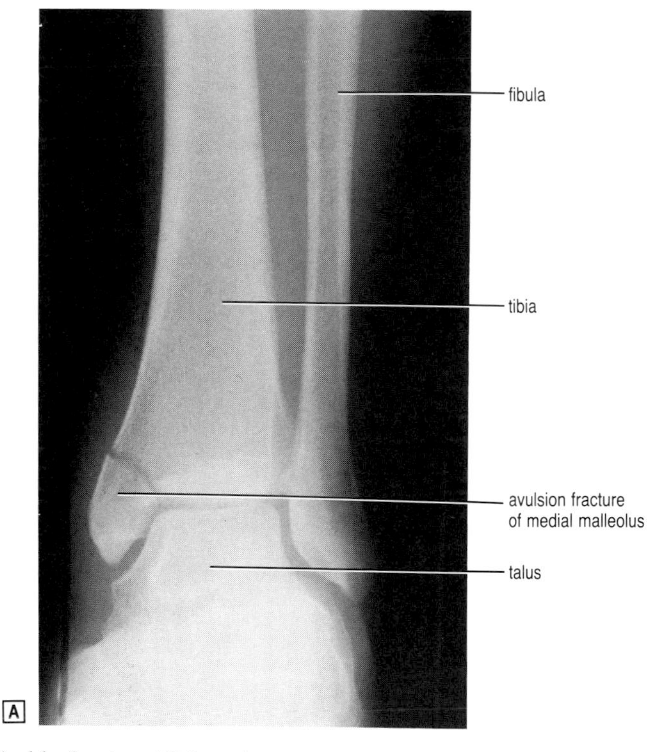

Figure 6.19. *A,* Ankle fracture/dislocation.

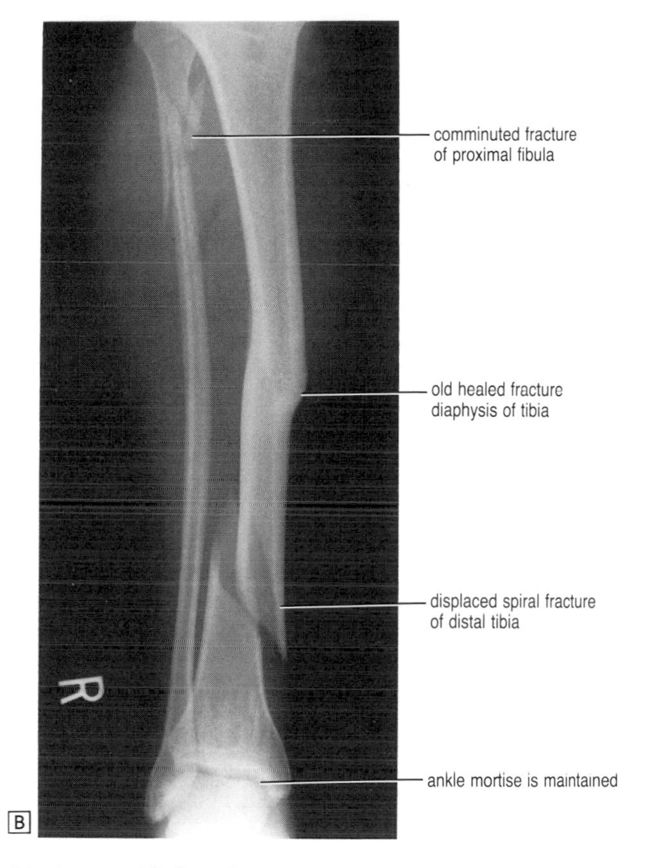

Figure 6.19. *B,* Ankle fracture/dislocation.

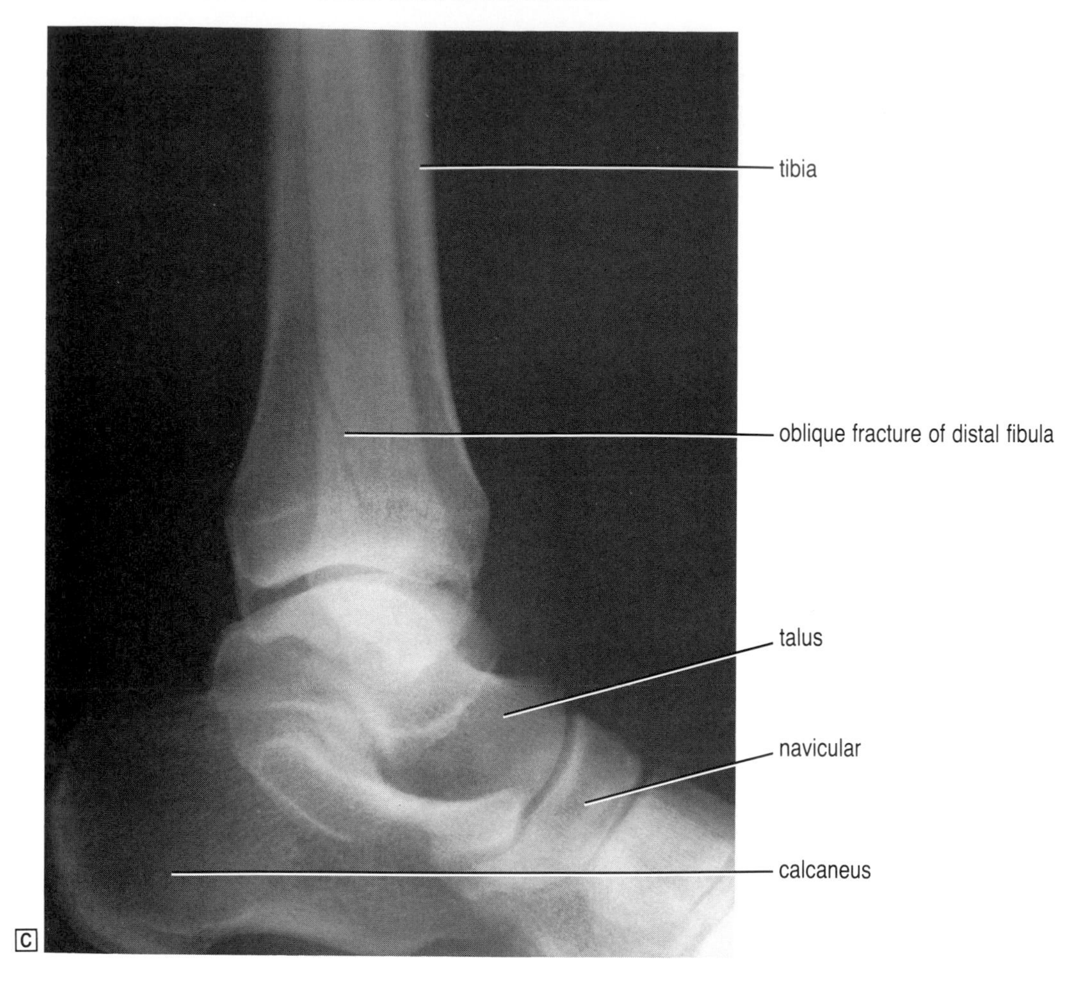

Figure 6.19. *C,* Ankle fracture/dislocation.

6.20 OS CALCIS FRACTURE/BOEHLER'S ANGLE

A. Most common tarsal bone fractured is the os calcis (calcaneus), and comprises 2% of all fractures. Frequently bilateral and associated with thoracolumbar spine compression fractures in 10% of the cases.
B. Usually the result of a fall from a height with the patient landing on his feet. The resultant downward force is transmitted through the talus to the calcaneus.
C. Most calcaneal fractures involve depression of the posterior facet of the calcaneus with flattening of Boehler's angle. Boehler's angle consists of two lines drawn along the anterior superior and posterior superior margins to the highest point of the articulating surface. Normal range is 20 to 40 degrees and is decreased in calcaneal fractures.
D. Lateral and axial views usually are sufficient in most injuries.
E. Extensive soft tissue injury is frequently seen with severe comminuted fractures of the calcaneus.

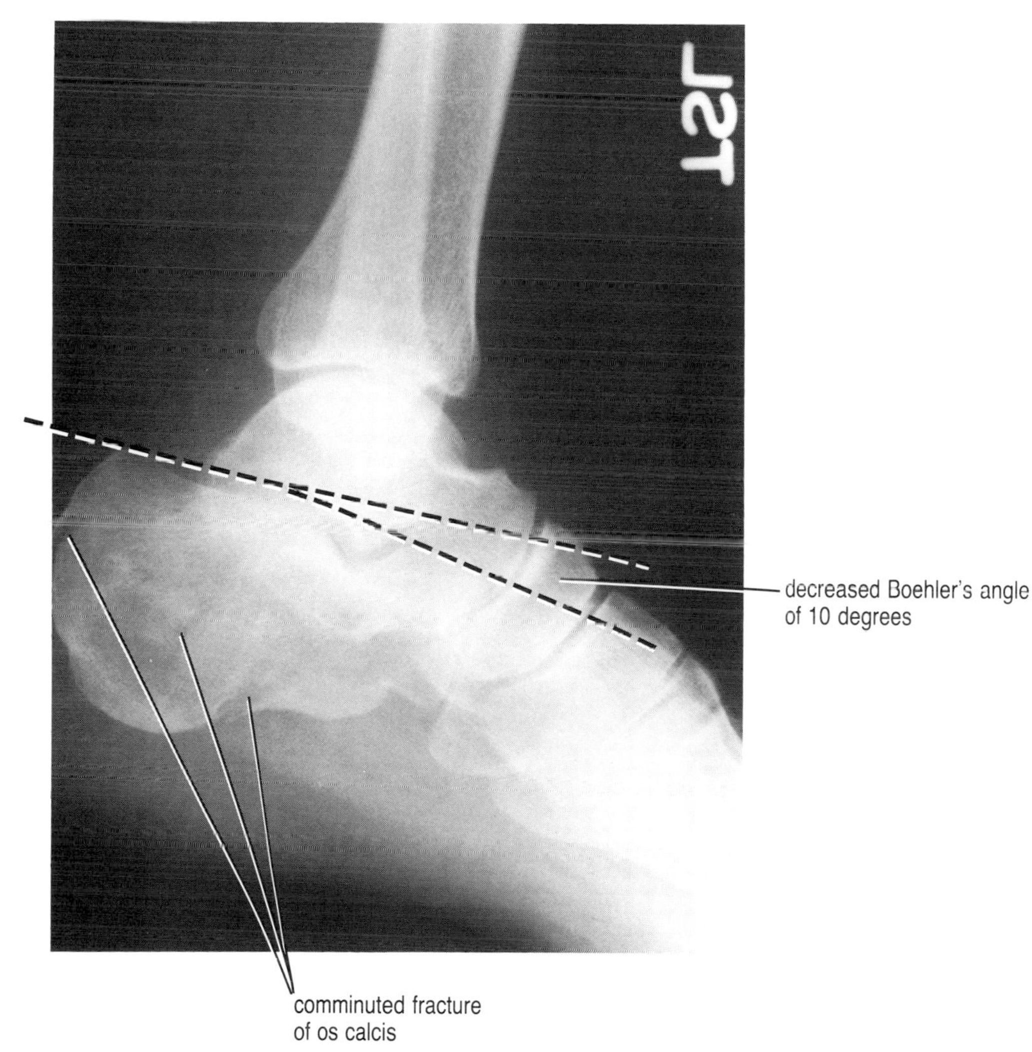

Figure 6.20. Os calcis fracture/Boehler's angle.

6.21 TARSAL/METATARSAL/PHALANGES FRACTURES AND DISLOCATIONS

A. Fractures of the tarsal bones occur infrequently with the exception of the calcaneus. Recognized by the cortical irregularity, buckling, or increased density at sites of impaction
B. Fractures of the base of the fifth metatarsal (Jones fracture) occur frequently and are the result of an inversion injury. Typically, the fracture line is perpendicular to the base and must not be confused with the developmental apophyseal line that parallels the lateral aspect of the base.
C. March, fatigue, or stress fractures commonly occur in the second to fourth metatarsal as the result of chronic activity such as walking, jogging, or marching. Initially the radiogram may be normal; however, films taken in 10 to 14 days will reveal periosteal callus and a fine nondisplaced transverse line of fracture.
D. Phalanx dislocations appear as loss of joint space with increased density superimposed on the phalanges. Usually occur in the anterior or posterior direction
E. Distal tuft fracture is a frequent injury involving the toes with associated soft tissue swelling of the phalanges.
F. AP and oblique views typically demonstrate injury.

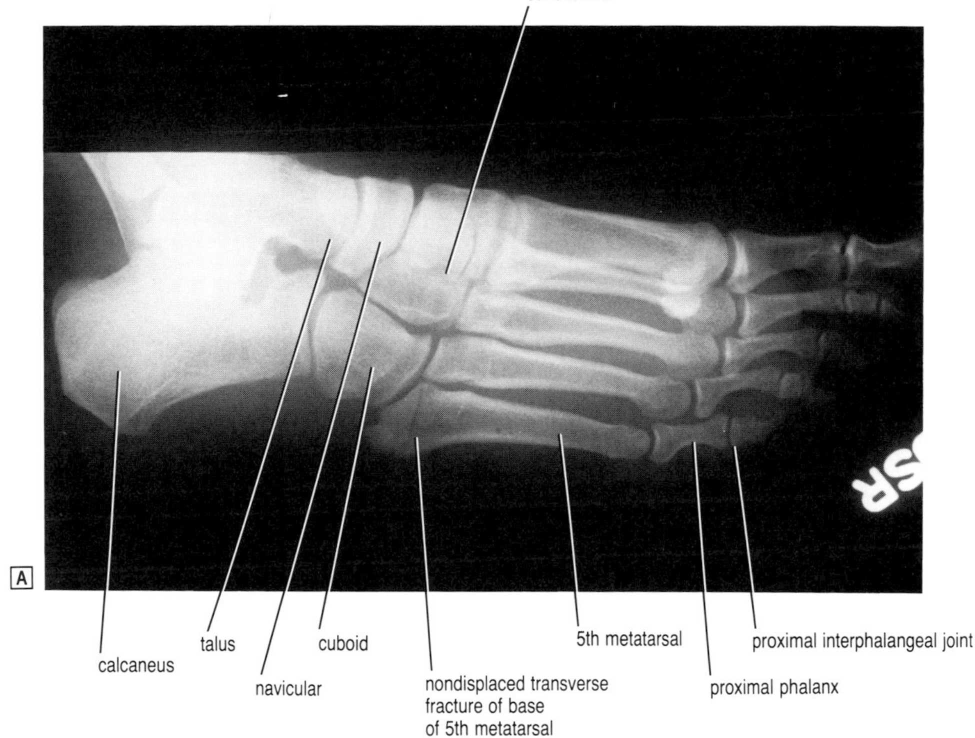

Figure 6.21. *A,* Tarsal/metatarsal/phalanges fractures and dislocations.

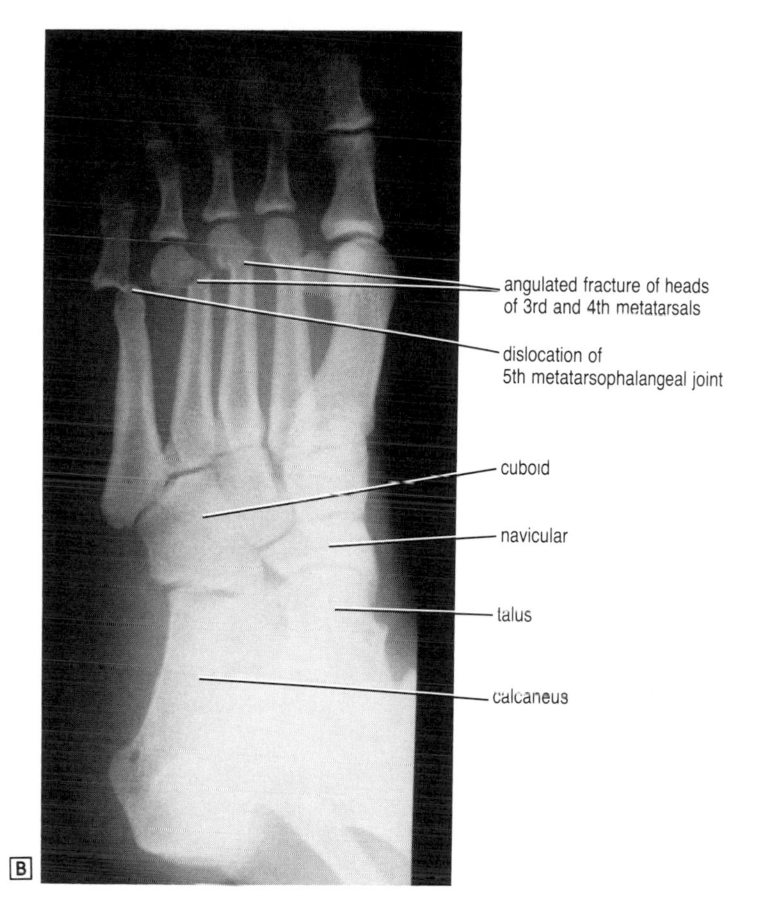

Figure 6.21. *B*, Tarsal/metatarsal/phalanges fractures and dislocations.

6.22 OSTEOLYTIC AND OSTEOBLASTIC METASTASIS

A. Primary malignant bone tumors are rare.
B. Most common cause of malignant bone tumors is metastatic disease
   1. Prostate
   2. Breast
   3. Lung
   4. Thyroid
   5. Kidney
C. Usual sites of metastases include spine, pelvis, skull, ribs, proximal aspects of humerus and femurs
D. Most metastases are of the destructive osteolytic type. The remainder may be osteoblastic or of mixed variety.
E. Radiographic features
   1. Osteolytic metastases
      a. Most common source of solitary lesion: kidney and thyroid carcinoma
      b. Most common source of multiple lesions: lung and breast carcinoma
      c. Tumor lesion begins in medullary canal, appearing lucent because of bone destruction; irregular margins without sclerotic rim. Enlarging lesion extends to destroy cortical bone. No new bone formation.
      d. When limited to cortex: usually bronchogenic carcinoma
      e. Spinal involvement results in pedicle destruction (see Sec. 2.14) as well as vertebral body and neural arch involvement.
   2. Osteoblastic metastases
      a. Most frequently secondary to breast and prostate carcinoma. Other causes include small cell carcinoma of lung, bladder carcinoma, and gastrointestinal carcinoma.
      b. Lesions characterized as ill-defined sclerotic densities with eventual loss of normal bone detail. Intramedullary bone density approaches that of cortical bone, e.g., characteristic "ivory" vertebrae. Variable size

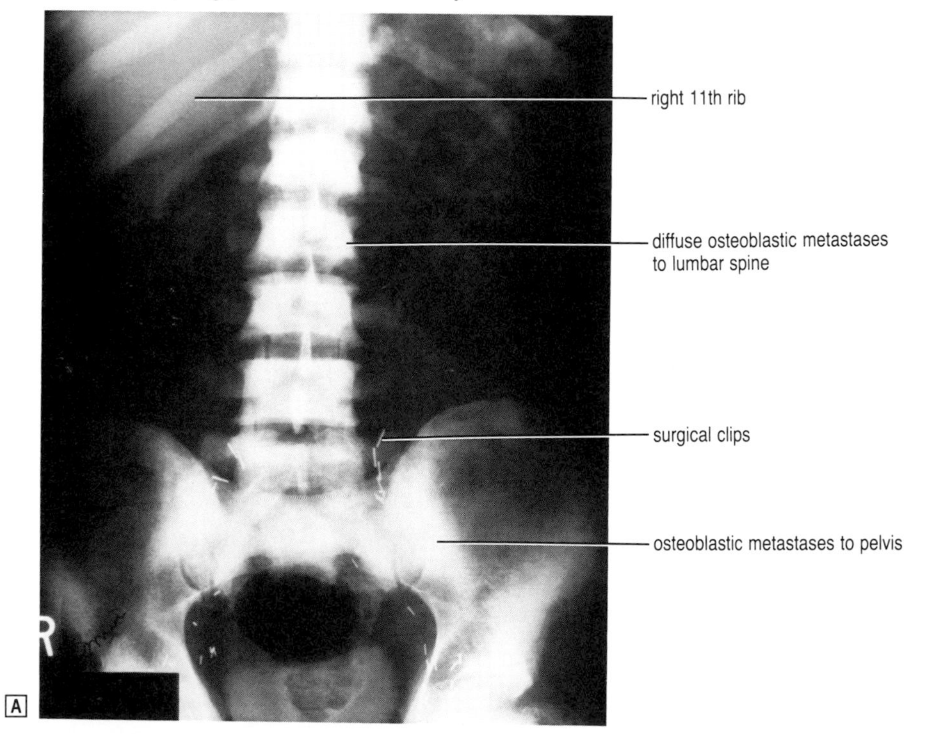

Figure 6.22. *A,* Osteolytic and osteoblastic metastasis.

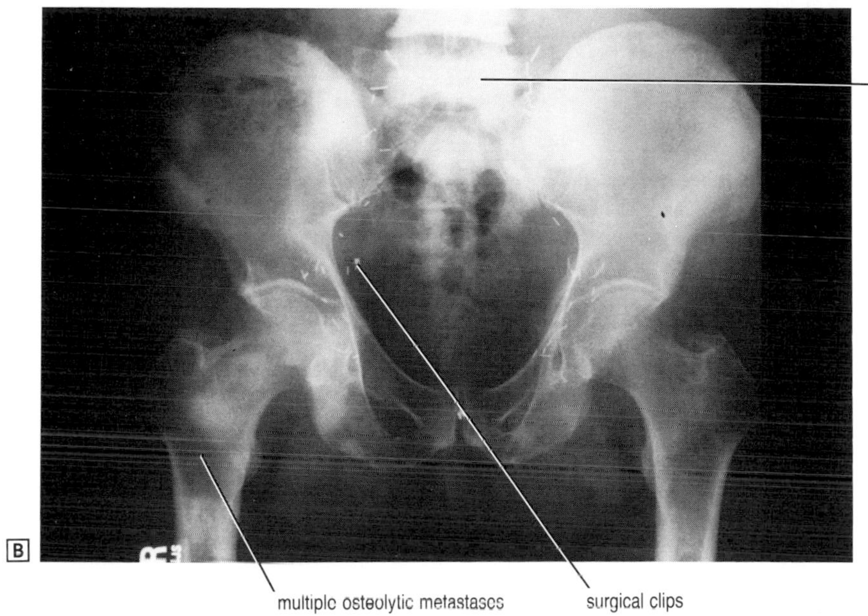

Figure 6.22. *B*, Osteolytic and osteoblastic metastasis.

6.23 OSTEOPOROSIS

A. Refers to a decrease in bone mass with a greater reduction in trabecular bone than cortical bone, allowing bones to be more susceptible to compression and fracture.
B. In general, 30 to 50% of bone density must be removed before it is visible radiographically.
C. Generalized osteoporosis is most frequently caused by senile, postmenopausal hormonal changes (decreased osteoblast activity). Other causes include Cushing's disease, exogenous steroids, idiopathic conditions secondary to alcoholism and cirrhosis, malnutrition (deficiency of vitamin C in scurvy), multiple myeloma, osteogenesis imperfecta, homocystinuria, hyperthyroidism, and hyperparathyroidism.
D. Regional osteoporosis results from disuse atrophy in an acute setting secondary to forced inactivity by fracture, Sudeck's atrophy (reflex sympathetic dystrophy syndrome), joint disease, or inflammation.
E. Radiographic findings of decreased bone mass and coarsening of the trabecular pattern, i.e., the thick larger trabeculae become more distinct because of the resorption of the smaller trabeculae.
   1. Spine: decreased trabecular pattern and bone density, with prominent dense cortex producing characteristic picture-frame vertebrae. Anterior wedging commonly seen at mid and lower thoracic (resultant kyphosis known as dowager's hump) and upper lumbar levels. "Codfish" biconcave deformity of the vertebral bodies results from expansion of the intervertebral disc into the softened vertebral body.
   2. Long bones and pelvis: thinning of the cortices from endosteal resorption, with decreased trabeculae in the spongy bone. Increased bone fragility of the thoracolumbar spine, pelvis, proximal humerus, femur, and distal radius are common fracture sites in elderly patients.
F. Bone density fracture threshold is less than 1 mg of calcium per cubic centimeter of bone. Evaluation may be done by single-dual energy photon absorptiometry and quantitative CT.

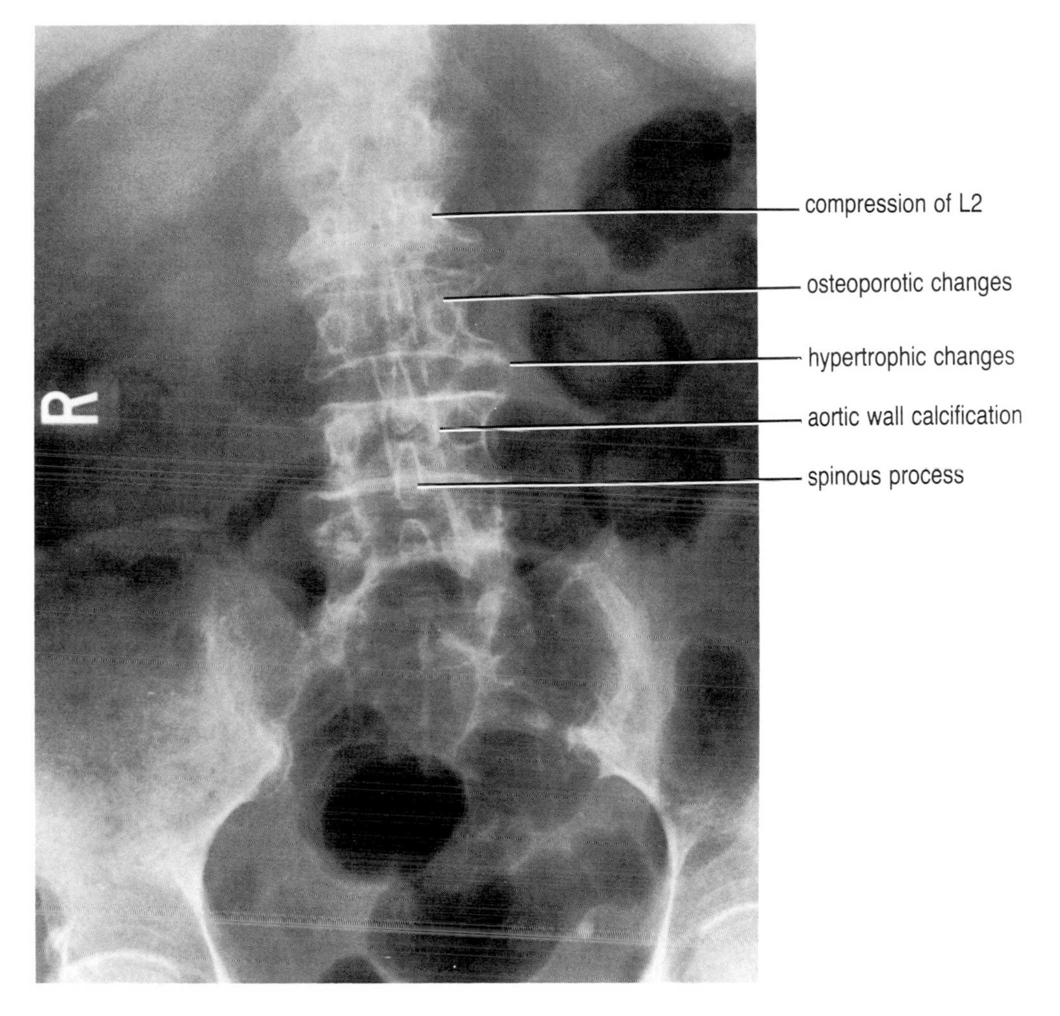

Figure 6.23. Osteoporosis.

6.24 MULTIPLE MYELOMA (MM)

A. A progressive neoplastic plasma cell disease occurring between 40 and 70 years of age, more common in men, characterized by abnormal spikes of monoclonal immunoglobulins (IgA, IgD, IgE, or IgG), presence of Bence Jones protein in urine, hypercalcemia, anemia, renal failure, and numerous osteolytic lesions.
B. Characteristic radiographic finding is that of multiple, discrete, round, osteolytic "punched out" lesions without surrounding area of osteosclerosis. These changes result from bone destruction and replacement by plasma cell tumors. Most frequently involve skull, pelvis, ribs, and spine.
C. Spinal changes may be generalized osteoporosis with compression fractures of several contiguous vertebral bodies and rarely affect the pedicle.
D. Long bone (proximal femur and humerus) involvement includes endosteal scalloping. The osteolytic lesions may coalesce, predisposing to pathologic fractures.
E. Radiographic findings and bones involved are frequently similar to those seen in metastatic carcinoma. Findings of larger nonuniform osteolytic lesions, pedicle destruction (see Sec. 2.14), or paraspinous or soft tissue masses are seen in metastatic carcinoma.
F. Bone scanning is of little value because there is no or little new bone formation in MM. A distinction from metastatic carcinoma where bone scans are sensitive to bone turnover
G. Ten percent of patients may develop amyloidosis.
H. Renal failure develops in about 20% of patients and is an unfavorable prognostic sign.

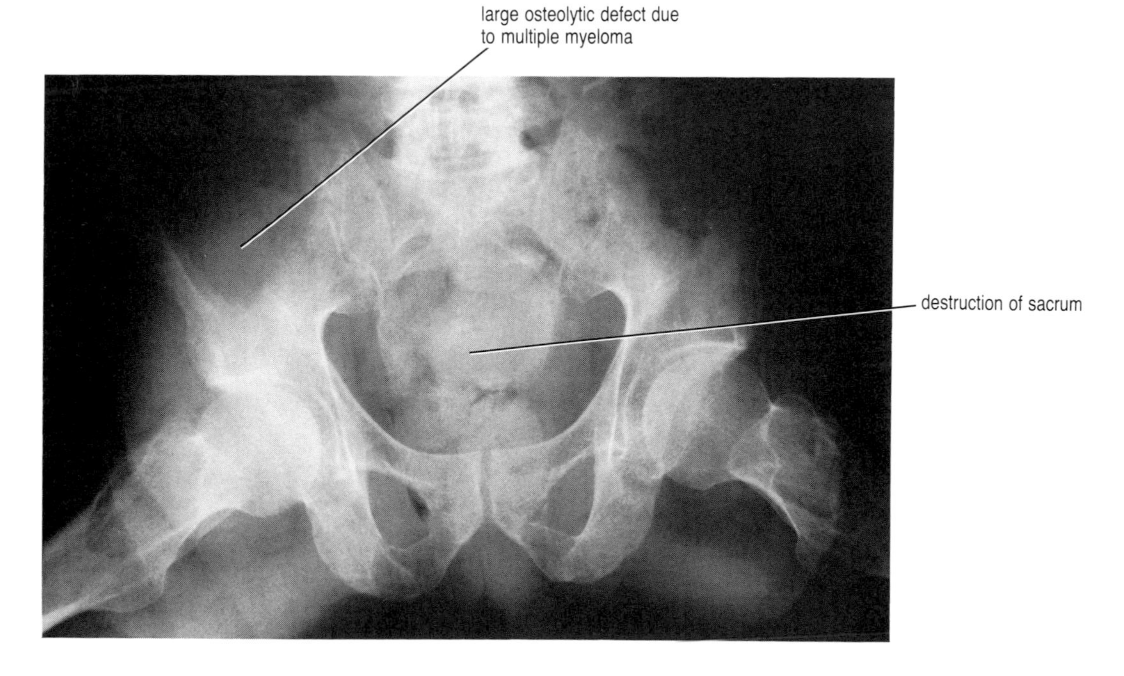

Figure 6.24. Multiple myeloma (MM).

6.25 PAGET'S DISEASE (OSTEITIS DEFORMANS)

A. A chronic skeletal condition of bone destruction followed by repair. Both conditions may occur at the same time.
B. Affects about 3% of the population; 20% are symptomatic (bone pain at involved site, headache)
C. Men affected twice as often, usually after age 40.
D. Bones frequently involved: pelvis, vertebrae, femur, skull, tibia, clavicle, humerus, and ribs. May involve single or multiple sites
E. Characterized by increased serum alkaline phosphatase, with normal calcium and phosphorus
F. Radiographically, bones markedly thickened with coarse trabeculation. Bowing may be present. Differentiated from osteoblastic metastasis, which lacks the coarsened trabeculae and thickened cortex.
G. Typical findings
   1. Pelvis most common site with widening and coarsening of the trabeculae of the pelvic brim. Cortex thickening best seen in the pubic bones
   2. Vertebrae: cortical thickening of the vertebral bodies presenting "picture frame" appearance on lateral view. Trabeculae are coarsened.
   3. Skull: initially begins at the outer table as sharply demarcated lytic areas with radiolucent centers (osteoporosis circumscripta). As repair begins, patches of sclerosis appear that resemble "cotton balls." Cranial vault is thickened.
   4. Long bones: initially destructive stage appears as a subarticular well-marginated V-shaped radiolucency extending along the bony shaft (blade-of-grass appearance). Reparative-stage findings of irregular thickened cortex and thick trabeculae with an increase in shaft diameter
   5. Flat bones: thickened with increased density
H. Complications associated with Paget's disease (secondary to softened bone)
   1. Pathologic fractures
   2. Basilar skull invagination with brain stem compression
   3. Sarcomatous degeneration in fewer than 1% to osteogenic sarcoma and, less likely, fibrosarcoma
   4. Nerve root deficits from vertebral compression

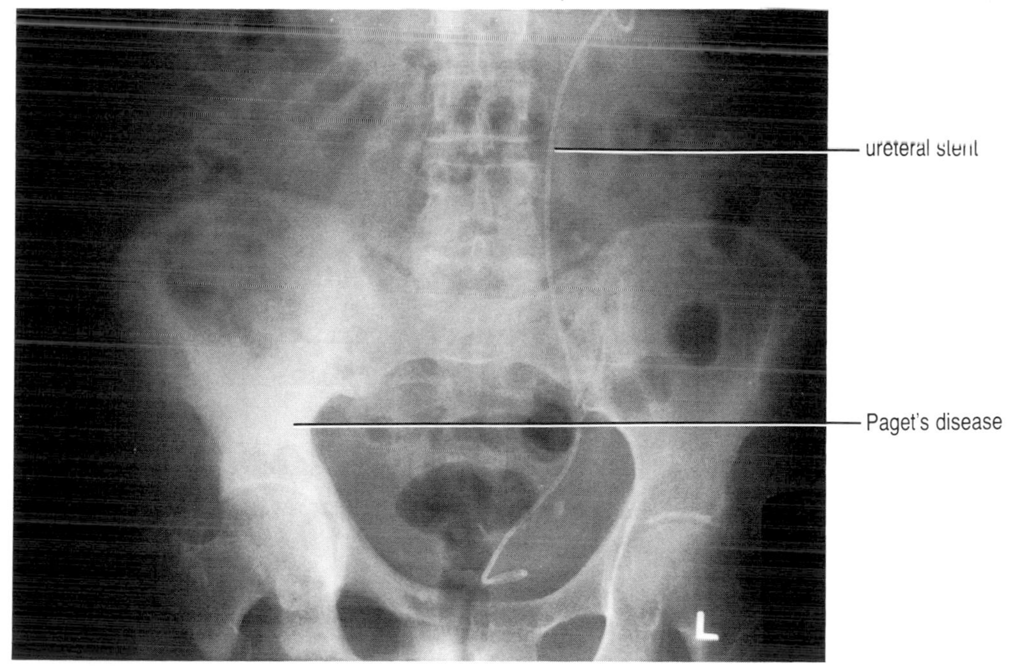

Figure 6.25. Paget's disease (osteitis deformans).

6.26 RHEUMATOID ARTHRITIS

A. A chronic disease with an insidious onset that begins at a synovitis of the peripheral joints. The disease may go into remission or be progressive with articular and periarticular destruction and may result in crippling joint deformity.

B. Onset most common between ages 20 and 60, with peak incidence at 40 to 50 years of age. Women affected three times more often than men. Approximately 1% of the general population is affected.

C. Classic clinical and radiographic signs of rheumatoid arthritis

1. Joint tenderness or pain with motion
2. Morning stiffness
3. Joint effusion, synovial inflammation, and edema in the early stages
4. Thickened and inflamed synovium produces a mass of granulation tissue called pannus in the region of the perichondrium. Pannus may cover the entire joint, interfering with bone nutrition, and results in destruction of articular cartilage and sclerotic marginal erosions at the joint edges. In advanced stages, bony ankylosis results.
5. Symmetric joint swelling of the same joint on both sides
6. Presence of rheumatoid nodules: subcutaneous nodules over bony prominences, on ulnar extensor surfaces or olecranon. Occur in about 20% of patients with rheumatoid arthritis and occur in no other disease
7. Bilateral symmetric joint space narrowing of the hips and pelvis without regard to weight-bearing stresses as in osteoarthritis. Femoral heads moved upward and inward: deepening of the acetabulum may occur (protrusio acetabuli).
8. Relatively symmetric joint space narrowing, soft tissue swelling, osteoporosis, and marginal erosions beginning at the proximal interphalangeal (PIP), metacarpophalangeal (MCP), and carpal joints of the hand and the fourth and fifth metatarsophalangeal (MTP) joints of the foot. There may be erosion of the ulnar styloid process.
9. Symmetric fusiform periarticular soft tissue swelling usually at the PIP joints.
10. Ulnar deviation of the phalanges
11. Phalangeal contractures and deformities: boutonnière and swan neck deformity
12. Periarticular osteoporosis: in the early stages is localized to the involved joint and is symmetric. Later on, generalized osteoporosis develops.
13. Cervical spine changes include odontoid erosion and atlantoaxial subluxation (increased predental space).

D. Felty's syndrome: longstanding rheumatoid arthritis, neutropenia, and splenomegaly

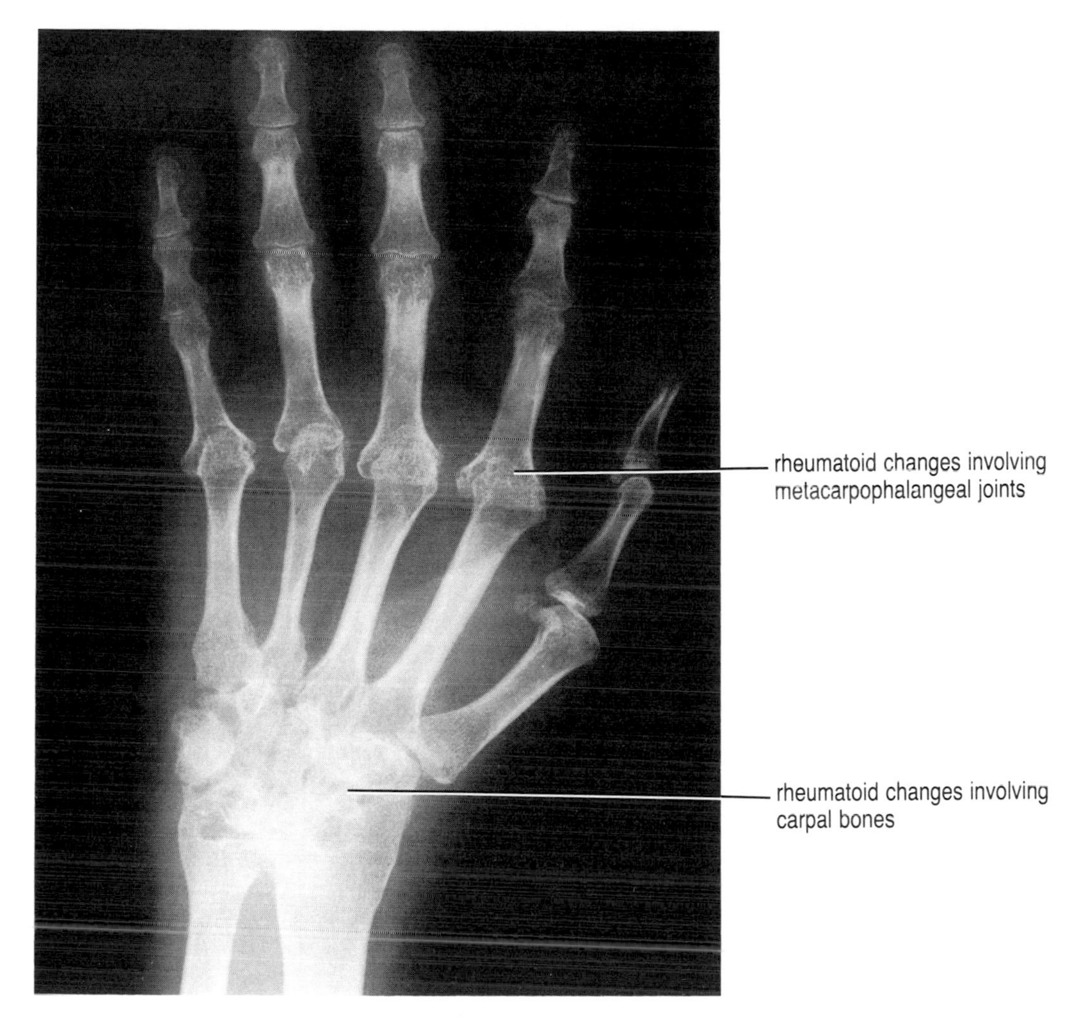

Figure 6.26. Rheumatoid arthritis.

6.27 HYPERPARATHYROIDISM

A. Refers to excessive parathyroid hormone production that results in increased bone resorption and elevated serum calcium and phosphate levels related to an increased number of osteoclasts. Serum phosphorus is decreased.
B. Primary hyperparathyroidism, usually caused by a single parathyroid adenoma
C. Secondary hyperparathyroidism, more frequent than the primary form, is related to chronic renal failure with associated parathyroid hyperplasia.
D. Renal osteodystrophy refers to the secondary form with associated skeletal abnormalities.
E. Bone mass reduction and nephrolithiasis are commonly associated.
F. Radiographic findings
   1. Subperiosteal bone resorption: earliest diagnostic and most sensitive indication of hyperparathyroidism. Involves the cortical bone resorption along the radial aspect of the middle phalange of the index and middle finger with irregular lacelike margins. Subungual tuft, acromioclavicular, sternoclavicular, symphysis pubis, sacroiliac, and proximal medial tibial resorption may also occur.
   2. "Rugger jersey" spine: characteristic of the secondary form refers to increased bone density (osteosclerosis), adjacent to inferior and superior vertebral body margins
   3. Generalized osteopenia: loss of bone density resulting in characteristic salt and pepper appearance of the skull
   4. Brown tumor: single or multiple. Usually occurs in pelvis, femur, and mandible but is not limited to these sites. Represents destructive expansile cystic lesions of varying sizes. Pathologic fractures may occur. Rare in secondary form
   5. Chondrocalcinosis: occurs in fewer than 50% in primary form
G. Preoperative assessment typically includes CT, arteriography, and/or venography. Ultrasound may be useful if adenoma is greater than 5 mm.

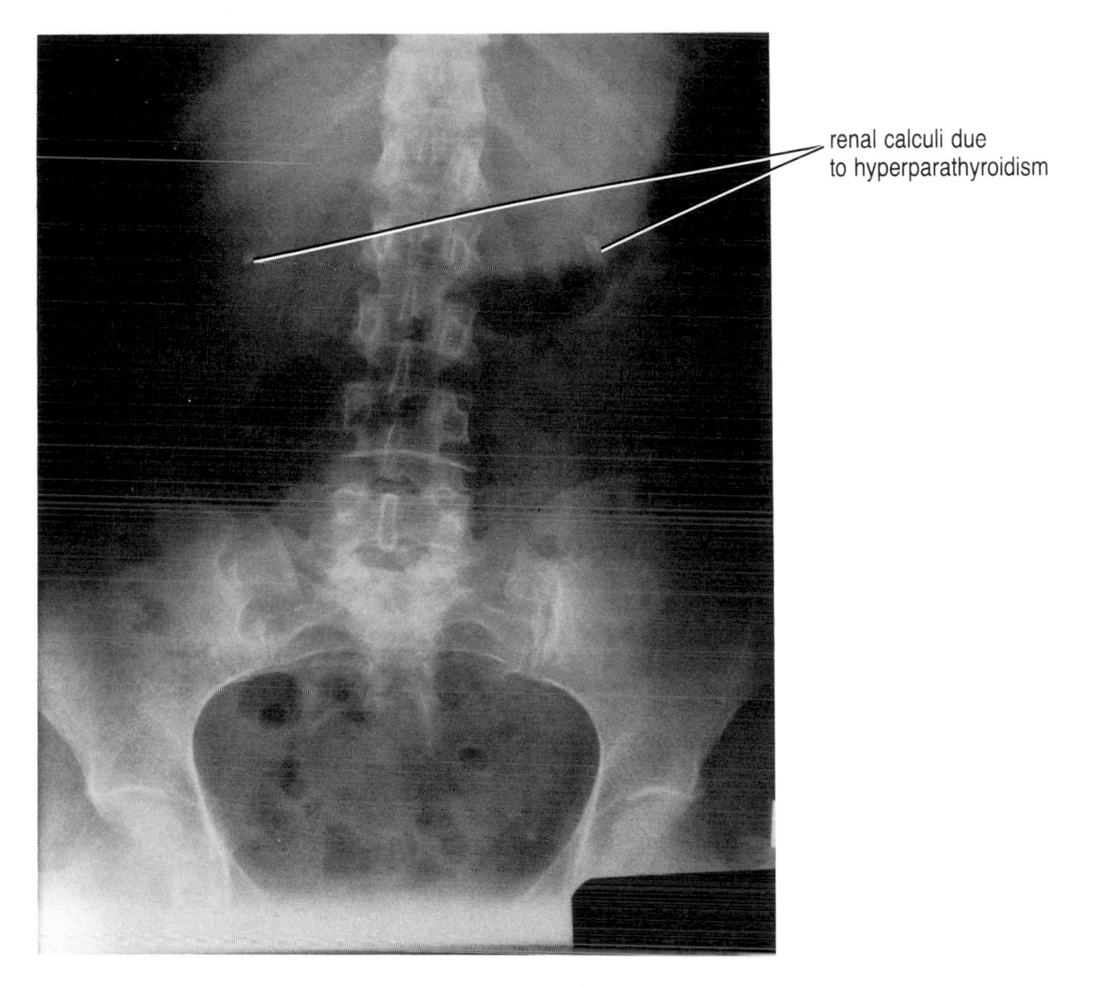

Figure 6.27. Hyperparathyroidism.

6.28 OSTEOARTHRITIS (DEGENERATIVE JOINT DISEASE)

A. Disease of older patients characterized by degenerative loss of articular joint cartilage with narrowing of joint space, subchondral and periarticular bony sclerosis, marginal osteophytes, and subchondral cysts
B. Primary form of the disease may affect any portion of the skeleton; however, is usually related to weight bearing and chronic wear and tear, affecting distal interphalangeal joints, hips, knees, and spine most frequently. Usually symmetric.
C. Secondary form is associated with intra-articular joint trauma (fracture or dislocation) or other bone disease. Usually asymmetric.
D. Radiographic findings
   1. Loss of articular cartilage and asymmetric joint space narrowing most severe along the superior lateral portion of the acetabulum, the point of maximal weight-bearing stress. Development of sclerosis (increased density) along the superior acetabular margin with osteophyte formation
      a. Differentiated from rheumatoid arthritis where there is more symmetric narrowing of the joint space
      b. Most commonly involved: distal interphalangeal joints of fingers and first MCP joint of the thumb. Proximal interphalangeal involvement may occur, but is not as severe as distal interphalangeal joint involvement. Osteophytes of the distal interphalangeal joints may enlarge to form clinically diagnostic Heberden's nodes.
      c. Knees: medial compartment narrowing is the earliest sign. Usually does not involve lateral compartment
      d. Spine: anterior and lateral hypertrophic spur formation. Some degree of intervertebral disc space narrowing and presence of vacuum disc in severe disease (radiolucency within the disc space) (see Secs. 2.12, 2.13)
   2. Osteophyte formation: involves fingers, hips, spine, and knees
   3. Subchondral cysts: usually associated with large joints. Extend into the articular space. Sclerotic margins with cavity-like appearance
   4. Periarticular sclerosis: increased density along the articular ends of the bones

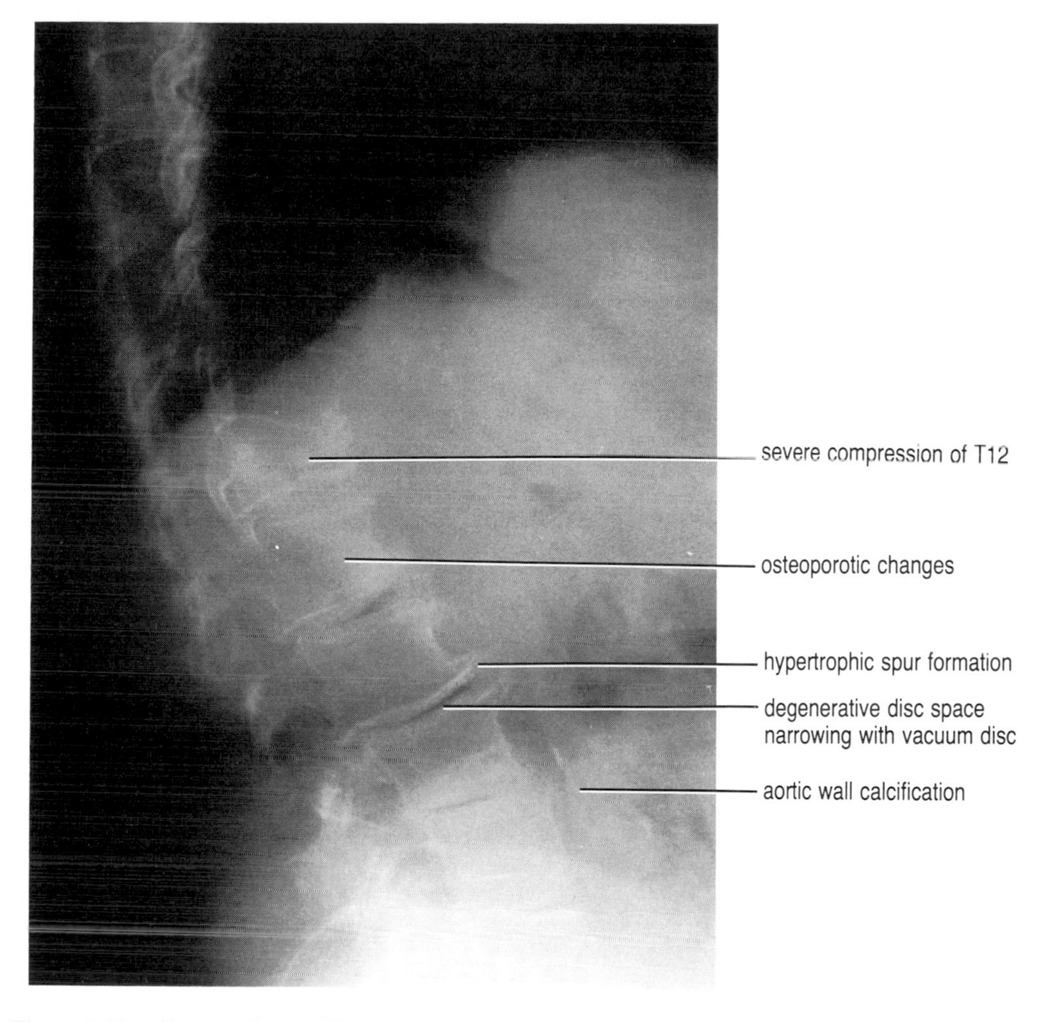

Figure 6.28. Osteoarthritis (degenerative joint disease).

6.29 OSTEOMYELITIS

A. Sources of osteomyelitis
   1. Hematogenous spread from cutaneous infections
   2. Extension to bone from a contiguous soft tissue infection
   3. Direct extension following open fracture, surgical procedure, or penetrating trauma

B. Staphylococcal aureus is most common organism. Streptococcus and Hemophilus are less common.

C. Metaphyses of the tibia and femur are the most common sites infected in infants and children by Staphylococcus or Streptococcus.

D. In adults, hematogenous osteomyelitis rarely involves the long bones and usually occurs in the vertebrae.

E. Radiographic changes do not occur until 10 days. Initially there is soft tissue inflammation and swelling followed by increasing bone destruction, periosteal bone reaction, and new bone formation.

F. Radionuclide bone scanning with technetium 99m pyrophosphate is used to evaluate early osteomyelitis. Typically, a three-phase exam, i.e., perfusion, blood pool, and delayed phase, is done. In cases of osteomyelitis, there is an increased perfusion phase with continued accumulation during the blood pool phase at the involved site. The delayed phase reveals intense focal area localized within involved bones, in contrast to cellulitis, which also has increased bone and soft tissue activity in the perfusion and blood pool phases and decreased bone activity on the delayed image.

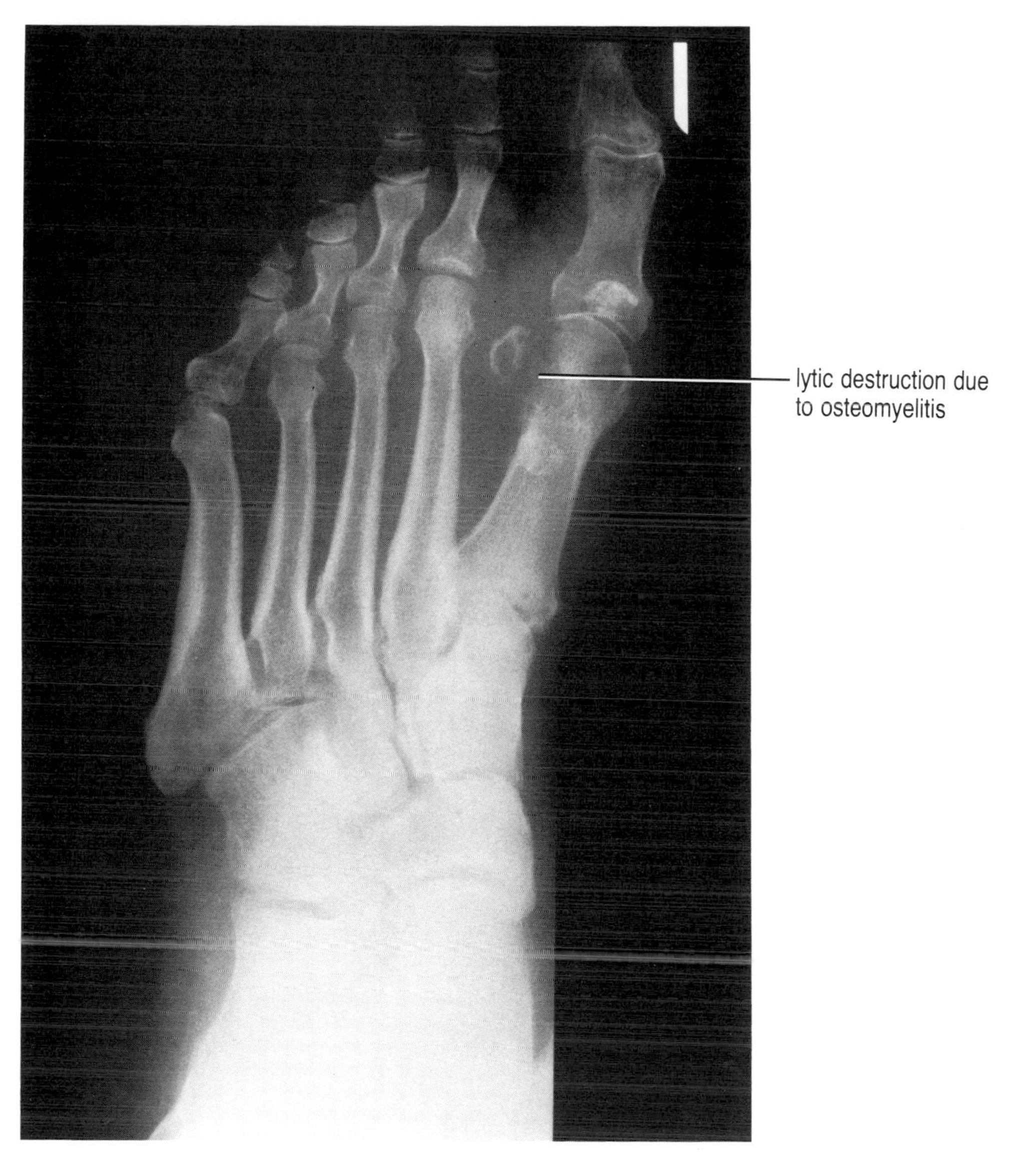

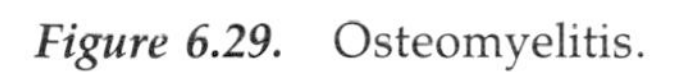
Figure 6.29. Osteomyelitis.

References

Eisenberg, R.L.: Diagnostic Imaging in Internal Medicine. New York: McGraw-Hill Book Co., 1985.

Harris, J.H., and Harris, W.H.: The Radiology of Emergency Medicine. 2nd Ed. Baltimore: Williams & Wilkins, 1981.

Juhl, J.H., and Crummy, A.B.: Essentials of Radiologic Imaging. Philadelphia: J.B. Lippincott, 1987.

Levy, R.C., Hawkins, H., and Barsan, W.G.: Radiology in Emergency Medicine. St. Louis: C.V. Mosby Co., 1986.

Mettler, F.A., Jr., and Guiberteau, M.J.: Essentials of Nuclear Medicine Imaging. 2nd Ed. New York: Grune and Stratton, 1986.

INDEX

Page numbers in *italics* indicate illustrations.

Bones and soft tissue Radiology

INDICations -

1. Pain
2. Trauma
3. Deformity

Preliminary workup

1. H+P
2. No prep needed (usually)

Types of Exams

1. Any bony structure
2. Need @ least 2 views.
3. Comparison views of uninvolved side.

Dislocations

1. Spine
2. Shoulder
3. Digits - (Tendon)
4. Knee
5. Elbow
6. Ankle and foot

Complication of fx's

1. Non-union
2. Aseptic necrosis

Soft Tissue Changes

1. FAT PAD Sign
2. FAT Fluid level
3. Hematoma
4. NOT related to trauma
   A) Sinusitis
   B) soft tissue calcifications (skull, other areas)

Arthritic changes

early or late

Osteomyelitis

Neoplasm.

SALTERS CLASSIFICATION of Epiphyseal fx.

Type I - Birth to 10 y/o - Epiphyseal separation

" II - over 10 y/o - Epiphyseal separation metaphyseal fracture.

Type III - Epiphyseal separation and fracture surgery. Periosteum intact

Type IV - Epiphyseal & metaphyseal fx. poor prognosis.

Type V - Crushed epiphysis Worst prognosis.